B

D1631226

ALONE WITH THE DEVIL

ALONE
WITH THE
DEVIL

Psychopathic killings that shocked the world

DR RONALD MARKMAN
AND DOMINICK BOSCO

PIATKUS

This edition first published in
Great Britain in 1990 by
Judy Piatkus (Publishers) Ltd of
5 Windmill Street, London W1

British Library Cataloguing in Publication Data

Markman, Ronald, *1936–*
   Alone with the devil: famous cases of a courtroom
   psychiatrist.
   1. United States. Forensic psychiatry
   I. Title   II. Bosco, Dominick
   614.1

ISBN 0–7499–1002–X

Printed and bound in Great Britain by
Butler & Tanner Ltd, Frome and London

DEDICATION

To my lovely wife, Nitza, and three wonderful children, Sharon, David and Michael, who provided me with support, assistance, and, above all, understanding through the gestation and birth of this book.

ACKNOWLEDGMENTS

Though this project spanned fifteen years, for the first decade, it lay dormant on a back burner, stifled by priorities, a lack of time, and a general tendency to procrastinate. The last three years required a dedicated concentration equivalent to that of a marathon runner in training. Completion of this book has made it all worthwhile.

Initial thanks must go to Larry Gordon, an artist in his own right, and a fellow Little League father, who lit a needed fire under me by initiating contact with a literary agent. Without his impetus, this book would still be on the drawing boards.

Although much of the data for this book came from personal files and public documents, a number of prosecutors and defense attorneys provided added information in many of the cases reviewed and to them I am appreciative. Special thanks are in order to Deputy District Attorney Al Locher of Sacramento, for his invaluable assistance in finding additional material in the archives on Richard Chase, and to Deputy District Attorney Jeff Jonas, who provided added information on Orlando Camacho.

Many colleagues, family members and friends assisted in reviewing the material. However, I would like to single out several who played a meaningful role either in my professional career or directly in the development of this book:

Russ Galen, my agent, who artfully led me through the literary mazes required to complete this project. Editors Ann Sweeney, who first expressed interest in the project, and Jim Fitzgerald and Ceci Scott, who despite entering the undertaking in midstream, provided valuable guidance and direction.

Dominick Bosco, with whom I spent hundreds of interesting hours, reviewing materials, discussing theories, and conceptualizing ideas, for converting the raw material into an understandable, interesting and readable treatise.

The late Seymour Pollack, M.D., a pioneer in Forensic Psychiatry, with whom I spent my early professional years.

Judges Jack Goertzen, Harry Peetris and the late Marvin Freeman, Commissioner Virginia Chernack, Deputy District Attorneys David Guthman and Dino Fulsomi, and Defense Attorneys Alan Simon and Bill Weiss: Heartfelt thanks for their friendship, interest and the many legal discussions over the years, both philosophical and practical, that stimulated my involvement in this field.

Finally, to everyone else who played a role in this endeavor, many thanks.

To Dr. Markman's acknowledgments I would like to add my appreciation to Russell Galen, who has guided us with unmatched patience and skill; Anne Sweeney, who first believed in this book; Jim Fitzgerald and Ceci Scott, who adopted us and made us feel wanted; my coauthor, who has always been generous, patient, and tolerant during the often demanding, tedious, and chaotic process of writing a book; and to the entire Markman family, for their warm hospitality in welcoming me into their home.

—D.B.

C O N T E N T S

ALONE
WITH
THE
DEVIL

A L O N E
W I T H T H E
M I N D
O F T H E
MURDERER

Logan, Utah, is not a very big city, especially when compared with Los Angeles, my home. Logan is neat, clean, and well lit. The first thing that caught my eye when I arrived was the crowd of people gathering around a policeman about a half-block away from my hotel. It reminded me of the crowds that movie location sets attract on the streets of Los Angeles. But even those events don't draw as much attention as whatever was going on down the street.

I looked closer and realized that the crowd was watching the policeman write someone a traffic ticket. Going through a red light was a crime worthy of drawing a crowd in Logan, Utah.

There was nothing psychologically unusual about this. People are curious about these events because they need to somehow integrate them into their experience of the world. The people of Logan were drawn to witness the policeman restore order in their community. The people of Los Angeles have a view that is, of necessity, somewhat less tidy than that of the people of Logan. Policemen giving traffic tickets in Los Angeles do not draw crowds.

I shook my head and smiled, and wondered how the good citizens of Logan would fit into their world the event that brought me to Utah.

I am a forensic psychiatrist—what many people would call a "courtroom shrink." It's my job to examine and evaluate people who have been arrested for various crimes. Often, that crime is the killing of another human being. In the more than twenty years I've been a forensic psychiatrist, I've evaluated hundreds of killers for the purpose of describing their state of mind. I guess you could say my goal is to get inside the mind of the killer. I do this by interviewing the person, usually across a small table, alone.

Living in Los Angeles, which has one of the highest homicide rates in the United States, I have plenty of work. I've interviewed mass murderers, serial killers, wife-killers, husband-killers, parent-killers, child-killers . . . every kind of killer you can imagine.

Some have been faces that have made the front pages of newspapers across the country. Some have made their way into our folklore. Others are mere footnotes in the legal journals. Names such as Bianchi, Manson, Corona, Pancoast, are names that are recognized by people everywhere.

It's unfortunate that, in our society, killers can become celebrities. Our morbid fascination with them is simple human nature —we're curious about killers, almost drawn to them. We want to know more. There is something inside them that is also inside us, and we are attracted to them so we can find out what that something is. That is not the unfortunate part—in fact, it is because of this curiosity that I have written this book. What is unfortunate is that, in turning killers into celebrities—if infamous ones—we obscure our view of them. By definition, celebrities are people who are different from us, distant, and somehow better for their glory. This gets in the way of satisfying the very curiosity that draws us to killers—that allows us to see our own reflection in their faces.

For this reason, although I have included a chapter about what I believe is an untold part of the Manson Family story, I have passed over such "celebrated" and much-written-about cases as Bianchi, Corona, and Pancoast. It is sometimes easier to get closer to the psychological and legal realities of the lesser-known cases, though the horror and brutality of the murders themselves may be even more intense than in the famous cases.

For example, I was one of the first psychiatrists to see the "Hillside Strangler" after his capture. Kenneth Bianchi and his cousin were found guilty of molesting, torturing, and strangling twelve women in California and Washington. But, in my opinion, the case of Lawrence Bittaker and Roy Norris (included in this book), though it received less nationwide fanfare, had at least as much impact and contains within it as grisly and horrific a vision of the dark depths of human nature. And perhaps a sharper view as well, since the story is not clouded by the folklore and controversy that often accumulate around famous cases.

In the Hillside Strangler case, the public's fear and horror were encouraged to build up gradually as body after body was found and reported in the press. Bittaker and Norris were so vicious, and their acts so cruel, that the hideous nature of their crimes was hidden from view until they were apprehended. And the horror still haunts the people involved in that case.

I also played a role in the Manson Family–Tate–LaBianca murder case. I not only evaluated three of the Manson Family murderers, but also Sharon Tate's husband, Roman Polanski, when he was charged with a sex crime years later. Charles Manson himself has become a folk figure in American culture, so I have not attempted to tell his story. However, less is known about Tex Watson and Leslie Van Houten, two kids who were "the boy and girl next door" if any ever were. I have found it more absorbing to explore how they became murderers—and what happened to them afterward, for I believe this gives us a better look at how close we all are to the act of homicide. It's easier to identify with Leslie and Tex because we are more like them than we are like Manson. By looking at their stories, we may get a keener feel for how Manson, himself, molded his flock and transformed them into killers. As for Polanski, I find his role as "celebrity victim turned sex criminal and outcast" powerful and gripping.

The case against Marvin Pancoast was perplexing from the start. The physical evidence was partly circumstantial: Vicki Morgan, the beautiful mistress of Alfred Bloomingdale, was found lying next to him with her head bashed in. The murder weapon, a baseball bat, was found nearby with Pancoast's fingerprints on it. Pancoast confessed, but then recanted. Then he claimed videotapes had been made of some of Vicki and Alfred's more tender moments. My interview with Marvin Pancoast supplied evidence of that most convoluted of all sexual worlds that Vicki Morgan, Alfred Bloomingdale, and Marvin Pancoast inhabited. But it was not more baffling than the world inside Orlando Camacho's head, a chaos that turned malevolent and ultimately led to the killing of his young wife. Camacho's crime was more bizarre and brutal in many ways, but it never reached national attention.

And while the deadly result of Pancoast's confusion was making headlines, to the north there was a young man whose own sexual confusion would eventually bear a deadly fruit. Yet Kevin Green did not come out of the underworld of Hollywood and the Sunset Strip, but out of a middle-class suburb in the Bay Area.

I was also called in on the Juan Corona case, after the farm contractor was convicted of murdering countless numbers of migrant workers and burying them in mass graves. Corona's original defense was that the evidence was circumstantial and that he hadn't committed the murders. When that didn't work and he was found guilty, the defense decided to explore the possibility of an appeal based on psychiatric grounds—that Corona was insane at the time of the murders. The prosecution called me in to examine Corona and to get my opinion on the viability of that defense. In preparation, I examined the material from the police records and trial transcripts and told the prosecution that, based on what I saw, there was no evidence—or psychiatric data—to prove that Corona suffered from a mental disability that would mitigate his responsibility for the killings. He may have been insane, but I said that unless I examined him or saw new information, for legal purposes there was no suggestion that he was mentally disturbed. After I presented my position to the prosecutor, the defense decided not to pursue a mental defense.

Clouds of controversy still hover around the Corona case, so I have not written about it. However, the story of Richard Chase, the "Vampire of Sacramento," is complete. And though our view of the mind of the murderer at work may be obscured in the Corona case, the grisly facts of the Chase case are chillingly clear.

Though John Zimmerman never made the national front

pages, his crime, too, was about as shocking and cruel a display of the mind of the murderous psychopath at work as any of the more famous cases, and because I evaluated Zimmerman face-to-face, I am able to bring *you* face-to-face with him, too.

The killing instinct does not spare close relatives; people who share bonds of love are not immune. Remember, the first crime in the Bible is a brother slaying a brother. As a matter of fact, of the twenty thousand or so homicides committed in the United States every year, a large proportion are between the closest of relatives—husbands and wives, parents and children. Nevertheless, despite the fact that husband-wife killings are common, when death came visiting the home of Lou and Laura Schindler, as you will see, the irony outstripped astronomical odds.

Torran Meier, Barry Braeseke, and Eric Chapman all have one thing in common: they all focused their deadly instincts on their parents. Beyond that similarity, their stories are as different as can be. Together, they demonstrate how demonic the legal system is. The boy whose crime was the most brutal came the closest to not being punished at all.

Fumiko Kimura, Norma Jean Armistead, Arlyne Genger, and Priscilla Ford are together in one chapter because their stories demonstrate how a murderous rage can arise out of an emotion as normally beneficent as motherhood.

As it can, as well, out of fatherhood. Which brings us back to relatively pristine Logan, Utah, where I was about to become involved in what may be the most bizarre case of my career.

Jason Nelson was a fourth-year seminary student in the Mormon Church. He was an excellent student, as well as an accomplished teacher. On the previous Friday a demonstration videotape had been made of his teaching an undergraduate class. I saw that tape. Though Jason was over six feet tall, his spare 142 pounds gave him the appearance of being smaller than he actually was. Jason was animated and skillful in handling the class. He was alert, lively, engaging—a very able and interesting teacher. His emotions were steady and positive, he engaged the class in dialogue to clarify issues, he knew what he was talking about, and easily won the class's attention and respect.

Jason was in his final year of school at Utah State University, planning to become a full-time teacher at the seminary. In addition to teaching, to support himself and his family he worked part-time as an attendant at two different service stations, one owned by his father and one owned by his father-in-law.

Jason was married and the father of an eleven-month-old son, Paul, whom he called the "light of my life." His wife Ruth was expecting another child in just two more months. She had miscarried her first pregnancy.

On Sunday, November 22, 1981, Jason, Ruth, and Paul spent the afternoon and early evening with Jason's parents, six brothers, and two sisters. One of his brothers was about to leave on a missionary journey to Sweden, and another had just returned from his missionary work in Taiwan. Jason, the oldest son, had already performed his missionary service, in San Diego. After dinner the young family left and drove to have dessert with Ruth's parents. There was nothing abnormal about the day, although Jason had been suffering from a migraine headache. These headaches had started when he was in high school. They didn't come that frequently, but when they did they often lasted a week. During his missionary tour of duty he had suffered three or four intense bouts of migraine. And just the previous Wednesday he had suffered what he described as "the worst" migraine of his life. Jason had gone to a chiropractor for these headaches and was told that they were caused by low blood sugar and a displaced vertebra in his neck. The headache returned briefly that Sunday, but it was gone by evening.

Jason and Ruth got along fine that day, as they usually did. The couple had met before he went away on his mission to San Diego. When he returned, they dated for a year and then married. Their marriage was not without disagreements, but they would usually end with Jason admitting that he was wrong to argue.

After dinner, the family sat down to watch *Mary Poppins* on television. During the movie, Jason realized that the story and characters had an important message for him concerning his faith. But his in-laws didn't seem interested in the movie, let alone its special message.

Jason had received these special messages before. Several

weeks earlier, for example, he had picked up some hitchhikers. The first boy he picked up reminded Jason of a foster child he and Ruth had taken into their home but had had to return to the juvenile authorities after three months because he would not obey their rules. Now Jason felt there was a spiritual meaning to this young man's hitchhiking. So he stopped his car and gave him a ride. Along the way, he talked to him and tried to help him.

Later that same week, Jason had picked up a second hitchhiker. This young man told him that his father paid a tithing to the church even though he wasn't a member. Jason felt there was a special spiritual meaning to this incident as well.

On yet another occasion, while suffering from a migraine headache, Jason was leading his Cub Scout troop in a newspaper drive. He became upset and yelled at one of the scouts for goofing off—but later felt badly about the incident and apologized. The boy refused to accept his apology, and Jason became convinced the headache would go away if only he could get the boy to forgive him. During the next week he went to see the boy to ask his forgiveness, but was unsuccessful. A few days later, the boy finally agreed to allow his penitent scoutmaster to help him on a scrap drive to collect aluminum cans. Jason knew this event, too, had special spiritual meaning.

So when the special message in *Mary Poppins* became clear to Jason, he suddenly stood up, summoned his wife and son, and said it was time to go home. Although Ruth thought this strange, she responded dutifully and did not argue with her husband. She gathered up her son, made her apologetic good-byes to her parents, and left with her husband.

When they arrived home, Jason and Ruth watched the rest of *Mary Poppins,* then talked about the movie for a while. Jason told her that he felt the movie had deep religious significance, and that the writers of the story might be the "Three Nephites," since the names of the authors of the movie were similar to the names of the apostles in the Book of Mormon.

Jason and Ruth said their family prayers, and as she prepared for bed he went into the living room to say his private prayers. While he was praying, he heard Paul start to fuss in his crib and went to help Ruth calm their son. While in the nursery Jason heard the front door open quietly. A spirit had entered the house: one of the Three Nephites who had written *Mary Poppins.*

Paul settled down and Ruth went to bed. Jason went back to the living room to finish his private prayers. He thanked the Lord for the special help He had given him in his seminary class. He prayed that he would have the spirit of the Lord all the time, and told the Lord how much he loved Him and how he would do anything for Him. As he was praying, he thought that maybe he could be a prophet. Abraham came to his mind. Jason wondered if he could love the Lord as much as Abraham did.

Jason went through the kitchen on his way to his son's bedroom and selected a large bread knife from a drawer. He thought it odd that no one else had heard the important message in the movie. It was a message about a test of faith. Perhaps that's why no one else had heard it, Jason realized: It was his test of faith. He had been putting it off too long. The angels of the Lord had spoken to him through the characters in the movie. The time for the test had come, and the Nephite who had come into the house was there for Jason's test.

Entering the nursery, Jason put the knife down on a chair. He picked up Paul from his crib and laid him on his back on the padded wooden dressing table one of Jason's brothers had built for them. He started to pray. He prayed that the Lord would know that his faith was strong, for he was being tested as Abraham had been tested, to see whether he loved the Lord even more than he loved his son. As he prayed, he closed his eyes and raised the bread knife over his son. Jason knew that the Lord had sent the Nephite to stay his hand. Silently he spoke to the Lord, professing his faith and at the same time asking for a sign . . . and then he thrust. The blade cut a neat slice in the mattress pad. Paul had turned and avoided the knife.

Jason saw that his son had moved and felt he had failed the test. Someone had moved Paul out of the way of the knife—but Jason had not brought the knife down far enough or fast enough. Had he done so, it would have proved there had been a spiritual intervention.

Guilty and disappointed in himself, Jason put Paul back in his crib, returned the knife to the kitchen drawer, sat on the couch, and began to pray again. He felt that he was afraid to sacrifice his own life for the Lord and decided to go to bed in order to think some more about his faith. But he remembered that Abraham had gone to bed in anguish, and then had gotten up and obeyed the Lord's command.

Jason moved faster this time as he retrieved the kitchen knife from its drawer, entered the nursery, laid the knife down, picked up his son out of the crib, and laid him on the table on his back. Jason prayed faster and with more intensity and again asked God for a message as he raised the knife and thrust. He missed again. But this was only a sign of Jason's lack of faith—for he had opened his eyes as the knife descended. He squeezed his eyes shut, prayed harder, raised the knife again, and thrust. Paul screamed.

Jason saw his son's blood and further intensified his prayers. But the blood kept spreading across the pad on the table. Awakened, Ruth called to Jason from their bedroom, but he didn't go to her. He knew that something was wrong. He had not wanted Paul to suffer, like Christ. Jason had to have an answer and he would get it from the Lord, Himself. As Ruth came running into the nursery, she saw Jason raise the knife again, and this time slice it across his own neck several times. Then he plunged the knife into his own belly.

Ruth saw Paul bleeding all over his nightclothes. In horror she called an ambulance and then ran downstairs and pounded on the door of an apartment rented by a couple. She screamed at them to come upstairs and help her. They offered to take Jason and Paul to the hospital.

But Jason said that what he and Paul needed was not an ambulance but prayer. The tenants succeeded in getting Jason into the car, but when they went back for Paul, Jason came back in and took a shower. Then Ruth asked the tenants to pray with her and Jason. They placed the wailing Paul on the floor in front of them as they knelt and prayed together. The phone rang, but no one answered it. As the four prayed together, Ruth felt an evil spirit leave her body. Paul continued to wail.

The phone rang again. It was the ambulance service calling to confirm the previous call for help. Jason told them that the ambulance call was in error, that no medical help was needed, and that everything was all right. Then he told the tenants that

they and Ruth were like the three witnesses in the Book of Mormon. He assured them that they had helped cast an evil spirit out
of him, and he tried to cast similar evil spirits out of them. Then
he told them all to go back to bed. The tenants, apparently unaware of the seriousness of either Jason's or Paul's wounds, left.

Jason then implored Ruth to have enough faith to understand that Paul was like Jesus Christ now, and that, as Jesus's
Heavenly Father had allowed His Son to suffer and die, they now
had to do the same with Paul. Then, after Paul had died, the Lord
would allow Jason to raise his son from the dead. Together, they
cleaned Paul's wound and wrapped one of his diapers around
Jason's wounds.

At about 3 A.M. Paul died. The knife had penetrated his liver
just below the rib cage and he bled to death. Ruth cleansed the
baby's body, put a Band-Aid over the stab wound, and dressed
him in clean nightclothes. She then washed Paul's and Jason's
bloodstained clothes, and buried the kitchen knife in the garden.

Jason and Ruth called their bishop, who came over at about
4 A.M. Husband and wife confessed to some minor sexual problems and asked for his blessing so that they might be healed.
Then they showed Paul to the bishop, and Jason asked him if he
had faith enough to raise someone from the dead. The bishop did
not answer him but, not suspecting foul play, did agree to anoint
Paul with oil. Jason and Ruth asked for the bishop's blessing,
which he gave. Before he left, he promised to call later in the
morning.

Jason and Ruth then went to bed. Jason was in great pain
from his wounds. He felt he was going to die and go to heaven,
where he could talk to Paul and the two of them would come
back for Ruth. At 6 A.M. Jason called his mother and asked her to
pray for him and Ruth and Paul.

At eight that morning, Ruth called Jason's father and asked
him to come over. When Mr. Nelson arrived he saw the blood on
Jason and told Ruth to call their doctor. But the doctor wasn't in,
so she called the chiropractor, who advised them to get Jason to
the hospital. Jason's father put a coat over his son and took him
there. He was not told of Paul's death.

Meanwhile, Jason's mother had her daughter drive her to
Jason and Ruth's house. She suspected something was wrong with

Paul because Ruth told them not to go into the bedroom. Eventually, she went in anyway and found her grandson lying flat in his crib, dressed in a diaper, plastic pants, and a blue terry sleeper. His quilted baby blanket was tucked in up to his chest. She touched the baby and the cold stiffness she felt in his arms, the paleness in his skin, seemed to spread up through her fingers and arms and over her own body. The baby's eyes were partially open. Horrified, she screamed that Paul was dead. Her daughter entered the room and said to call an ambulance. Ruth followed her in and said it was too late.

The visitors assumed Paul had died a crib death, but they asked Ruth if Jason had hurt Paul. Ruth replied that they all knew that Jason loved Paul so much he would never harm him. Mr. Nelson and Ruth's father arrived and a mortician was called. The mortician called the police, a routine procedure.

Back at the hospital, Jason was silent. He lay like a stone on the gurney, his eyes shut. He did not respond to questions, withholding as much as a nod. Examining emergency-room personnel found that Jason's neck wounds were not serious, but that the puncture in his abdomen was. The bread knife had penetrated at least five inches into his abdomen and had sliced his large intestine.

When the police arrived at the Nelson home, there was no sign of blood or foul play in the house. Paul was lying peacefully in his bed. Ruth was there with her mother- and father-in-law and her own parents. The police took photographs of Paul and the room. Ruth told the police that when she had awakened that morning, she found her baby dead and her husband lying on the floor, bleeding from his stab wounds. The police officers assumed it was a case of sudden infant death syndrome, and Ruth said nothing to correct that assumption. The mortician arrived to take the baby's body to the mortuary. The police left, marking in their reports another tragic crib death.

When the police were gone, Ruth took the mortician into the nursery, undressed the baby, and showed him the Band-Aid. As soon as he arrived at the mortuary, the mortician saw that there was a serious wound under the Band-Aid. He called the police. The cause of death was determined to be the stab wound. Search warrants were issued, the Nelson home was searched. The in-laws, the bishop, and the tenants were questioned by police. Soon thereafter a warrant was issued for Jason's arrest for the murder of his son. Ruth was arrested for obstruction of justice.

I was in Logan to evaluate Jason for the court. As I had done countless times, I was asked to get inside the mind of a killer and then tell the court what I found there in a way that would help not only the court, but the families involved, Ruth, the spectators in the courtroom, and the city of Logan make sense out of this. If, indeed, making sense out of it was even remotely possible.

To do that, I was going to be alone with Jason. Although some psychiatrists and psychologists request police guards when they interview killers, I never do. I prefer to be alone with the killer. Only then can I be free to ask the kinds of questions I need to ask. Only then can the accused feel free to answer them.

I thought about the crowd out on the street, and wondered how their curiosity would extend to Jason. Some of them might believe I was there to somehow absolve Jason of his crime, to "get him off easily," without punishment. Many of them would probably attribute his crime to demonic forces, and think that, in examining Jason, I was going to come face-to-face with a mind possessed by the devil. That might be the only way they could fit this killing into an orderly universe, the only way they could feel any sense of peace or security—believing that a force of incredible evil had suddenly and without warning possessed this good and loving man and turned him into a killer.

There have been times when I've felt that too, when I've found myself alone in a tiny room, across a small table from someone who has brutally taken a life. But I didn't know what I would find this time. As I watched the videotape I didn't see a psychopath or a psychotic. I saw a good teacher, a man who loved his work, his students, and above all his family—a man who was obviously quite good at what he had chosen for his life's work.

And yet his infant son was dead by his hand.

I was there to gauge the magnitude of Jason Nelson's mental disorder, as if his act was not measure enough of his madness. Ultimately, I was there not to absolve Jason Nelson or help him escape punishment, not even to explain what was going on in the deepest recesses of his mind, but to fit his behavior and his mental processes into the severely limited framework of the criminal justice system. The court would have some very specific questions for me to answer. Of course, all my years of training and experience had prepared me to answer such questions, to evaluate and describe the event in more elaborate terms, in words that sounded scientific—words that made it sound predictable and even part of some kind of order. I was there to help the criminal justice system render justice and restore order. That's what the people of Logan expected of me and of the system—what they expected of the policeman who was writing the ticket. In so doing, the chaos inside Jason's mind that had loosed itself upon his innocent son would somehow be vanquished. Order would be restored.

I wasn't sure the legal system was up to it, and I was not optimistic. For as seemingly demonic as this man's act had been, I knew the legal system could be equally demonic. I was there to do a job, to muster as much professional coolness and detachment as I could to perform the psychiatric evaluation—not a hostile interrogation, but a meeting not unlike a friendly initial therapy session between doctor and patient.

I'm not going to finish this story yet, however. Because the Nelson case and its remarkable disposition challenges our conventional notions of justice, mercy, religion, social order, and family love, I am going to frame this book with it. At the end of this book I will return to Logan, Utah, and Jason Nelson and his family and tell what happened after I arrived on the case.

I am telling my story in this way because when I went to Logan to meet with Jason, I knew that I would see more, illuminate more dark secrets than the court was prepared or equipped to handle. I want you to know that, too, and be able to see those secrets. I want you to see and feel what I see and feel when I expose the mind of a murderer. To say that Jason Nelson's son— and perhaps Jason himself—had been alone with the devil for those few moments, and that now it was my turn, is not saying enough. For I knew that the mind of the legal system could be at least as chaotic, disordered, and cruel as the wildest killer's.

I've explored the minds of hundreds of killers, I've lived the last twenty-odd years within the legal system as a psychiatrist and an attorney, and seen and felt and been part of its madness. I want you to see and feel that madness too. I want you to experience what it's like to learn—during the progress of a long career doing the very best you can to tell the truth according to your medical training and skills—that not only was Jason's son Paul alone with the devil, but that we all are.

C H A P T E R

1

Extramarital

Mayhem

John Sweeney's earliest memory of problems between his parents was the image of his father's hands squeezing his mother's neck. Later, there were times when he would come between them and try to stop his father from beating her. But the drunken rages were too powerful to stop, and John himself was often battered too.

Set on escaping, as he grew up, John learned to cook. He figured that was the ticket he needed—and he was right. Ambitious, skillful, and anxious to excel, John was hired as a chef at Ma Maison, a fashionable Hollywood restaurant. After a year of training in France, he became head chef in 1981, a position once occupied by Wolfgang Puck. He was now invited to Hollywood parties. At one of them he met rising young actress Dominique Dunne. Though Dominique was twenty-one, the petite, dark-eyed actress appeared much younger and regularly played the roles of teenagers. Her most recent one had been in the hit movie *Poltergeist*.

Their love affair was intense and stormy. They moved into a small West Hollywood house only a few months after meeting. Dominique loved the house especially because it had a yard big enough for all her many pets. She was also in love with John Sweeney. When his temper would explode and he would demolish furniture and hurl dishes, Dominique endured. Though she wept and complained to her mother about the outbursts, she defended Sweeney, too. She believed he would never hurt her.

But Sweeney did hurt her. John Sweeney had come a long way from Hazelton, Pennsylvania. But though he escaped the poverty-ridden coal town, he did not escape the imprint of his violent past on his mind. In one of his rages he tore out handfuls of Dominique's long black hair. She escaped, weeping, to take refuge at her mother's home. Fitting the classic pattern of wife-beaters, a contrite, repentant Sweeney showed up with flowers the next day, begging her to return, promising never to lay a hand on his beloved Dominique again.

But the pattern continued in a spiral of increasing violence. One night, after a pleasant evening spent with a houseguest, the fearful image of Sweeney's father's hands around his mother's neck was played out again. During a violent argument, Sweeney attacked Dominique and left bruises around her neck. Dominique survived the attack, and in a chilling case of art imitating life, she was able to play an abused young woman on TV's "Hill Street Blues"—without makeup.

As far as Dominique's family and friends could tell, she and Sweeney broke up at that point. Sweeney moved out of the house. But he went back one last time, the night of October 30, 1982. Dominique was rehearsing a scene with another actor when Sweeney arrived. He had come to try to change her mind and let him back into her life. But Dominique had taken enough abuse. They began to argue—and Sweeney picked up where he had left off after the last fight.

Almost a year later, when the prosecutor opened his case against John Sweeney, he pulled out a stopwatch and held it before the jury. He let the watch tick off four minutes—and told the jury that this was the amount of time John Sweeney kept his hands in a viselike grip around Dominique Dunne's neck. And when the four minutes were over, he let her slump to the ground in a coma from which she never awakened.

Dominique's family visited her every day at Cedars-Sinai Medical Center. But there was nothing they could do but hold her hand. After five days they made the agonizing decision to allow the doctors to remove Dominique from the life-support system. They buried their daughter two days later.

Today, John Sweeney is a free man. He was found guilty of manslaughter and given the maximum sentence: five years. Although his old job at Ma Maison was not waiting for him when he walked out of a minimum security prison after serving three years, seven months and twenty-seven days, he quickly found a job at an equally fashionable Los Angeles restaurant.

Dominique Dunne's family was enraged and embittered. They felt punished. As well they should, because they *were* punished, by a system that protects the guilty and punishes the innocent. In this case, the judge refused to allow evidence of John Sweeney's history of battering women. It was a pivotal ruling and ultimately molded the jury's decision.

The law allows the introduction of past crimes if these crimes show the same modus operandi, or mode of operation. John Sweeney's history of battering was clearly relevant, as far as the prosecution was concerned. It demonstrated that he knew he was potentially dangerous, that his personal lack of control was lethal. And because he knew how dangerous he was, he was guilty of killing with malice—culpable of at least second-degree murder.

The judge defended his decision by claiming that the introduction of the previous incidents of battering would have been inflammatory and prejudicial. This is the classic legal dichotomy between what's relevant and admissible versus what's inflammatory, emotional, and excluded.

Sweeney's attorney argued that Sweeney did not know how dangerous he was, and that he was acting in the "heat of passion," which—when established—sharply reduces the legal responsibility for a homicide.

I was retained by the D.A. to review the records of the case, with an eye toward testifying as to Sweeney's state of mind at the time of the murder. The defense refused to allow me to interview Sweeney and I was never called to testify.

John Sweeney is now in his early thirties. True to the form of a compulsive wife batterer, John is contrite and resolute. He claims that the "real" John Sweeney is in control now, not the one who was responsible for killing Dominique Dunne.

Unfortunately, the problem that society must deal with—and that the criminal justice system has lost sight of—is that the "unreal" John Sweeney happened to kill the real Dominique Dunne.

And the real Dominique cannot be brought back as easily as the "real" John Sweeney.

The system often seems to identify more strongly with the male criminal—almost to the point of sharing his compulsion to punish women. Just as John Sweeney was reliving his father's abuse of his mother, and was so blinded by his intense desire to reenact his father's violence, the system was blinded by its own compulsions—blinded to the real harm done to the victim. Just as he would then, and now, state that beating a woman was wrong and that the "real" John Sweeney had not done it, so would the system say it was a reprehensible crime. But in those moments when real and unreal exchange identities, and chaos takes the form of flesh and blood and muscle and strength—a woman is killed. And in those same moments in the courtroom, that woman is beaten again, and killed, and her killer is protected.

Has there been justice for the Dunne family? The real question is: Does the criminal-justice system care whether the Dunne family has received justice? And the answer is no.

Though the criminal-justice system tries to create the illusion of order and justice, it routinely ignores the needs of the victim, or the victim's family, for justice. Not only does it often not work to protect us and maintain order, but it also loses touch with any reality beyond its own confusion, much the way a mentally disordered person does. The system renders what it considers justice. Just as John Sweeney did, and just as a man named Orlando Camacho did, in the cold-blooded brutality of his rage against his wife Elizabeth.

Orlando Camacho began to feel jealous of Elizabeth Guzman from the first moment he met her. He had come to the United States from Ecuador when he was sixteen. Elizabeth and her family were from Bolivia. They were attracted to each other from the start, and saw each other every day on the campus of California State University at Northridge. Soon they were spending as many as six hours a day together. Elizabeth told the tall, slender, almost gaunt young man with the dark mysterious eyes that she loved him. To Orlando, Elizabeth was the "purest girl" with the "purest heart." She was a virgin, and refused to have sex with him. Orlando loved to play with children, but Elizabeth was the only adult he would allow to get close to him, because he felt good when he was with her.

Yet the lovers' path was not strewn with roses. After they'd been going together four years, he asked her to marry him. But her family did not want her to marry Orlando, and they talked her into changing her mind. Although he had done well in school while at the university, he had since quit and now worked as a janitor. He was a very sensitive young man and had chosen this kind of work because it allowed him to be by himself. "I am a very nervous person. I am a good person," Orlando said. He felt uncomfortable and suspicious around people. "I am too good, which is not good. . . . Her family didn't like me," Orlando complained. "They wanted her to marry someone else. I was supposed to marry her a year ago, but her family kept making excuses. I was afraid of losing her that year. I'm just a janitor and they wanted someone with money."

Elizabeth and Orlando didn't get along too well, either. They always seemed to fight about the same thing: Orlando wanted her to have oral sex with him, and she usually refused. He believed that she did it with other men. And when she refused to even kiss him, he was convinced it was because she was afraid he would be able to smell other men on her breath. "A couple of times before we were married I smelled genitals on her mouth," he claimed. "It was different than my smell. She did not want to do it with her mouth with me. But she did it with somebody else."

Elizabeth became very angry when Orlando accused her. Often, she would simply refuse to talk to him. On at least one occasion, he flew into a rage and almost strangled her. Finally, she did agree to have sex with Orlando. But even then he was not satisfied. "She wasn't a virgin. She had sex with somebody else. I could still feel that she was tight, so she was a half-virgin."

One day Orlando gave Elizabeth a gift—a miniature guillotine.

Convinced that she was "fooling around with someone," Orlando felt that if he married Elizabeth, she would be faithful to him. So on August 6, 1976, Orlando Camacho and Elizabeth Guzman were married in a Catholic church in the San Fernando

Valley. Both families attended. "My honeymoon in Monterey was beautiful," Orlando said.

After their marriage, Orlando and Elizabeth made love every day. They also fought. When Orlando came home from work, his wife did not want to cook for him or talk to him. She just wanted to play her records over and over again and lie down on the bed or the sofa in what seemed like a stupor. "We fought the whole time we were married. I was irrational," Orlando confessed. "She denied doing anything. She'd stop talking every time I faced her."

Two days after their marriage, when the fighting began again, Orlando began drinking heavily. "Every time I drank, I'd get drunk. I get vicious, in fights. Everything hits me in the wrong way," he admitted.

One of the things that hit Orlando the wrong way was his wife's coyness when he came home from work. "I kissed her before work and her mouth was clean. I came back from work and my wife wouldn't let me kiss her. I forced her to kiss me, and she had the smell of genitals in her mouth. It was like rubber. It destroyed me. It hurt my heart. It meant she was with someone doing these things. She had gone down on me before we were married, so I knew what it smelled like. After that my insides were torn apart. It was the only thing in my mind. She told me she wasn't doing these things. I couldn't think of anything else."

Orlando was obsessed not only with the changing aroma of his wife's mouth, but also with the size of her vagina. He convinced himself that she was growing "more widespread down there" because of her multiplying infidelities. Finally, one night as they were lying in bed, he asked her how many men she had before, or in addition to, him. To Orlando, "She was telling me it wasn't one man but ten men. If I'd look at her she wouldn't tell me nothing. It was only when I was looking away from her that I would hear it, so I wouldn't look at her. She was whispering in my ear, 'There were ten, Orlando—one, two, three, four, five, six, seven, eight, nine, ten—vamos, come on, let's do it again.' Then she started counting again.

"I said, 'Did you charge money?'

"She said, 'No.'

" 'Did they use rubbers?'

" 'They did it without nothing,' she said.

"I said to Elizabeth, 'Do you know what you're saying, you've been to bed with ten men?'

"She started crying and started packing to leave home. She said the first time she was with ten men was the past Thursday. She came home and she couldn't walk—like she was really hurting. Her family came and they saw her that day. I didn't do anything to her but other people might have thought I did because of the way she looked."

Elizabeth went to work at six-thirty the morning of the sixteenth, not knowing what to do. She came home at 9 A.M. She said she felt sick and refused to talk to Orlando. He asked if he could use her car to go to work, and she refused. Elizabeth told him that she had to go to her mother's house and get some pills to calm herself down. She asked him how long he'd be at work, and then told him she'd be gone when he got home.

Orlando was now convinced that she was going to abandon him. "Before I left, she said she'd be gone, that she would leave me."

He decided to come home early and catch his wife in the act of being unfaithful. "I wasn't supposed to come back until eleven-thirty that night, but I came home at six. The door was unlocked. She had a candle burning. I saw her laying on the sofa half-naked, wearing a negligée and panties. I could see her breasts. She used to undress only at night."

He locked the door and sat down next to her. She said, "Don't lock the door." Her voice was very faint. "Why don't you go to work?" she asked Orlando.

But to Orlando, "she stops talking when I face her." And when he turns away, he hears her say, "They're coming, Orlando, go, go to work."

"It meant that five or ten people were coming to see her and she was naked," Orlando said. "I thought I'd kill myself. I went to look out the windows. There was a Mexican man standing outside looking at my window and gesturing, like, 'What's going on?' and 'What's taking so long?'

"They were playing music outside—I heard it. She said, 'They're here now, Orlando.'

"The music went away—then it came back real loud."

"They are here now, Orlando, please go to work," he heard her say.

"I wanted to tell them that she's married and to give us a break. They took off. I was infuriated. I kept saying to myself: I really love her. I don't want anyone to be with her. I will kill her and myself.

"I turned on the stereo and the air conditioner, so if she screamed they wouldn't hear her. I grabbed her neck and started choking her. She looked sick. I moved her arms. I choked her for ten minutes as hard as I could and she gasped. It was the only thing she did the whole time I was killing her. She did not struggle at all. Her face was blue."

Orlando put a pillow over Elizabeth's face.

"I could still hear her breathing. I put her on the floor and pressed my knee on her neck because my hands were tired. I could still hear her breathing. I took a pot from a plant and broke it on her head. Then I hit her with the candle holder. I could still hear her breathing.

"Finally, I thought of a knife to kill her. I only had a butter knife and I tried to stab her in the stomach and chest, but the knife didn't go in. I almost gave up. She looked too sick, pale, and bloody.

"She said to me she wanted a crazy guy to kill her.

"I took the butter knife and stabbed her in the neck many times. I got a big hole in her neck and the knife bent. Her neck bones cracked. I finished cutting the veins and had her head out.

"I changed my clothes. I was ready to leave and I heard her voice telling me, 'Don't leave me here, Orlando.' When I walked into the living room, she was looking at me."

"Take me with you, Orlando," he heard her say.

"I put her head in a bag, and put her next to me in the front seat of the car. She kept on talking. She asked me what I was going to do. She wanted to know what I was going to do with her head."

With his wife's head in a bag on the seat next to him, Orlando drove to a liquor store, bought a half-pint of whiskey, but didn't drink it. Then he drove to Malibu, while Elizabeth "started telling me how much she hated me. She wanted me to take her head to where the ten men lived. She gave me the address on

Roscoe Boulevard and I got mad and thought, 'You're crazy, why should I take you there?' "

"They really love me," Orlando heard her say. "They're coming now because I'm calling them. They're behind you in the white car."

Orlando got mad and said, "You're trash."

"Then she told me she was a gypsy girl and had special powers."

"Do you see that Market Basket?" she said.

Orlando saw the Malibu supermarket. "I said 'Yes.' "

"Leave me in one of those trash cans," she said.

Orlando took the bag with Elizabeth's head and dumped it in the trash can outside the market. "I left her in the trash can. Then I went to the beach to swim out and drown."

But Orlando did not swim out far enough to drown. As he walked back toward his car, he heard Elizabeth talk to him from the trash can: "I'm going to tell the gypsies about you," she said.

Orlando got in the car and fled. He drove to his parents' neighborhood but didn't go in the house. Instead, he parked the car nearby, drank the whiskey, and slept in the car.

Elizabeth called to him through the night.

"My head is feeling warm," she said. "Come and see me, Orlando."

In the morning Orlando drove back to the trash can in Malibu. Elizabeth told him of the ten other men, and Orlando tried to drown himself. "I went in the water, but I was too tired so I came back out. She was talking to me."

When he approached the trash can, Elizabeth begged him, "Take me to where they live, Orlando."

"I got mad and said, 'I won't take you anywhere.' "

Orlando got back in the car and tried to drive away. But he was stopped by a California Highway patrolman, who noticed his erratic driving. The officer was attracted to Camacho for possible Vehicle Code violations and driving under the influence. Orlando was given a field sobriety test, which he passed. Because the car was registered in his wife's name, the officer asked about Mrs. Camacho. Orlando said she was "at home." During the entire thirty-minute encounter, Orlando and the CHP officer were just yards away from the trash can where Elizabeth's head lay. There were bloodstains on the red seat cover that the officer didn't notice. He let Orlando go, satisfied that nothing was wrong.

Then Orlando drove away, but the car broke down. He left the car and started walking. No one stopped to pick him up, so he got on a bus, wet clothes and all.

Her voice followed him: "I don't want to talk to him," she said. "I don't want to have anything to do with him."

Orlando went to a bank to withdraw money to buy a gun "to shoot myself." Elizabeth called to him even inside the bank and told him the ten men were now in the trash can with her. "They came to pick her up and now they wanted to talk to me," Orlando said.

The ten men started accusing Orlando, two, three, four or more voices at a time. "What have you done? What have you done? What have you done?" They told him they were going to kill him before the day was out.

"I said it was their fault. I really loved that girl. For five years. That's why I killed her. If I can't have her, no one will."

Finally, Orlando telephoned his brother.

Meanwhile, Elizabeth's parents had gone to their daughter's apartment to check on her. She had visited her mother the day before and told her about her problems with Camacho, so they were worried. Mr. and Mrs. Guzman walked into the apartment and found their daughter's headless body in a pool of blood.

Orlando's family brought him to a mental hospital and called the police. The admitting physician noted that he didn't have much to say and seemed to be deep in thought about something. Most of the time Orlando stared at the door. In the afternoon he was released into the custody of two Los Angeles police officers. In jail, Orlando continued to hear voices: "I've been hearing the voices of the ten people in jail. Only two of them stay with me. I hear Elizabeth's voice. They tell me who they are, what their name is. All of the people are saints. They all come to jail and make big noises. One says he's God, and the other is part of the gang of ten. Since then I've been hearing and seeing all kinds of things. My wife is talking to me, and there's God, and his wife, and she's very friendly. There's two more from the gang of ten who have been talking to me. They scream and cry and call me names. They insult me and read what I'm thinking. Yes, I know she had sex with ten guys a week after she married me, because she couldn't walk because they hurt her.

"I'm in jail because of a bad break. It was bad luck that I killed her. Now I'm in jail for years and it's ruining my life. I don't have her no more—it was nice. I bet her family really misses her.

"She was sick. She said she wanted to die young. Maybe she's happy where she is. It's hard for me to be in jail. People insult me. I take everything personally. It put my heart out of pace. It was the worst time in my life. I think the court should let me go. Anyone in the same situation would have done the same thing."

I was first called in to examine Orlando Camacho on October 22, 1976.

The idea of a court's being interested in the mental state of an accused person dates back to the beginning of civilization. The Code of Hammurabi (1850–1792 B.C.) provided that "the strong shall not injure the weak." Presumably, the "weak" included the mentally infirm. Courts have long been wrestling with the distinction between people who have committed crimes because of willful misconduct and those whose state of mind impaired their understanding of their criminal behavior. The Roman Empire's Twelve Tables accounted for the reduced competency of mentally ill persons. The Roman courts also appointed expert witnesses to give nonpartisan advice to judges.

European courts before the Middle Ages regularly sought the advice of physicians wherever medical matters might impinge on a verdict. In the Middle Ages, bishops presiding over church courts usually decided issues of guilt, innocence, madness, and sanity. They believed that an insane person did not know what he was doing, was lacking in mind and reason, and was "not far removed from the brutes."

During the sixteenth and seventeenth centuries, physicians

sometimes went to the defense of people accused of being witches. By this time, physicians were beginning to urge the courts to draw a finer distinction between people who committed crimes willfully and those who did so because of a "troubled spirit." At the beginning of the seventeenth century, British law established that someone who was either insane or "an idiot" should not be put to death for having committed a murder or other serious crime, provided the crime was not committed during his "lucid moments."

In the eighteenth century, physicians urged that the "criminally insane" be treated rather than punished. In 1724, a "wild beast" test was created in English courts. And by the nineteenth century, doctors were testifying in court that some people committed crimes out of an "irresistible impulse" or a "psychological drive." This issue of an accused person's state of mind, and responsibility for his crime, was argued time after time in case after case. Still, no definitive rule was established in English law until the middle of the nineteenth century. Finally, in 1843, the furor over an insanity verdict in the case of Daniel McNaghten brought forth a landmark decision that remains applicable today as the insanity standard in many jurisdictions in the United States. Known as the McNaghten Rule, this guideline was formulated by the Common Law Court judges of England, sitting as an advisory council, following the concerns expressed by both Parliament and Queen Victoria. It is ironic to consider that today, McNaghten would have a difficult time being found insane using the rule that bears his name.

Daniel McNaghten, a Scot, felt that he was being persecuted by the Prime Minister of England, Sir Robert Peel. He attempted to shoot Peel, but missed and killed the Prime Minister's secretary, Edward Drummond, instead. He was caught, tried, and found insane by a jury of his peers, who relied on unanimous medical testimony. In the uproar that followed, the judges ruled: "To establish a defense on the grounds of insanity, it must be clearly proved that at the time of committing the act, the party accused was laboring under such a defect of reason, from disease of the mind, as not to know the nature and quality of the act he was doing, or if he did know it, as not to know what he was doing was wrong."

Though it was coarse and primitive, the McNaghten Rule, a purely cognitive test, was also simple and seemingly workable, so the precedent was adopted by most British and American courts over the next century. In California, where statehood was achieved in 1849, six years after the McNaghten trial, the insanity issue arose in an appeal of a murder case in 1863. The Supreme Court of California held that the McNaghten standard would apply.

As with Daniel McNaghten, who remained confined in a mental hospital for the rest of his life, the insanity verdict initially led to a lifelong incarceration despite its not guilty aspect. With the evolution of a more humane approach to the mentally ill criminal defendant, there has been a move to release insane people back into the community when it is determined that they are no longer dangerous to society.

However, in the intervening years, the McNaghten ruling did not settle the issue permanently. It merely became a target for all sides within the adversarial system. Prosecutors fought to narrow the standard, while defense attorneys sought to expand the criteria. In the past twenty-five years, because of the evolution and increasing sophistication of psychiatry, the American Law Institute test, which incorporates both a cognitive and volitional, behavioral leg, has been adopted in many states. California experimented with this standard for a brief period of time, but following the furor over the Dan White murder case, there was a return to the McNaghten standard, imposed by a vote of the people via the initiative process. Other jurisdictions have changed to modified standards, such as "irresistible impulse," the mental illness "product" rule, and "guilty, but mentally ill." Regardless of the standard used, however, psychiatrists are increasingly called into the courtroom to provide guidance on insanity, as well as other issues, for the trier of fact.

I was asked by the court to evaluate Camacho's ability to stand trial. For this purpose, a defendant must be capable of understanding the nature and purpose of the proceedings, aware of what's going on, and capable of cooperating with his attorney in conducting a defense. He must also be capable of answering questions relevantly and carrying on a rational dialogue with his attorney.

It didn't take long to find out that Orlando was unfit to stand trial. It was my opinion that he was actively psychotic. Psychosis is a medical condition in which the person loses contact with reality in a profound manner. Thoughts, perceptions, feelings, and behavior become severely disorganized, and the personality begins to deteriorate. The psychotic person displays distorted perceptions, delusions, and hallucinations, and is compelled by these misperceptions to respond to people or situations in a bizarre, disorganized, "crazy" fashion. Camacho was almost a "textbook" case. He was unable to carry on a rational conversation, and became totally mute and unresponsive. He was detached and out of touch with his environment. In fact, my examination of Orlando Camacho had to be ended because of his lack of response. Whatever awareness he had was at best superficial. It was my opinion that he required intensive treatment, including antipsychotic tranquilizing medication.

Psychosis comes and goes. A person who seems perfectly normal one minute can deteriorate into a psychotic "episode" within minutes—and vice versa. If he commits a terrible crime during a psychotic episode, he may believe he is actually doing his victim a favor. When the episode is over and his mind returns to some semblance of normal organization, he may either forget what he has done or, if he remembers, find it as reprehensible as everyone else does. Occasionally, he may then try to commit suicide. Three weeks later, Orlando tried to strangle himself in his jail cell. He was found unconscious.

Since discovering her daughter's headless body in the apartment, Mrs. Guzman had been having severe emotional distress and her health was deteriorating. Finally, in November 1976 she was admitted to a community hospital in the San Fernando Valley. She spent two weeks in the hospital, and was released shortly before Thanksgiving. On the day after Thanksgiving, she decided to confront Orlando Camacho, not only to express things she had on her mind, but also to find out why he had murdered her daughter.

So about 5 P.M.—normal visiting hours—on November 26, she and her husband went to the county jail on Bauchet Street and requested to see Orlando Camacho. She told jail personnel that she was Camacho's mother-in-law. Orlando agreed to meet with his in-laws. They spoke entirely in Spanish.

"Why did you kill my daughter?" she asked him.

"Oh, I thought that she had other boyfriends," Orlando replied. "She did not let me make love the way I wanted to."

Orlando went on to describe to Mrs. Guzman how "she was hurting down there," and so he "tried to do it by the mouth but your daughter refused and I told her that she doesn't love me." When Mrs. Guzman related this part of the conversation to the D.A., she broke down and cried for several minutes. She said that her daughter was a virgin before marriage and she was sure that Elizabeth was either shocked or horrified at Orlando's request.

Orlando told Mrs. Guzman that a week before the murder, one night when they were sleeping, he asked Elizabeth how many men she had had before him. He understood her to say, somewhat drowsily, the Spanish word for ten, *diez*. Mrs. Guzman told the D.A. that the last time she had seen her daughter alive, on August 16, around 6:30 P.M., Elizabeth had come to her house and told her about this conversation and her husband's reaction, which apparently resulted from a misinterpretation. Elizabeth told her mother that she had never said *diez,* but had actually said *Dios.* She had been awakened by Orlando asking the question and had not said "ten," but "Oh God," in Spanish.

Orlando told his mother-in-law that "Monday she was weak," and asked her if she had given Elizabeth pills to relax her nerves. Mrs. Guzman said that she had. Camacho told her that he and his wife quarreled almost all night about the same issue—oral intercourse and sex. At the end of the argument Orlando had said, "I'm leaving you and not coming back." Elizabeth had replied, "I'll leave you, too."

Orlando told Mrs. Guzman that he then left the apartment and did not return until six-thirty in the evening. Mrs. Guzman corrected him, since she knew Elizabeth had been at her house at six-thirty. Orlando admitted it could have been later. He told her that when he got home he found her lying on the sofa, asleep in her negligée. "Why did you come back? Go away," Elizabeth had said to him.

Orlando told his mother-in-law how he then searched all

over the apartment to see if anyone was there, and how he saw the Latin man passing by the window. The man waved. Then the music started. "I then proceeded with my plan to kill her," Orlando told his mother-in-law. "I turned up the music and the air conditioner so no one could hear. First I strangled her very hard —she was still breathing so I got a vase and struck her with it."

Mrs. Guzman asked Orlando if it was the vase with the candle in it. He said that it was, and he "struck her in the head," but she was still breathing after that, too.

"Why did you cut her head?"

"Because I was very nervous," Orlando answered her.

"Did you know my daughter loved you so much," Mrs. Guzman said as she handed Orlando a poem that Elizabeth had written to him.

Orlando read the poem to himself and then asked, "Where did you find it?"

"In her book in the car."

"Oh, she was beautiful," Orlando said.

Mrs. Guzman then told Orlando that Elizabeth had come to her and asked her for money. She did not give her daughter any on Monday evening, but she had planned on giving the newly-weds $3,000 as a wedding present.

Surprised, Orlando said, "Oh, I did not know."

Mrs. Guzman later showed the D.A. a small folder containing $3,000 in $100 bills. She confessed that what had been bothering her was the feeling that if she had only given her daughter the $3,000 Monday evening, Elizabeth might still be alive.

During the entire confrontation, Mrs. Guzman was surprised Orlando could talk about the murder so calmly. "You're cold-blooded," she finally said to him.

Then her husband, who had been silent the whole time, added, "And you're not afraid to kill?" Mrs. Guzman started to cry.

In a very calm, cool voice, Orlando said, "I killed before. So what?"

Mr. Guzman became angry and said, "Just wait until you come out of jail. I'll kill you."

Mrs. Guzman's conclusion was that Orlando "hates us," meaning her and her husband. She said she always felt that Orlando did not want them to interfere or allow Elizabeth to remain close to her mother and father. She concluded that in addition to the horror of the act itself, the method by which her daughter had been killed was a means of showing hate and disrespect to her and Mr. Guzman.

In December 1976 I examined Camacho a second time at the Department 95 holding tank. This time he was able to talk with me. He answered all my questions, remembered killing his wife, and was able to tell me all about it. Though obviously on medication, he was fit to stand trial.

Meanwhile, in part because of all the delays in the case, and in part because they were dissatisfied with the way the district attorney's office was handling it, the Guzmans launched a letter-writing campaign. They wrote to everyone from the governor to the attorney general, and they enlisted relatives, friends, and acquaintances to write letters, too. The letters narrated the details of the case, and made special mention of the fact that Orlando had confessed to the murder and that there was not the least shred of doubt as to his guilt. Then they went on to plead for justice, which—since they regretfully acknowledged that California at that time had no death penalty—meant a first-degree murder charge and a life sentence for Orlando. Finally, the letters complained that the district attorney's office was simply not moving quickly or vigorously enough in prosecuting the case. They asked that a new, more aggressive, prosecutor be appointed.

But the delays continued to postpone Orlando's date with justice. In April 1977 his attorney told the court that he could not communicate with his client, and that Orlando claimed he was hearing the voices of five to ten people, including that of his wife Elizabeth. The voices lived in his head and told him not to testify. On April 20, two other psychiatrists and I reexamined Camacho and found that he understood the nature of the proceedings against him, but that was about all. The other physicians felt that he could not rationally and meaningfully cooperate with counsel because he was suffering from delusional behavior and auditory hallucinations. The court once again pronounced Orlando Camacho unfit to stand trial. He was committed to Patton State Hospital, to remain there until he could cooperate with his defense counsel.

California law says that the guilt of the defendant must be decided before his sanity at the time of the offense can be determined. This is what's called a "legal fiction." Actually, it's two fictions strung together, but they're necessary for the criminal justice system to untie itself from its own illogical loopholes. In the first place, the law says that if a person is insane he cannot be guilty of a crime. But the law also requires that before it can be decided whether he's insane or not, he must first be found guilty of a crime!

Standing alone, each of these rules makes some sense. But when you actually have to apply them, you've got to suspend logic to make them work. I should also point out that insanity and psychosis are not interchangeable terms. Psychosis is a medical term or diagnosis. Insanity is a legal concept or determination. Whether one is psychotic is up to a physician to determine. Whether one is legally insane can be determined only by a court of law, though physicians will give expert testimony to help the judge or jury decide. A defendant may be judged insane for a variety of mental conditions, only one of which is psychosis.

At this point in Camacho's case, the district attorney's office made a strategic decision. They decided to accept a plea of guilty to second-degree murder in the guilt phase and then go on to try the sanity phase. So the first task—finding Camacho guilty of murder—was accomplished. Next, there would be a trial to determine his sanity at the time of the crime. If he was found insane, then legally no crime had occurred. But by virtue of the plea bargain, we had already agreed he was guilty of a crime.

If the system seems confusing, hold on, because it gets worse. Before the trial to determine his sanity could proceed, his competency to stand trial still had to be determined. None of the mentioned legal fictions can be argued until the defendant is found competent to stand trial.

In October 1977 I examined Orlando a fourth time. For approximately three months, he had been in Patton State Hospital, one of the state mental hospitals in the California system. Along with Atascadero State Hospital, it's used by Los Angeles

County as a reception and holding center for defendants who are awaiting psychiatric evaluation and/or treatment.

Camacho had been given major tranquilizing and antidepressant drugs in high doses, and he was responding favorably to the medication. Many times when a person is given high doses of tranquilizers, most, if not all of the symptoms, can be eradicated. A person can seem quite rational until you discontinue the drugs. Then the psychosis will return. Yet despite the high doses Camacho was on, there still were clinical signs of an underlying mental disorder. Nevertheless, he was now improved to the point where he was competent, and a trial date was tentatively scheduled.

Meanwhile, the Guzmans' letter-writing campaign continued. As before, the letters complained about the delays and pointed out that Orlando was trying to get away with the crime by pleading insanity and that the district attorney's office was going along with it. They begged, urged, and demanded that a more vigorous prosecutor be appointed. The Guzmans received many replies from state officials, including one from the attorney general, who said that the Los Angeles district attorney's office was "acting within its broad discretionary powers," and that "they are vigorously prosecuting the matter to the fullest extent possible under the circumstances."

Although the family's letters expressed legitimate feelings, their authors did not know enough about the law. Actually, the D.A. *was* prosecuting Orlando Camacho to the full extent of the law—and then some. A prosecutor is ethically bound not to try to convict a person of a higher crime than he really believes the law will allow. In plea bargaining, the rules of the marketplace hold sway, but in the courtroom, the prosecutor is ethically bound not to ask for more than is warranted by the evidence.

In this case, the second-degree murder conviction was a legitimate goal. And when you understand a little about the limitations and intricacies of the law, it becomes clear that second-degree murder was perhaps a bit more than they should have expected.

Let me explain. The brutality or method of the killing does not, in and of itself, classify the state of mind of the killer. Neither does it automatically classify the degree of homicide with which the killer is charged. The more serious the homicide charge, the more severe the punishment and the greater the degree of mental sophistication required of the defendant at the time of the killing to sustain the charge. First-degree murder requires three mental states indicating a guilty mind: premeditation, deliberation, and malice aforethought, a man-endangering state of mind which incorporates the intent to kill. If premeditation or deliberation are not present, but malice is, the highest charge that can be sustained will be second-degree murder. If malice is absent, but the killer mentally had the intent to kill, then the crime is voluntary manslaughter. If intent to kill is absent, involuntary manslaughter is left—provided there is a reckless disregard for human life.

What level of homicide should Camacho have been charged with? Even second-degree murder was stretching it, because three psychiatrists, including me, had already determined that at the time of the murder Orlando was incapable of premeditating, deliberating, or harboring malice. Furthermore, at the time California was operating under "expanded" definitions of premeditation, deliberation, and malice. Thanks to some controversial—and eventually rescinded—California Supreme Court decisions, premeditation and deliberation had to be "meaningful and mature." The definition of malice was expanded to include the ability to "conform one's conduct to the requirement of law." Actually, these new definitions opened a cavernous loophole through which countless killers escaped first- and second-degree murder charges. The loopholes were ultimately closed by the passing of Proposition 8, which was known as the "Victim's Bill of Rights."

But Orlando Camacho was tried under the expanded definitions, and the prosecutor knew there was no way he was going to get a first-degree murder conviction. How could he hope to prove that Camacho had "meaningfully and maturely deliberated and premeditated" beforehand? A man who believed that his wife of ten days had been having sex with ten other men? It was equally amazing that a second-degree murder conviction was ever sustained. How could anyone believe that Camacho was capable of "conforming his conduct to the requirement of law"? A man who beheaded his wife and then carried the head around with him, having a conversation with it!

The fifth and last time I examined Orlando Camacho was the day before his trial, November 22, 1977. He was taking two

tranquilizers and an antidepressant in high maintenance doses—
doses so high that it's very rare to have someone receive such
amounts unless hospitalized. A normal person would be highly
sedated and possibly in a coma if so dosed. It is, in fact, a good
indication that a patient requires those drugs when they fail to put
him to sleep. Camacho was now fit to stand trial. Since the second-degree murder conviction had already been established by
plea bargain, this trial was only to decide whether he had been
sane or insane at the time. The outcome of the trial would presumably determine what to do with him—send him to prison or a
mental hospital.

As the trial began, the prosecutor's basic strategy was to try
to demonstrate that Camacho was not insane, that he had killed
his wife because "if I can't have her, no one else will." My conclusion was that he was legally insane. I found a continuing
mental disturbance, requiring massive doses of antipsychotic
medication over the year he had been in custody. The prosecutor
claimed that Orlando was malingering, or faking his madness. I
found that while he was exaggerating some of his symptoms, he
was not faking his fundamental illness. I did not find Camacho
overly sophisticated in terms of his understanding of psychiatric
principles. He did not show, as I see in many malingering cases, a
haphazard assortment of crazy behaviors. He did not look too
crazy to be crazy.

This information, in addition to that about his obvious delusional behavior and the hallucinations, added up to my evaluation
of him as psychotic. That was my opinion. It was subject to error
as all medical opinions are—but all I could do in court was stand
on it.

Both the prosecutor and I were basing our opinions on our
interpretations of the McNaghten Rule, which says that to be
determined insane, a defendant must be "laboring under such a
defect of reason, from disease of the mind, as not to know the
nature and *quality* of the act he was doing, or if he did know that
as not to know what he was doing was wrong" (emphasis added).
In my opinion, while Orlando *may* have understood the nature of
the act, known it was wrong and even have intended to kill Elizabeth, he did not understand the quality of it, owing to his mental
illness and his delusions.

You could argue that in plain English nature and quality mean the same thing. But there's no such thing as plain English in a court of law. In ordinary prose two similar words joined by "and" suggest either nuances or a writer who loves adjectives. The law prides itself on placing a very high value on each word, and this supposed stringent economy with words requires that any time two words are used to describe something, they must each be different. So we're obliged to interpret them differently, to distinguish one from the other. We're also required to ignore the fact that this dedication to economy and clarity invariably leads to hopelessly confusing legal battles fought with millions of superfluous words.

In my opinion, to understand the nature of the act is to understand that when one strikes another person with a vase, or stabs with a knife—or chops a head off—extreme harm will result. Understanding the quality of the act requires deeper comprehension. It requires being able to ask "Why do I have to do this?" or "What are the ramifications of my act?" or "Could it be done in a different way?" Understanding the quality of the act means being capable of a more humanistic thought process and comprehending the act on a deeper level.

If a man discovers that his wife is unfaithful, decides to kill her, and fabricates an elaborate scheme to carry out the deed, chances are good that he understands both the nature and the quality of it. However, if under the same circumstances he walks in and, before killing her, accuses her of having sexual affairs with the Pope, the Premier of Russia, the President of the United States, or some similar cast of characters that would suggest a grandiose delusional system—under those circumstances, although the superficial act of killing may be the same, the basis for the act changes. I interpret that as an impairment in the understanding of the quality of the act. Camacho's belief that his wife was having oral sex with ten men all at the same time was just such a delusional system.

As the prosecutor kept picking away at my evaluation of Camacho as psychotic at the time of the murder, he pointed out the fact that Camacho turned the stereo up louder and the air conditioner higher so no one could hear what was going on. Yes, that clearly indicates that he knew that what he was doing was wrong, and that he didn't want to be detected. But this was never a totally clear-cut case. If his level of impairment were total, I would have evaluated him as unable to distinguish right from wrong. But Orlando Camacho was not totally impaired. Only the higher levels of thought and understanding were impaired. He could understand the nature of his act—that doing what he did would result in his wife's death, and that it was socially wrong.

On a very primitive level, in human terms, Camacho knew exactly what he was doing: he was debasing Elizabeth as well as killing her. The Guzmans understood this. The problem was that the law in the State of California demanded a higher notion of human understanding and a more refined interpretation of understanding the quality of an act. You might say that the law demanded that Camacho be judged as we might judge the best and brightest among us, as if everyone were truly capable of a deep, human level of understanding.

Nevertheless, Prosecutor Jeff Jonas relentlessly argued that Orlando was sane. Just before the trial was scheduled to begin, the D.A.'s office received a letter from the president of the Bolivian Association of Los Angeles. The letter stood out because it gave a reason why Orlando Camacho may not have been quite so crazy as everyone assumed he was:

> The fact that the defendant gave the victim a miniature guillotine before they were married, and made an unsuccessful attempt on her life before decapitating her suggests to us that it was unquestionably premeditated murder. In the Anglo culture murder by decapitation is committed only by the insane; but it is not a sign of insanity in the Latin cultures. In the culture of Ecuador, from where the defendant came, decapitation is not an abnormal method of murder. It was a traditional practice to decapitate the victim and shrink the head, which was displayed as a sign of courage and prowess. We, of the Bolivian colony, knowing the psychology of people of Latin descent, assume that the murder was the consequence of lengthy disagreement between the victim's family and the suspect. We also believe that the "machismo" factor is involved and motivated the crime, because the suspect's ego would have been hurt by being repeatedly rejected by

the girl's family. It is not uncommon in our countries that a man whose machismo has been threatened commits a crime to get even. This does not mean that the person is insane. As a matter of fact, they believe it is a normal and proper thing to do in order to prove their manhood. The decapitation, which in the defendant's culture is closely associated with machismo, supports this conclusion.

So the prosecutor argued that Camacho's crime might be considered crazy in this country, but that in Latin America, where he came from, beheading was actually the accepted form of "macho murder."

Although the prosecutor was trying to interject this fact into the trial, the system was really forced to ignore it. The prosecutor was using it to show that the brutal manner of murder did not, in and of itself, demonstrate a mental disorder. He was right. In deciding whether someone is psychotic or not, the method of killing is immaterial. The more bizarre process doesn't necessarily correspond to the more bizarre behavior or the degree of impairment. The fact that Camacho beheaded his wife was not, to me, a major factor in determining his state of mind. It may, in fact, have been his cultural heritage that was operating to inspire him to cut off her head, not his madness. His madness may have enabled him to do it, but the specific form his madness took was dictated by his cultural ideas.

Camacho was behaving in a basic macho way: a woman was an object. If she strayed from acceptable behavior, it was the man's job to put her in her place. All races and ethnic groups suffer from this. It was as much a part of Sweeney's relationship with Dominique Dunne as Orlando Camacho's relationship with Elizabeth Guzman. Both men assumed control over the woman's behavior. The moment she wanted to leave, he refused to allow it. Neither man was willing to let his woman go.

The macho attitude relegates a woman to the status of property, or chattel. In some states a man could once get away with shooting his wife's lover, but not his wife—notwithstanding the fact that the wife was in bed with her lover of her own free will. Why should the lover be more responsible than the wife? Because the macho thinking was that the woman *didn't* have as much

free will or responsibility as the man. She was not a full person—
she was property. Chattel.

The psychological irony of macho behavior is that it derives
from very strong, deep feelings of inferiority. Camacho unconsciously considered himself inferior. People who suffer from seriously low self-esteem, as he did, manifest it in a number of ways,
most of which are misinterpreted by society. Camacho's tendency
to stand off from other people might be misinterpreted as a "ro-
mantic lone wolf" thing to do. Actually, he felt himself incapable
and inferior to others. His extreme jealous outrage might be misinterpreted as macho courage. Actually, it was extreme inner
weakness. The more jealous a person is, the less self-esteem and
self-confidence he has. There would be no need for these intense
feelings of jealousy if he truly felt strong and secure within.

Orlando was, in effect, saying to Elizabeth, "I'm not good
enough for you. That's why you relate to 'them' better than to
me." Camacho's jealousy, given rhyme and reason by his machismo misogyny, was intensified to murderous proportions by
his mental illness. His jealous fantasies grew into delusions—and
finally exploded into hallucinations. His jealous fantasy was that
Elizabeth was unfaithful to him. His delusions caused him to hear
his wife say "ten men" when she'd actually said "Oh God," and
to fundamentally misinterpret just about everything she said and
did as some kind of attack against him. In his hallucinations, his
wife's severed head spoke to him, and was finally joined by a
chorus including the ten men, God, God's wife, and others.

Finally, in trying to prove Orlando sane, the prosecutor
brought up the possibility that Orlando's insanity came on after
he killed his wife. His insinuation was that Camacho was legally
sane at the time of the act, "standing on the line of sanity," as he
phrased it, "and he has brutally murdered—let's say killed rather
than murdered—his wife, and he has cut her head off and he
knows that he's loved this girl. He just married her. And then in
the process of evaluating what he has done, he steps over the line
and now looks back and says: A sane person couldn't have done
that."

I agreed that this was a reasonable possibility. It's conceivable that a person by committing an act, can protectively deteriorate into a psychotic state as a result of the act itself. But, as I

testified in court, I have seen it work the other way, too. I have seen disturbed people commit a crime, and then improve as a result. So it was possible that Camacho was even more psychotic before killing Elizabeth.

Although his condition when I evaluated him suggested that he most likely had a chronic psychotic condition, Camacho had never had a documented psychotic episode before. I assumed that the killing of his wife had been the first such episode. There always has to be a first time—and it's usually associated with a definable, specific stress. You can always find it if you look long and hard enough. In this case, I think the marriage was the stress that precipitated his downfall into psychosis. Marriage is a stress in anyone's life. In psychiatry we see many serious personality disruptions occur after marriage. As long as there were no commitments and no involvement, I believe Orlando Camacho was able to function reasonably well—until the marriage. Then began the precipitous disintegration of not only his sanity, but also of the internal barriers to violence.

Let us assume that there is a series of steps the mind goes through on the way to killing another human being. Let us assume that those steps exist in us all, but that at one point some people go in one direction and some go in another. Some kill and some don't. In the case of John Sweeney, for example, if what Sweeney did in strangling Dominique Dunne was not first-degree murder, you have to assume that he went to her house not intending to kill her. He did not premeditate or deliberate.

But at some point he took a certain deadly step, crossed a line, and made a choice to kill her. What went on in his mind— and in Orlando Camacho's mind—that wouldn't have gone on if he hadn't killed her, if either man had instead simply broken down and cried, or driven away, or done any of a number of things? What actually happened in their minds to make them take that deadly step?

In most cases of this kind, there are options along the way. The person may not necessarily think them through. Indeed, he may not be capable of thinking them through, as Orlando certainly was not. Nevertheless, the options are there. Some are acceptable and some are not. Some are devastating. Usually, the options that lead away from the killing are the most devastating to the killer's psyche, so he chooses the path that take him in the other direction. In the case of Sweeney or Camacho, crying, going away, letting go of their women was so devastating that they couldn't make those choices. So painfully impassioned were they, that these choices most likely didn't even occur to them.

The heart of the issue is control. Power. Both Camacho and Sweeney simply could not handle the loss of control over their women—which was equated in their minds with power over the "situation" of their own lives. Sweeney and Camacho had made Dominique and Elizabeth into such integral parts of their lives that when the women threatened to break free the danger was not one of loss of love, but a loss of control that was psychically interpreted as a potential loss of life itself. The anxiety created by this anticipated loss could not be dissipated by running away or "letting go." In fact, both of these steps would only heighten the anxiety.

Unfortunately, violence usually is just what is needed to dissipate the anxiety as well as restore control. The wife batterer usually does regain power over his woman through his violence, while at the same time calming his inner rage and fear. When Dominique Dunne wanted to leave him, John Sweeney would beat her up and she would stay. Finally, Dominique got to the point where she said she didn't care if he beat her anymore, but that she was leaving anyway.

Such defiance is devastating to the ego of the wife beater because it signals a total loss of control. It was as if Dominique had her hands tightly around the neck of Sweeney's ego and was choking the life out of it. As far as Sweeney was concerned, losing control over her was like becoming nonexistent, and it produced an anxiety level that was intolerable.

Psychically, the killer kills out of self-defense. The only way he can preserve his psychic integrity and discharge the explosive anxiety within is to restore control through the most extreme violence.

But not everyone in a provocative, ego-threatening, anxiety-producing, control-relinquishing situation takes that step. Not everyone kills when faced with a destructive loss of control. What is it that keeps most of us from taking the final steps necessary to kill another human being? Is it because we're fundamentally more peaceful? Do we lack some inner "heart of darkness" that pushes killers over the edge?

No. We all share the inner forces that drive people to kill other people. We're all capable of murder, which is why all religions contain specific commandments against it and why it's against the law. If we weren't all capable of it, there would be no need to forbid it. But the reason why some of us are more likely to do it than others lies in the makeup of the individual psyche.

Though all of us (except sociopaths) have inner, psychic restraints against killing other people, we are all capable of killing if we feel our existence is profoundly and imminently threatened. In some of us, however, this instinct for self-preservation is provoked at lower levels of danger than in the rest of us. While most of us must be placed in a situation in which our lives are immediately and clearly threatened in order to kill face-to-face—the way Sweeney and Camacho killed—some of us can be brought to that point much more easily. Mental illness, in and of itself, does not necessarily predispose someone to get to that point sooner. It's not necessarily a matter of the kind or quality of one's mind, but the quantity of inner and outer forces that the mind is able to keep in balance.

If people who have murdered are different from those of us who have not, it is only because the forces in their lives and within their psyches have brought them to the point where the instinct for self-preservation has gone into action in a violent, aggressive manner. (This is not true of sociopaths, who kill not because they feel threatened, but because they totally lack inner restraints, or conscience, in the first place. Sociopaths kill when the outer restraints—policemen and other restricting circumstances—are missing and the death of the victim means removing an obstacle or enjoying a godlike rush of power over another person.)

In my opinion, Orlando Camacho's killing his wife was an instinctive act of self-preservation he couldn't control. It was a measure of how threatened he was by the very thought of losing her love. It emerged from the whole morass of usually prohibited behavior that we, in the requirement to become socialized, suppress and bury in our subconscious.

We see this kind of response in most psychotics, although it is not always aggressive. Psychotics often behave just like little children. They are instinctively doing what they want to do without control, without reflection, without concern, without interest, without deliberation, and not doing all those things that we demand of an adult in our society.

But we're *all* born with a real Pandora's Box of these same self-preserving instincts that can provoke us to kill. And the instincts are so pervasive that even parents feel them toward their children sometimes—though they usually don't act on them. Children feel them toward their parents—though they usually don't act on them. And husbands feel them toward their wives—though they usually don't act on them.

But Camacho and Sweeney, two very different men, did act on them, striking out with vicious brutality.

Unfortunately, the Guzman family—perhaps because of the same cultural reasons the prosecutor was trying to interject into the trial—felt as though no one was on their side, or their daughter's side. To some extent they were right. No one had to tell them that this was an assault not only on their daughter and her dignity, but on *their* dignity, too.

But the state ignored that, and also, in effect, ignored the assault on Elizabeth. As a matter of course, the state steps in for the crime victim—and essentially removes the victim from the process, stepping in as alter-victim. The way the law is set up, the state interprets the murder as an attack on its own integrity, not that of the victim or the victim's family. All crimes are considered crimes against the state. The trial was "the State of California *v.* Orlando Camacho," not the Guzman Family *v.* Orlando Camacho. Presumably, the state acts as the wronged party in order to use the resources of society against the person who committed this outrageous act. But if the state doesn't get the result the people it stood in for think it should—which is more common than not—the victims feel they've been wronged by the state as well as by the criminal.

The criminal justice system may have originally been set up to put itself between the criminal and the victim to supersede personal vengeance. It was thought that the state could more effectively render justice as well as maintain order by preventing a blood feud from developing between families like the Camachos and the Guzmans. Eventually, however, the rules of the game evolved so as to protect the defendant, while still ignoring the victim. In order for the state to step in, the victim has to step aside —and out of the process—if not totally out of the picture.

The system—in the form of the judge, the attorneys involved, the doctors called to testify, and sometimes even the jury —is so intent on creating an emotional distance from the actual event, that even the most serious trials are never too serious for some humor. In the Camacho trial, within a few minutes of talking about Orlando Camacho's brutal murder and decapitation of his wife, the judge broke up the courtroom with a joke.

PROSECUTOR: When you say that he was just an average student, is that based upon what he told you or based upon your belief as to what his IQ was?

MARKMAN: No. He told me that. And I could, once an examination capability existed in him, it was evident that his intellectual capacity was no better than normal.

PROSECUTOR: Would you consider a person who got an A in inductive logic just a person of normal intelligence?

MARKMAN: In today's college world, possibly.

PROSECUTOR: I guess it would depend upon the instructor and the course and so forth.

MARKMAN: I think there is an inflation in college grades.

JUDGE: Depends on whether you can buy a term paper or not. Gentlemen, we are going to break with that happy note. Let the record indicate that there was laughter, Miss Reporter. We will stand in recess until one-thirty this afternoon. The admonition not to form or express is in full force and effect. . . .

The Guzman family was present during that exchange. Were the professionals being disrespectful? Perhaps. But it has always impressed me how the judge, the attorneys, sometimes even the witnesses, will tell jokes in a trial as serious as this. It's done to maintain a certain amount of order, to add some levity to a serious case, and to keep it in perspective. Otherwise everyone becomes too immersed in the seriousness. Of course, another explanation is that our attempts at levity are really to shield us from the horror of what actually happened.

But nothing could shield the Guzmans from the horror. They felt wronged—by the state as well as by Camacho—and they wanted justice. They wanted retribution and revenge. As far as they were concerned, the system failed. From their point of view, Orlando had obtained South American justice for himself in the matter of his wife's alleged behavior. Now the Guzman family wanted the same kind of justice for themselves, and they were distinctly uncomfortable with the rules of this country's criminal-justice system.

I really can't blame them for not tolerating the obstacles running rampant through the system. From my vantage point, with my decade of experience, and by virtue of my legal training, I was aware of more perversity than they were.

For example, the defense was arguing that Camacho was insane at the time of the crime, and the prosecutor was arguing that he was sane. It seemed to me that each could have just as easily done his job—and perhaps better served his client—by arguing the opposite side. If the defense had simply accepted the second-degree murder conviction, the highest sentence that Camacho could have received would have been six or seven years with the possibility of parole in three. On the other hand, if the prosecution had gone along and accepted the NGI plea (not guilty by reason of insanity), Camacho would have been committed to a state mental hospital for at least the same six or seven years, yet with the distinct possibility that he would stay longer if he were found to be a continuing danger.

But prosecutors are trained to go after convictions, even if an insanity verdict would keep the defendant off the streets longer. And defense attorneys are trained to go after "not guilties," even if a conviction would free their client sooner.

As it turned out, Prosecutor Jonas relentlessly argued against a verdict of not guilty by reason of insanity—and won. Despite the fact that other doctors and I testified that Orlando Camacho was insane, he was found sane. More than seventeen months after

Orlando Camacho murdered his wife Elizabeth, he was sentenced to five years in prison.

The Guzmans' letter-writing campaign intensified after the trial. They charged that the Los Angeles County district attorney's office had been "bought by the defense." They even offered to pay for a special prosecutor, who would somehow order a new trial, convict Camacho of first-degree murder, and sentence him to the death they felt he deserved. They declared that they would not cease their efforts until their daughter's death had been avenged.

The D.A.'s office sent a Spanish-speaking investigator to the Guzmans to explain to them "the function of the district attorney's office and the state constitution regarding the district attorney's power." The investigator tried to tell them that "people received the best possible disposition available, and that their efforts were without merit and that the case would remain closed" as far as the district attorney's office was concerned.

The investigator came away from the Guzmans convinced that the family would continue their efforts, keep track of Orlando's whereabouts, and try to have him killed when he was released from prison. He believed they might even have him kidnapped and taken to Bolivia, where he could be tried for the murder of a Bolivian national and given the death sentence.

In September 1978 the D.A.'s office received a request for information about the case from the Quito, Ecuador, office of Interpol. The D.A. sent them a narration of the events in the case, including the investigator's suspicion that this case was not yet really closed.

It wasn't—and isn't. Orlando's craziness has served to keep him in prison longer—so far. He was originally scheduled to be released from prison on August 3, 1984, less than six years after he killed Elizabeth. However, Orlando attacked a security guard at Atascadero State Hospital, was tried, and found NGI. In October 1984 he was charged with another offense, and his sentence was extended again. He is currently serving his sentence at Atascadero State Hospital, and is now scheduled for release on August 3, 1989. In this case, the criminal-justice system seems to have, so far, done its job—by accident.

DON'T BOTHER ME WITH THE FACTS, MY MIND'S ALREADY MADE UP

It was very early in my career that I became aware of just how unjust and immoral the system could sometimes be. My first "big" case put me on the witness stand with testimony that not only defied the perversions of the system, but also cast me in direct opposition to a legendary, razor-sharp district attorney who was trying to close the book on a horrible sex crime.

Anthony David Dontanville was born March 26, 1933, the oldest of three brothers. He went to Catholic schools and was class president in grammar school, but later came to be known as a "loner" who, nevertheless, liked to talk. He followed his father into the landscaping profession by studying landscape construction and design for two years at Pierce College in the San Fernando Valley. In 1955 he went to work for the City of Pasadena Parks Department as a landscape draftsman, and eventually was promoted to construction supervisor. Dontanville was drafted into the army in 1956 and spent almost two years in uniform. When he came back from the service, he took up where he left off working for the City of Pasadena, and also took on private landscaping jobs. He was known as a hard worker, and the men he supervised liked him. He owned property in the Pasadena area, including an apartment house and some vacant land.

Dontanville had a problem with alcohol: he drank ten to fifteen bottles of beer a day and finished off at least a fifth of whiskey each week. He had once been engaged to be married, but his drinking interfered and the engagement was broken. His job was periodically in danger because of the drinking, and he was also beginning to experience some health problems.

But Dontanville's problems began in earnest in mid-September 1967, when the thirty-four-year-old landscaper was arrested for the rape-murders of two sisters aged six and seven. The police investigation had established that around August 9, 1967, the little girls had been kidnapped near Pasadena, sexually molested, and strangled with scarves, and that their bodies had been driven to Watts and dumped. The case received a lot of media coverage in the Los Angeles area. The police were stumped until a woman stepped forward and told them a friend of her husband's had bragged to him in a bar that he had molested and murdered the girls. The police and district attorney's office were certain they'd found their man when they arrested Dontanville, who was in a drunken stupor at the time.

At Dontanville's first trial, in October 1967, he claimed he didn't remember the incident. Later, he did recall that he and the friend were quite drunk and the other man was causing trouble in the bar. Dontanville, in trying to get his friend out of the bar, said to him, "You think you have troubles? What about the family whose two little girls in Altadena were murdered?" The friend thought Dontanville said he had killed the girls. He later told his wife, who called the police. Evidence such as this is always dubious, and Dontanville was convicted primarily on the evidence supplied by a chemical analysis of some hairs found in his truck. The test indicated that the hair belonged to one of the murdered little girls, and the first trial took only two days.

But in a strange twist, the prosecutor moved for a new trial immediately after the guilty verdict. Why? Because during his trial, though Dontanville was "on the wagon" for the first time in years, his court-appointed attorney, ironically, smelled of alcohol throughout both days of the trial. The prosecutor and the judge didn't want to risk having the conviction reversed because of inadequate representation by the defense attorney, so they immediately set the wheels in motion for a second trial. Everyone, from the judge to the D.A.'s office, on down to the news media, considered it an open-and-shut case anyway. They figured it would be easy enough to convict him a second time.

But Dontanville's new attorney, Charles Hollopeter, did not see things that way. He conducted a very able defense. While cross-examining the pathologist whose testimony had identified the hairs, Hollopeter stumbled onto a fact that completely turned the trial around.

Hollopeter certainly had the odds stacked against him and his client, so it was not unusual for him to ask some routine questions hoping to pick up a detail that would help his case. He asked the pathologist whether any additional tests could have been performed on the damning hairs.

The pathologist said that a complete sequence of tests had *not* been performed, because of time constraints, and then went on to name a few.

A less able attorney might have let that detail go by, but not Hollopeter. He picked up the scent of an important fact and went after it. First, he wanted to confirm what he had heard. Hollopeter asked the pathologist if, indeed, all of the possible identification tests had been performed to confirm the identity of the hairs.

The pathologist confirmed that all the possible tests had *not* been performed. More tests could have been done.

Were the tests that had been performed always 100 percent accurate, Hollopeter asked.

No they were not.

Could other, more accurate, tests come up with different results?

Yes, they could.

The courtroom exploded. When the judge quieted things down, the trial was adjourned until the remaining tests could be performed.

Several days later the trial reconvened and the pathologist was put back on the witness stand.

Had the additional tests been performed?

Yes, they had.

According to the results of these new tests, did the hairs belong to the victims?

No, they did not.

Once again the courtroom exploded.

It was decidedly downhill from there for the so-called open-and-shut case.

Still, the prosecutor, the police, and the judge thought they had their man, regardless of the pathologist's report. When the jury brought in a verdict of "not guilty," two fascinating things happened—both somewhat questionable legally and ethically.

First, the judge got angry at the jury. He called the twelve men and women who had decided that Dontanville was "not guilty beyond a reasonable doubt" into his chambers and, according to newspaper accounts, chewed them out for forty-five minutes for bringing about this "serious miscarriage of justice." His shouting could be heard through closed doors in the courtroom.

Maybe they had and maybe they had not made a mistake, but, in any case, a judge, like a ship's captain, is allowed such liberties.

But things went still further downhill from there. J. Miller Leavy, the prosecutor, immediately moved that Dontanville be held in custody until it could be determined whether or not he was a "mentally ill person." According to Leavy, Dontanville was dangerous and should be "put away." Indeed, if Leavy's strategy succeeded and Dontanville were found to be legally mentally ill, he could be locked away in a mental hospital, possibly for life.

Although Leavy's action might be considered a bold, unprecedented move on the part of the prosecutor, legally it was akin to a baseball team asking for an extra inning in which to try to win a game they had just lost.

One of the sharpest legal minds and most expert prosecutors in the country was arguing that a man who had been acquitted of a crime should be "put away" because he was likely to commit that crime again. Leavy was shooting baskets after the final buzzer.

Leavy argued that Dontanville should be committed on the grounds that he was mentally ill and, therefore, in need of hospitalization, supervision, care, treatment, or restraint. This tactic was legal only if there was a basis in Dontanville's behavior to suggest that he was suffering from a debilitating mental disorder that rendered him either dangerous to himself and others, or unable to care for himself. In view of Dontanville's acquittal, there was no legal basis for bringing up this question. By all legal expectations, Dontanville should have walked out of the court-room a free man.

More than the law and the fate of Anthony Dontanville were at stake now. Some very powerful egos were on the line. In pros-ecuting his "overtime" case, Leavy argued that Dontanville's de-meanor during the trial was evidence that he was severely men-tally disturbed. Certainly, Dontanville *had* appeared somewhat disturbed during the trial. He sat passive and motionless and made eye contact with no one, including the more than twenty witnesses who testified on his behalf. All he did was stare at the walls, the table, and his hands. Dontanville did not speak, except to call one of his own witnesses a liar.

Dontanville's attorney resisted this attempt to railroad his client into a mental institution, but there wasn't much he could do. Hollopeter agreed that Dontanville needed treatment, but he said it should be done voluntarily, not by the order of the court. To support his plea that Dontanville be committed, Leavy cited a previous psychiatric evaluation of Dontanville, which found that he had hallucinations, was overwhelmed by anxiety, could not remember anything about the day of the crime, and that he was psychotic. The irony was that Hollopeter himself had provided that evidence to the court, and was put in the awkward position of justifying his strategy in a case he had *won:* he had to admit that he did not put Dontanville on the witness stand in his own behalf because he knew his mental condition was unstable. Still, Hol-lopeter argued that Dontanville's mental problems came from his alcoholism, not from any underlying mental illness. The halluci-nations and other mental symptoms he experienced were in large part caused by his withdrawal from alcohol during his trials.

The judge took his time making a decision. He listened to lengthy arguments for and against, and spent hours consulting law books. Finally, he came back with his decision. Dontanville was to be held in custody and sent over to Department 95, the mental health court, for psychiatric evaluation. The judge named two psychiatrists to do the evaluation: Blake Skrdla and me, Ronald Markman.

Forensic psychiatrists are called many things, not all of them kind. We're called forensic experts, courtroom shrinks, apologists for criminals, doctors for hire, voodoo doctors, magicians. . . . We're maligned, mistrusted, vilified, and courted by attorneys. Judges generally don't like us because they often find our testimony confusing or difficult to understand. If we consistently testify for only one side, we're thought of as prostitutes, bought and paid for. In many cases we are just that—although many psychiatrists who testify mostly for one side do so because they are supporting a personal political agenda or cause, not necessarily their bank account. For those who work both sides of the courtroom, as I do, the contempt can be universal.

Although conventional psychiatrists do occasionally have to make decisions regarding diagnosis and treatment, for the most part they can listen to their patients' complaints and analyze the problems in the quiet solitude of their offices. Many psychiatrists will see a patient once or twice a week for years and never have to make a definitive diagnosis or design a complex treatment plan. This is standard accepted medical practice for psychiatry.

But a forensic psychiatrist must be prepared to do something no other doctor ever does as part of standard procedure: make a diagnosis that he may be required to defend in a court of law. Physicians, as a rule, do not enjoy having their decisions challenged. But to have them challenged on a regular basis is a nightmare for most doctors.

Why would any self-respecting, highly trained physician-psychiatrist subject himself to such abuse? I can only speak for myself: I don't know what draws other physicians into forensics, but in my case it was a matter of being in the wrong place at the wrong time. After my residency at UCLA, I was teaching at the University of Southern California and serving as Assistant Clinical Director of Postgraduate Education, Department of Psychiatry, at the L.A. County–USC Medical Center. I was not formally in the forensic program for the courts, whereby psychiatrists were made available for evaluations and testimony. Nevertheless, I had al-

ways been interested in psychiatry and the law. Most of the forensic psychiatry work was done at Department 95, the mental health
court of Los Angeles County. Although Department 95 eventually got its own building, in the late 1960s it was still based in the
psychiatric ward of the County–USC Medical Center. It was not
far from my office, so I got to know the people working there.

There were four psychiatrists regularly consulting for Department 95. Not long after my residency was completed, one of
the doctors there died suddenly of a heart attack. The mental
health officer for the court knew me and my interest in forensics.
He asked if I wanted to take this man's place at Department 95. I
said I did.

From then on I evaluated all manner of criminals, from the
most pathetic petty thieves to the most vicious of murderers.
Though I had previously seen only the victims of violent crimes
as they were wheeled into the emergency room or the morgue, I
now was seeing the people who had committed the acts of violence. And there were plenty of them. Department 95 eventually
became recognized as the largest mental health court in the country. A great percentage of the defendants in the Los Angeles
County criminal-justice system were evaluated at Department 95
at least once.

I say "at least once" because many suspects or convicted
criminals are evaluated more than once. The first evaluation can
come about merely to determine whether the person is competent to stand trial. If a person is found competent, he or she may
still be returned to Department 95 for further evaluations. For
example, if someone is convicted of the crime, he may be returned to Department 95 for evaluation as to his sanity at the
time of the crime.

Most lay people suspect that forensic psychiatry exists to help
criminals get by with less punishment. Most lay people also suspect that many forensic psychiatrists want it that way. However,
even though it gets a lot of press, from a practical point of view
insanity is very, very rare as a successful defense. Only about
1 percent of all defendants plead it, and probably only 5 to 10
percent of those who do, do so successfully. So out of a thousand

cases only one case may result in an NGI verdict. Nevertheless, its use in a lot of high-profile cases gives it a notoriety out of proportion to its actual use. As a matter of fact, the insanity defense has historically been avoided by defense attorneys simply because of the reality of sentencing. In most cases, an NGI defendant is held in custody longer than a person merely found guilty of the same crime and sentenced to prison. Many states have, or once had, laws that allowed them to keep an insane person in custody for life, even though the crime that was committed may have carried a prison sentence of only four years.

Ultimately, the states identified hospitalization as incarceration similar to jail time, and now an insane person can be kept only as long as if he had been convicted and sentenced to prison —unless he remains a danger. But people in mental hospitals don't get time off for good behavior, so a person who is found insane generally is kept longer than a person who is simply convicted and sent to jail.

Nevertheless, it is true that most attorneys view the forensic psychiatrist as someone who can potentially reduce the level of culpability and punishment for a client. This is not completely the fault of forensic psychiatrists. It is true that many forensic psychiatrists use the courtroom and the expert-witness stand as a place where they can win ground for their particular cause, whether it's one or the other side of an issue: capital punishment, prison reform, institutionalization, or one of the many esoteric controversies in psychiatry. Attorneys know that there are certain psychiatrists and psychologists who can be counted on to find the least shred of evidence to allow either a defense of limited mental capacity or a full-blown defense of insanity. The public is often appalled at the kind of results this testimony can bring about. So am I.

I must confess that, as a citizen, I am sometimes appalled at what I know will be the results of *my own* testimony. However, the only issue at stake in my mind when I testify is the medical accuracy of my evaluation. Unfortunately, other players in the criminal-justice system often misuse that testimony for their own purposes.

If I try to make up for the deficiencies of the system by coloring my testimony, as some psychiatrists do, I run the risk of becoming as confused as the system is. The system may be mad, but no doctor tries to heal the patient by catching the patient's disease.

In the Dontanville case, however, I found out right away that the system was extremely ill and that the pressure was going to be on me to blink, sneeze, and cough right along with everyone else. I was aware that Dontanville was on his way over to us. The trial judge had signed the papers. The receiving judge at Department 95 had dutifully acquiesced and done the same. Now, the only people standing between Dontanville and commitment to a mental institution were the two doctors set to evaluate him, and I was one of them.

We had a meeting with the judge, who asked us to undertake a complete examination and to be sure of our conclusions. Somehow I got the feeling that the system was trying to use psychiatry to achieve what it had been unable to do legally. I said I didn't see the point in examining Dontanville. To say that I was rather new in this job was an understatement, and I figured I could avoid the problem by politely bowing out. Perhaps my relative youth and inexperience worked against me, in that the prosecution believed I would play along and be easily caught up in the mounting enthusiasm to railroad Dontanville. But I was not about to be part of this quasi-legal conspiracy. Maybe Dontanville did kill the two girls. Maybe the pathologist didn't analyze the hair properly. Maybe the jury's verdict was a miscarriage of justice, as the judge had charged. Taking all that into consideration, I did not believe that psychiatry or medicine should be used to undo the law. It's not the way the system should work.

The judge smiled in a fatherly way and nodded his head. He told me to go ahead and do the evaluation. "I know you'll do the right thing," he said.

I sat down with Anthony David Dontanville and explained what I was there to do. Dontanville was an average man, friendly, congenial, and somewhat passive. I told him that my interview with him was not confidential, because it was court-appointed. As a "friend of the court," my analysis of him would be public and available to all sides in the case. I told him that I had been appointed by the judge to make a psychiatric evaluation and diagnosis and then to evaluate the level of impairment associated with that diagnosis. Finally, I was supposed to transpose that diagnosis into the legal framework. In other words, I was going to try to find out whether he was a mentally ill person in need of supervision, treatment, or restraint.

I do not use a standard test in evaluating people. There are standard tests for intelligence and personality development, and I do incorporate parts of them into my evaluations. But like any medical diagnosis, the physician needs to rely on more information than is supplied by answers to an objective test. This is particularly true for a psychiatric diagnosis. The quality of the interaction often tells me more than the specific answers. In Dontanville's case, he exhibited no elements of a major mental disorder at the time of my examination. He was congenial, cooperative, and intellectually sound.

I wrote up my report, which said that Dontanville was not a mentally ill person. Normally, the written report would be enough to dispose of the case. Dontanville should have been released as soon as the reports were filed. But the district attorney's office insisted on a hearing during which I would have to defend my evaluation against hostile cross-examination. Normally, when a case is sent for a hearing at Department 95, one of the prosecutors assigned to the department takes over the case. But this case was too important. Leavy was going to see this thing through himself.

J. Miller Leavy was a legend. He had long before established himself as a prosecutor of mythic proportions by winning the L. Ewing Scott case—the first conviction in California of a murder *without a corpse.* Throughout his trial, L. Ewing Scott professed his innocence in the murder of his wife. And defense attorneys made much of the fact that the woman's body was never found. According to legend, at one point in the trial the defense attorney said that because there was no body, Scott's wife was alive and could walk right into the courtroom at any minute. As he spoke he dramatically pointed to the back doors of the courtroom—then noted that every person in the jury looked when he pointed. This was supposed to indicate that there was, indeed, a reasonable doubt that Scott had killed his wife.

Yet Leavy prevailed. He took up where the defense attorney left off and told the jury that every head in the courtroom had turned to the door—except one. Ewing Scott hadn't turned his head, because, Leavy said, he knew his wife was dead. Scott was convicted.

Even as he went off to prison, all the time he was in prison, and after his eventual parole, Scott held on to his claim of innocence. He sang the same tune for more than thirty years: he had been wrongly accused and unjustly punished.

Had Leavy railroaded Scott? No. Just before he died, Scott confessed that he had killed his wife. I'm sure Leavy would not have felt vindicated, since he was sure of Scott's guilt from the start. If asked, he would have said that after thirty-five, forty years of working at this, you develop a gut feeling if a man is guilty.

Leavy's gut feeling was that Anthony Dontanville was a murderer and a menace. He pledged to "exhaust all legal remedies to protect the public." The force of his personality and his legendary skills had convinced two judges and several other attorneys—not to mention the news media and their audience—that Dontanville ought to be put away, regardless of the violence done to the law. Everyone seemed to forget that a jury had not shared this feeling, and had acquitted the man.

The day of the hearing, all attention was focused on Department 95's makeshift mental health court. We normally used this room at the hospital as a conference room. Even when we pressed it into service as a courtroom, there were only about half a dozen people in it at once. For Dontanville's hearing, we had upwards of eighty—reporters, attorneys, spectators—most of them standing.

And here I was, the young doctor, fresh out of my residency training, and it was my first time at bat. I knew I was rendering an opinion that was, to put it mildly, unpopular. I confess I was more apprehensive about being cross-examined by J. Miller Leavy than I had ever been evaluating a murderer face-to-face.

Leavy came on very strong. It was apparent from the very beginning that he wanted to impress upon the court that Dontanville was, in fact, guilty of the crime, and that the decision of the jury in the previous trial should be ignored. He wanted the judge to "require proof other than that of the doctors" that Dontanville should be put in a mental hospital. In other words, Leavy wanted the judge to make his decision based not on medical testimony alone, but on the *assumption* that Dontanville had raped and murdered the little girls. Leavy even wanted to call the judge from the previous trial as a witness who would testify to Dontanville's guilt.

The judge reserved his decision on calling the previous judge as a witness and began the proceedings by formally asking Dr. Skrdla and me about our evaluation. Both Skrdla and I stated that we found no evidence of psychosis or mental illness in Anthony Dontanville. Then Leavy was allowed to cross-examine Dr. Skrdla. In his questioning, Leavy bore down hard and repeatedly tried to establish his assumption that anyone who could commit such a crime must be mentally ill.

LEAVY: Well, Doctor, assuming any person had murdered two little girls last August 9, would such a person who strangled and raped two little girls be considered, in your opinion, a mentally ill person?

HOLLOPETER (Dontanville's defense attorney): Objected to, immaterial, on the basis that this defendant was acquitted of those charges.

JUDGE: It is a hypothetical question?

LEAVY: Yes.

JUDGE: Overruled.

Hollopeter's objection was sound. Hypothetical questions must be based on evidence that can and will be introduced in the trial. In this case, what Leavy was introducing could definitely not be used because Dontanville had already been acquitted of that charge. The judge, however, was apparently bending over backward to allow all points of view into evidence, so Dr. Skrdla had to answer the question anyway.

SKRDLA: No, a criminal act, Counsel, doesn't necessarily mean that a person is mentally ill. A few mentally ill persons perhaps do perform criminal acts, but many of them are perpetu-

ated by sociopaths or character disturbances, so I wouldn't conclude on the basis of the criminal act alone that a person is mentally ill. I would have to examine them first.

Leavy now took another tack—but he was aiming for the
same conclusion.

LEAVY: Well, wouldn't a person—any person in your opinion, who strangled and raped two small children six or seven
years old—would, in your opinion, such a person be a mentally
disordered sex offender?
HOLLOPETER: Objected to as wholly immaterial, irrelevant.

Hollopeter was right again. According to the law at the time,
a person could be sent for evaluation as a mentally disordered sex
offender (MDSO) only if he had been convicted of a sex crime.
Since Dontanville had not been convicted of any crime at all,
there was no legal basis on which to even think of evaluating him
as an MDSO. But, once again, Leavy was not to be denied.

JUDGE: Overruled.
SKRDLA: I would assume if that is a hypothetical question
that it would be a logical conclusion that one might be a mentally
disordered sex offender under those circumstances.

Under the weight of Leavy's pressure, Skrdla had opened the
door to exactly the misinterpretation that Leavy wanted to make.
Leavy pressed on, trying to rewrite the law and bring in the judge
from the previous trial as a witness to state that Dontanville was
guilty beyond a reasonable doubt—the jury be damned.
Hollopeter objected, and this time the judge sustained the
objection. But Leavy would simply not relax his assault on the
supposition that if only he could bring in the previous judge to
convince the doctors that Dontanville was guilty, they would
change their minds and find the defendant mentally ill.
Leavy had apparently dismissed two very important facts:
first, that Dontanville had not been found guilty of any crime;
second, that guilt or innocence was not relevant to the psychiatric

evaluation. Now he was trying to get everyone else to forget the same two facts.

Skrdla was excused and Leavy focused his attack on me. I was fresh out of my residency training, and he tried to make the most of that. To say that my adrenalin was flowing would be an understatement.

LEAVY: Doctor, did you read the portions of the transcript that were made available to you through the court?
MARKMAN: I did.

Leavy was referring to a version of the previous trial transcripts, both of which had been edited by him to demonstrate Dontanville's guilt.

LEAVY: Well, you have rendered your opinion that he is not at the time of this hearing a mentally ill person, is that correct?
MARKMAN: Correct.
LEAVY: Well, in considering the material that you read that was made available to you from the first and second trials and the preliminary hearing, did you consider it in light that Mr. Dontanville did or did not murder the two little girls?
MARKMAN: I considered it in both lights.

Leavy was going after me with the same tactic he'd used on Dr. Skrdla. He wanted to know whether I would have made a different evaluation if the previous trial had found Dontanville guilty. Leavy was trying to mold my testimony. But I wasn't saying Dontanville did or didn't do what he was alleged to have done. The jury already had done that. I was merely asked to determine whether or not he was mentally ill, according to the definition supplied by law. I had examined Dontanville and found that he was not mentally ill. It had nothing to do with whether he committed the crime or not.

LEAVY: Well, when you considered it that he did actually murder the two little girls, did you consider that such an act was an act upon his part which would indicate that he is dangerous to other persons?

MARKMAN: A person who has done this is dangerous to other persons, yes.

LEAVY: And might repeat?

MARKMAN: Possibly.

LEAVY: Well, that is as far as you can go. You can't predict for certain, is that what you mean?

MARKMAN: Correct.

LEAVY: But that would indicate a predisposition, wouldn't it?

MARKMAN: Oh, definitely. (If he repeated.)

LEAVY: That is right?

MARKMAN: Definitely, Counsel.

LEAVY: To commit such offenses, is that right?

MARKMAN: True.

Leavy was trying to get me to say that the commission of a sex crime automatically made a person a mentally disordered sex offender. But I held my own as he kept hammering away.

LEAVY: Well, assuming that any person, including Mr. Dontanville, strangled, raped, and murdered two little girls, such a person, if they could repeat, would be a mentally ill person, wouldn't they?

MARKMAN: No, not necessarily.

LEAVY: But they could be, couldn't they?

MARKMAN: They aren't mutually exclusive. They could be, yes.

J. Miller Leavy was getting livid, and grew increasingly testy with each succeeding answer. The more questions he fired at me, the calmer I got, the more secure I felt. It was really quite simple, once I realized that Leavy's whole strategy was to try to force on the court a misinterpretation of the law and the medical facts. All I had to do was stick with the simple fact that I evaluated Dontanville and rendered sound conclusions. Mine was a very limited determination that Dontanville was not mentally ill. If you concluded that he committed the crime, he did it while in a drunken stupor, not because of a mental illness.

I suddenly found myself not only defying Leavy's onslaught, but turning it on him, as well.

LEAVY: Isn't a person who would repeatedly rape and strangle young children, isn't such a person a danger to other persons?
MARKMAN: He is a danger, yes, but not necessarily mentally ill. . . . You are throwing in a second speculation. I am saying that they are not necessarily mentally ill and then you are saying they could be mentally ill if they could repeat.

Here, Leavy was using grossly faulty logic. On the other hand, I was sure about what I was saying. There was no question in my mind. Leavy really thought he had a just case, and he was pulling out all his best tricks to try to win. I didn't realize until I went to law school a decade later, and learned how lawyers are trained, that Leavy was demonstrating a classic difference between medicine and law. Leavy was trying to make one and one equal three, by saying that rape plus murder equal mentally ill. And I was defending my medical position that one and one is two, that rape plus murder equal rape plus murder. As lawyers are taught to do, he was trying to go 100 percent of the distance with only 50 percent of the information needed to get there.

Leavy then launched into another attempt to persuade the judge to allow him to call Judge Brandler, from the previous trial, as a witness who could testify to Dontanville's guilt. The presiding judge said he could call Judge Brandler, but only as a witness to Dontanville's personal conduct during the previous trial. He could not call the judge as an "expert witness" to offer an opinion, based on the previous trial, that Dontanville was, in fact, guilty. Rebuffed but not defeated, Leavy went on to ask that his edited version of the two trials be submitted as evidence and that it be reviewed by the present judge.

Hollopeter objected, on the grounds that Leavy had carefully edited eighteen volumes of trial testimony down to what would show only the prosecution's side of the story. Leavy's answer to the objection revealed his disdain for—or maybe just his frustration with—psychiatrists:

LEAVY: I think it is admissible, if the Court please, because the psychiatrists said they have used it and Your Honor well knows *psychiatrists can use most anything to support their position or opinion,* and properly so (emphasis added).

Hollopeter pointed out that it had already been established that Skrdla and I had seen the material Leavy was trying to introduce as evidence. The judge directed the issue to me.

JUDGE: Dr. Markman?
MARKMAN: Counsel, if all those statements in the court transcripts that I read, and I am talking about trial one and trial two and, I think, the pretrial hearings, were true, I today would find Mr. Dontanville is not mentally ill.
JUDGE: What criteria did you use in reaching the conclusion that Mr. Dontanville is presently not mentally ill?
MARKMAN: The manner in which he conducted himself during the interview.
JUDGE: Was that appropriate? Was his manner appropriate?
MARKMAN: Totally appropriate, Your Honor. He was guarded, but I thought that was appropriate also. His responses were relevant. They were coherent. He was cooperative. He was appropriately anxious. He was aware of what was going on around him. There were no signs that I could discern of psychotic thought activity or behavior.
JUDGE: That would include delusional material or hallucinatory material?
MARKMAN: Correct. His concentration span was adequate. He was tense, and that was evidenced by his tense facial muscles. He grimaced occasionally but tried not to show it, and I felt that he exhibited adequate judgment and was able to abstract adequately.
LEAVY: Did he indicate to you that he heard voices?
MARKMAN: He did not.
LEAVY: Did you read the social evaluation?

The evaluation Leavy was referring to was made by an official of the court, and though it called attention to the fact that

Dontanville was experiencing hallucinations, it concluded that he was not a mentally ill person.

MARKMAN: I did. I read Dr. Pollack's evaluation, which is part of the hospital file also, or his continuing report.
LEAVY: Did you learn in one of those evaluations that Mr. Dontanville heard voices two or three times a day?
MARKMAN: Yes, I did.
LEAVY: Isn't that hallucinatory?
MARKMAN: It is, yes.

Then Leavy tried to make headway by pointing out Dontanville's behavior during the trial. Dontanville was extremely nervous, and constantly folding and unfolding his arms and fidgeting. At times he started shaking and trembling and could hardly steady his hands long enough to gulp water from a paper cup. But these were signs of profound anxiety, not necessarily mental illness.

At this point, M. B. Thale, an assistant district attorney who was normally assigned to Department 95, interrupted with a question. By this time Leavy was growing tired, so the "bull pen" was relieving him. Normally, only one attorney per side is allowed to cross-examine a witness.

Hollopeter objected on the grounds that it was improper and that it would eventually lead to having me cross-examined by the entire staff of the district attorney's office, many of whom were present in our crowded makeshift courtroom. The judge, however, allowed Thale to cross-examine me. This was the first time in my career that I had been double-teamed. Because he had more experience in mental health issues, Thale went after me with a sharper line of questioning.

THALE: Doctor, what is your definition of danger?
MARKMAN: That an individual can inflict physical harm upon the person or property of others or upon themselves.
THALE: Is Mr. Dontanville capable of inflicting such injury upon the person or property of others?
MARKMAN: We are all capable of that.
THALE: Did you find him not mentally ill because he didn't

have a mental condition or did you find him not mentally ill because he was not dangerous?

MARKMAN: On the basis of my examination, I could neither find him dangerous nor mentally ill.

THALE: Even assuming, as you did before under Mr. Leavy's question, the fact that he might have committed the act?

MARKMAN: Yes. Now, on that basis, if he did commit the act he would be dangerous but he would not be mentally ill.

THALE: And did you notice anything unusual in your observation of Mr. Dontanville at that time?

MARKMAN: Nothing unusual.

THALE: Did you notice his affect? (Moment to moment display of emotion)

MARKMAN: Yes.

THALE: How was that?

MARKMAN: He was anxious. For the most part he presented a bland, expressionless face, but there was obvious anxiety as evidenced by his tense facial muscles.

THALE: Now, bland—you mean he showed no emotional tone according to the material that was being discussed at the time, is that true?

MARKMAN: Yes.

THALE: Isn't that a case of mental illness, Doctor?

MARKMAN: No, it is not.

THALE: In other words, when you give the same material, the same affect, regardless of what you are talking about, no change in the facial expressions, that does not mean a condition of mental illness?

MARKMAN: It is a condition, but it is not a *sine qua non*.

THALE: It is one of the conditions that are considered by psychiatrists in evaluating a mentally ill person when they show no facial or tone of voice regardless of the material being discussed?

MARKMAN: Correct.

THALE: You took that into consideration?

MARKMAN: I did.

THALE: You felt that there was insufficient (evidence) to show a mental illness at this time?

MARKMAN: Correct.

Thale ultimately wound up asking the same question Leavy had asked several times: If Dontanville had committed the crime, would that make him a mentally ill person? And the answer was still no. Whether he had committed the crime or not, whether he had been convicted or not, Anthony Dontanville was not mentally ill.

In effect, the proceedings were stopped. Although the judge could have taken our testimony and discarded it and ruled that Dontanville was a mentally ill person, he chose not to climb out on that limb. Dontanville was found not to be mentally ill and was not involuntarily hospitalized.

Afterward, one of the assistant district attorneys came up to me and said, "You know the guy is guilty. Why didn't you help us put him away?" I got crank phone calls from both sides. Someone called me the "embodiment of Christ," while others actually threatened me with death.

Though there have been times in my career when I have been upset at the consequences of my testimony, this was not such an instance. Dontanville was not a mentally ill person, nor was he a threat to society because of a mental disorder. I've often been asked whether I believed Dontanville actually committed the rape-murders. My answer to that is that I didn't, for certain, know the answer. But even if Dontanville had committed the crime, he had not done so because of a mental disorder.

My responsibility within the system is to provide psychiatric information that I can support within the boundaries of my profession and the requirements of the law. I can only report what I see and hear as a physician—and only within the limits of the answers to the questions the system asks me. What the system does with those answers is sometimes deeply disturbing. But distorting what I know to be the medical truth is no way to cure the system.

The psychiatric route was not the right way to handle this case. After all, if merely committing a crime brands one as mentally ill, why do we need psychiatrists? Let the crime determine the medical diagnosis.

Our society is leaning awfully close to the idea that you have to be mentally ill in some way to commit a crime. This is not so. Most crimes—even grisly murders—are not committed by mentally ill people, but by people just like you and me. Furthermore, most mentally ill people are not dangerous. It's a recurring theme in my career that serious crimes are mistakenly associated with mental illness—not only in the public mind, but in the legal system as well. The legal system is in large part to blame for this. Ironically, in the Dontanville case, psychiatric testimony prevented a man's detention by stating that he was *not* mentally ill— rather than the other way around.

J. Miller Leavy finally won his crusade against Anthony David Dontanville. Leavy was determined to put Dontanville away. As far as he was concerned, Dontanville was guilty, and the hair that ultimately didn't match up was a meaningless artifact. Within moments of the judge's pronouncing Dontanville a free man, sheriff's deputies stepped forward and arrested him on charges of child molesting and lewd conduct with a six-year-old girl in an area park.

Though the ordeal was not over for Anthony Dontanville, he maintained a poignantly hopeful attitude, looking toward a day when it would be over: "After all is over I intend to take some time to adjust. I want to get used to not being ordered around again. I may go into landscape work again. I may go into design. I will have to get my feet on the ground. It will probably be in California. I have been receiving all kinds of advice."

This time, the district attorney's office didn't bother trying to nail Dontanville with a "mentally ill" ruling. They tried him on sexual misconduct charges, convicted him, and sent him to prison. However, before sentencing was carried out, he was sent to Atascadero State Hospital for psychiatric evaluation. Apparently he did not make a very good impression on the people at the hospital. Actually, in looking at his records, all that can be found of a negative nature is that he was uncooperative during group therapy sessions and that he continued to deny the crime. Every other detailed description of his behavior does not seem out of line for a man who has been wrongly sent to a mental hospital. Yet Dontanville was sent back with an official diagnosis of "mentally disordered sex offender" and a recommendation that he be returned to prison because he was dangerous and not amenable to treatment. In March 1969 Anthony Dontanville was sent to prison.

California state authorities continued to receive letters from a contingent of over two hundred friends, acquaintances, and former fellow employees of Dontanville who maintained that he was not guilty of any of the charges filed against him, that the evidence at his child-molesting trial was not sufficient to convict him, that the judge at his murder trial showed prejudice, and that he was being persecuted by the L.A. County district attorney because he was not convicted of the murders.

More than twenty years have passed since I interviewed and evaluated Anthony Dontanville. I am still a forensic psychiatrist, and during these years I have been involved in thousands of cases, both criminal and civil, involving the famous, the not-so-famous, the has-beens, and the never-weres. In many instances my contribution was pivotal. In others it was disregarded and of no consequence. About ten years ago, I went to law school, obtained a law degree, and passed the bar. Why? Although medicine has always been my first love, I have also been fascinated by the law. Forensic psychiatry was, for me, a way to combine both disciplines and prove to myself that I could take the heat of being a physician who was always on the firing line. I also felt it was time to learn about what made lawyers tick—from the inside. Admittedly, I was also coaxed and cajoled into it by my friends in the legal profession who were tired of my complaints about the system.

There is still plenty to complain about—but now I can criticize with a much sharper edge because I know both professions from the inside.

J. Miller Leavy tried to put Dontanville away by using limited psychiatric information. Eventually he succeeded. I have been involved in similar cases, where prosecutors or police intent on solving a case have tried to use bits and pieces of evidence to construct a case, as well as cases where the system utterly failed to put dangerous criminals away because it refused to use information that was readily available.

I even played a key role in a case where the system tried to do both. I was called out of California on a case I call the "Solved Unsolved Murder Case," where a prominent citizen and his wife were found murdered in their bed. I can't identify the place any more specifically, for reasons that will become apparent. The man was about to be appointed to a very important position, so there was great media interest in the crime. But the police didn't have the slightest clue. That didn't stop them from coming up with a suspect, however. They arrested a young, slightly retarded man, who was known to wander around the neighborhood and look in windows. There were a few instances where the police were called in because he had just calmly walked into people's houses without being asked.

It seems he was particularly friendly with the woman who had been murdered. He had been seen with her several times, helping her around the house and yard with chores such as carrying her groceries, and other odd jobs. And he had been seen in the vicinity on the morning of the murders.

So the police had pieced together a scenario implicating him. They felt very strongly that he was the killer, and called me in to examine him.

Once I got a look at him and talked with him, it became clear to me that he was not the killer. As in Dontanville's case, this kid had been in the wrong place at the wrong time and got caught in the authorities' drive to put a thorny case to rest. Also like Dontanville, he was odd enough to appear to be a criminal—and hapless enough to be unable to defend himself against a powerful system. I told the police that in my opinion he was not the killer. But they were adamant. As in the Dontanville case, the official attitude was, "Don't bother me with the facts, our minds are already made up!"

I suggested they give him a polygraph test. They did, and the kid passed. As a result, they reluctantly let him go—although he remained their prime suspect. I returned to California, leaving behind some police officials who were not too pleased with the results of my consultation.

A few months later, a minister came forward and informed the police that someone had confessed the killings to him, and he knew the person's identity.

The case was solved—but it had to remain officially unsolved. The information obtained by the minister could not be used in court: it's inadmissible, privileged information, and is treated legally the same as information between a psychiatrist and a patient. So the police know who the killer is but can't do anything about it except keep an eye on him until some usable evidence is uncovered. Until then, the killer is walking the streets, a man whose body and soul, presumably, are free.

Unfortunately, no such confession ever emerged in Anthony Dontanville's case and he remained in custody until 1976, spent one year on parole, and was fully released on December 21, 1977, more than a decade after he was arrested.

3

THE FRUIT OF
THE FORBIDDEN TREE

As I saw in the Dontanville case and in all too many cases afterward, the truth often takes a beating in a court of law. Moreover, in the search for truth that a trial is supposed to be, the unfortunate fact is that certain truths are inadmissible. Truth is often the "fruit of the forbidden tree"—a biblical metaphor that is actually used in legal parlance. Hence we have cases like the one in the Midwest where a man murdered a young woman, was arrested and charged with the crime, but refused to tell the authorities where he had hidden the body. The murder had occurred between Thanksgiving and Christmas. One night, just before Christmas, the state police were driving the killer to the state prison to be held before his trial. The officers remarked to him that it would be nice if the family could bury their daughter before Christmas. The murderer relented and showed them where the body was.

At his trial, this evidence was not allowed. Why? It was "fruit of the forbidden tree" because the officers had not properly "Mirandized" the killer (read him his rights) *immediately before* asking him where the body was hidden. Though the man had been properly Mirandized when he was arrested and interrogated originally, the court ruled this new evidence inadmissible because the officers' talking to him in the car constituted a "new interrogation."

It's not unreasonable to protect the defendant, except that in doing so we often forget the victim. When we forget the victim, we lose touch with what the entire system is set up for in the first place. The system can be so perverted, however, that quite often the very protection afforded the defendant by the truth is the last one considered.

In the Chatman case I was brought in by the court to evaluate a man who was arrested for rape. The victim had positively identified Kenneth Chatman, a twenty-two-year-old welder, in a lineup. He had been arrested weeks after the rape and had been held in custody at a mental institution for three years because he was determined to be incompetent to stand trial. When I evaluated the man, I recognized him too. I knew I had seen him before. I checked my records and found that I had indeed evaluated him before. On the very day he was supposed to have committed this rape, he was in custody in the psychiatric unit of the county jail! Although this information was, to say the least, vital, there was no formal way I could provide it. I was limited to reporting on his mental state. I was being asked only whether he was insane or not—not whether he committed the crime. I had to strain the English language to its limits to make it a part of my official report. I said, in essence, "Kenneth Chatman was insane on the date of the crime, and was, in fact, in custody and being treated for his mental illness."

Though this fact was in plain view in all of Chatman's records, nobody noticed it until I brought it up. Belatedly, the charges against Chatman were dismissed.

In the case of John Zimmerman, I played a similar role, only in reverse. Because of facts I uncovered during the course of my evaluation, evidence was discovered that was vital to the conviction of a heinous killer.

Monday, April 17, 1978, began like any other day for the Dean family of Santa Monica. The house was in some disarray because of the repainting and remodeling the family was doing in some of the rooms. But Jim and Martha Dean, their eighteen-year-old son Brian and their twelve-year-old daughter Vriana, began the day pretty much the way they began every day. At six-thirty in the morning, Jim left for his job as a regional sales manager for an insurance company across town in central Los Angeles. Martha left for work at seven-thirty, and the children left for school around eight o'clock.

Brian got out of school early and stopped by his friend Stan's house for a while. Stan was mowing the lawn when Brian got there. They talked for about a half-hour and Brian left for home, which was not far away, saying he was going to mow his lawn, too. At around two-thirty that afternoon Brian called his father from the phone in the kitchen. He wanted to get a passport because he was planning a trip to Europe with a friend during the coming summer. He needed his birth certificate and asked his father if he knew where he might find it. Jim told him to look in the file cabinet in the master bedroom, which is exactly where Brian found it. The conversation lasted about five minutes.

About half an hour later, Vriana was leaving Lincoln Junior High School with her best friend, Monica, and another girlfriend, Jennifer. Doing more talking than walking, the seventh-grade girls took their time strolling from the grounds of the school, at Washington and Fifteenth Street, straight down Fifteenth Street until they arrived at Jennifer's house. Jennifer was going to let Vriana borrow some phonograph records. During the short time the girls were there, Monica drank a glass of water and Vriana had some Pepsi-Cola and tried on a pair of pants. Monica and Vriana left together at three forty-five. They walked to the corner of Fifteenth and Carlyle, and then split up. Monica walked off toward her house, and Vriana headed to hers. As they said good-bye, Vriana said she had some homework to do.

Two and a half hours later, the first unusual thing Jim Dean noticed when he arrived home was that the lid on the secretary desk in the living room was closed. He didn't give it much thought, but simply opened it. As he was looking through his mail, he glanced out the window and noticed a police car pull up near a neighbor's house. He went back to his mail before he could see exactly which house the policeman entered.

But then he noticed something else out of place. A small blue felt pouch, which was usually stored in the dining room hutch to protect the silverware, was lying empty on the floor. Jim walked over to the hutch and opened the three little drawers

where the silverware was kept. The drawers were empty. Then
he discovered more things out of place: dishes and several items
of silverware were strewn about the floor.

Jim realized that his home had been burglarized. His first
thought was to check if the microwave oven and the TV set were
taken. He walked from the dining room to the kitchen, and found
that the microwave and, from where he could see into the den,
the TV were still there. But he could also see beyond the den into
the family game room. And there he saw his son Brian's legs
sticking out from under the pool table.

Tentatively, Jim called his son's name. Then he walked over
to the pool table and saw that Brian was lying on his back with his
hands tied behind his back and his feet bound by the same cord of
speaker wire. His head was crushed and a hammer was embedded
in his skull. He was gagged.

Jim touched his son's leg and found that it was so cold that all
he could think was "Oh my God, oh my God." He got up and
ran out of the house and over to the next door neighbors' house.
Frantic, he rang the doorbell. Jim would not remember that it was
his neighbors' daughter who answered the door. When she did,
he asked if the police officer was there. She said he was.

"Please tell . . . please get him! My son has been murdered!" he stammered.

The policeman came to the door and followed Jim back to
his house, through the dining room, kitchen, and small den to the
pool table. The officer lit up Brian's body with his flashlight and
immediately said, "Let's get out of the house." The two men
started to walk out of the house when Jim remembered his daughter. He bolted from the policeman's side and ran into Vriana's
room. Her room was one of those that was in disarray from the
remodeling. All of the furniture had been pushed in the center of
the room, to allow them to work on the walls. Nothing appeared
to have been disturbed.

But on his way back down the hall, Jim could see into Brian's
bedroom. Before he even entered the room he could see that the
bed was saturated with blood. The room had been ransacked.
Dresser drawers were lying open and their contents strewn about
the room. Vriana was lying on the bed, naked and bloody. All Jim
could say was, "Oh no, no, no!" He started toward his daughter

but the policeman grabbed him and said, again, "Let's get out of the house."

The officer held on to Jim and walked him out of the room. As they were passing through the living room, the officer had to hold on tight and struggle with Jim a little when he thought of his wife and said, "Let's look in the rest of the house. My wife may be here."

"No, let's get out of the house," the officer repeated as he wrestled Jim Dean out the front door. While the officer called for back-up assistance, he left the stunned, horrified man leaning against the outside wall of his house.

A little while later, Martha Dean arrived home to find policemen all over her front lawn. Jim was waiting for her there, too. When he told her she couldn't go in the house, and why, she broke down, hysterically crying and screaming, "It can't be! It's a mistake!" Jim and another officer tried to comfort her. They took her to a neighbor's across the street, where they sat for a few moments. But it soon became apparent that Jim and Martha Dean were in shock. They were taken in a police car to the emergency room of the Santa Monica Hospital.

Witnesses to a murder, or people like the Deans, who happen upon loved ones who have been murdered, will remember only certain stark details of their discovery. Their minds may perfectly record every detail of the gruesome scene, yet they will "forget" all but a few. The police, however, must not only inspect the scene of the crime, but examine and record every minute detail—on paper—no matter how gruesome.

When the police inspectors reentered the Dean house, they found that all the lights in the house were on and that all of the rooms appeared to have been ransacked. They examined Brian Dean's body under the pool table. His blue-and-white tennis shoes, socks, and tan shorts were soaked or splattered with his blood, as was the floor around him. Brian's hands were tied behind his back with speaker cord, which then extended down to his feet, which were bound together, and up to his neck. He was tied in such a way that any movement would tighten the cord around his neck. He had been alive when he was tied, because he had bruises from the tight cord. He was also, in part, tied up with some drapery cord torn from some nearby drapes. The curtain rod lay on the floor.

Brian had not died of suffocation or strangulation, however. A blue-handled claw hammer with white paint spots was embedded in the boy's smashed right temple. He had been hit on the head at least 15 times. Pieces of his brain were splattered on the floor and on the side of his face, which was also almost completely covered with dark blood. His hair was matted with blood. The handle of what was later found to be a pickle fork was sticking out of the side of Brian's head. He had been gagged with one of the many blue-and-white strips of cloth that were lying around from the family's remodeling efforts.

Brian's blood was all over his neck, chest, and stomach, as well as in dried pools on the floor. In the midst of the blood there were several stab wounds and lacerations. There were three fingermarks in the blood on his chest, but no defensive wounds on the body. Brian's eyes were closed. Police noted that there were no signs of life.

Not far from his body were some barbells that had not been disturbed. In the dried spot of blood to his right there was a paring knife with a broken blade. The broken-off portion of the blade was never found. A few inches away there was a screwdriver. A little farther away there was an overturned portable cassette player with blood spots all over it. A bloody blue towel partially covered the player. A white cloth next to Brian's head was saturated with blood.

On top of the pool table was a pile of freshly laundered clothes, some of which had been neatly folded. Some of the laundered shirts hung from the center pocket of the pool table down to the floor near Brian's head. They were splattered with blood, and some of the laundry had been strewn around the room.

The sliding glass door beyond the pool table had pry marks on the outside. A lock had been removed from the inside of the door, enabling escape.

In the bathroom washbasin a blood-soaked blue towel was found and a fork. The toilet seat showed that someone may have vomited into the toilet. A young woman's clothes were lying on the floor.

In the kitchen, there was bloody water in the sink and spots of blood on the counter around it. A step-chair had been pulled over to the front of the refrigerator to enable someone to check the higher cabinets. Among the large carving knives hanging near the sink, one hanger was empty.

In Brian's bedroom, Vriana lay on her back across Brian's bed, naked except for a blood-soaked red knit jacket that was loosely draped around her shoulders. There was a red cloth around her neck. Her hands had been tied behind her back with speaker cord. There were at least twenty-five stab wounds in her neck and chest, many of which had merged into larger wounds. She was gagged with a strip of sheet torn from the bed. Vriana's face was covered with blood and the bed was soaked with her blood. There was blood and semen in and around her vagina. She had been alive when she was raped. Her head had been hit by an ax and a hammer at least eleven times. Vriana's skull was crushed and pieces of her brain had splattered here and there on her blood-soaked hair. Under her head and neck were her own blood-soaked panties. Her eyes were closed.

Lying across Vriana's right shoulder was a large stainless steel carving knife. The handle was nestled in the crook of her neck, and the blade extended down across her right breast. A two-inch splinter of wood lay on her right breast. Investigators were never able to trace the source of the piece of wood.

The walls and the lamp near the bed were splattered with blood. A blood-spattered blue blanket lay across her legs and a blue towel lay across her stomach. The night-stand drawer was open. A box of coins inside had been opened, and some papers from the drawer were scattered on the floor. On top of the night stand was an open jar of cleansing cream. Police found that the jar had some cream in it, two spots of blood, and one more thing: John Zimmerman's fingerprints.

Police inspectors canvassing the Deans' neighborhood found several people who had seen a blue or black Volkswagen in the area around the time of the murders. Two young men had been walking down the street when a black Volkswagen pulled up to the curb and the driver asked them where they lived and if anyone was home. The driver of the car told them that he "repaired houses." The Volkswagen was an older "bug" model, dull black, with dents front and back on the driver's side, and the rear windows darkened. The young man described the driver as a young adult white man, with the stubbly beginnings of a beard, black hair, wearing a tan ski cap. Other witnesses who saw the driver when out of the car said he was of medium height and build and was wearing faded jeans and a red shirt. He was apparently alone in the car. The boy and his friend saw the car drive up an alley. When they walked up the alley, they saw that the car was parked behind the Deans' house, and it was empty. They walked up to the car and wrote down the license number. The number was traced to Merrilee Zimmerman, John Zimmerman's wife.

While Zimmerman's latest address was being traced, it was learned that he had been arrested before for burglary.

At seven o'clock the next morning, nine police officers (five detectives and four officers) went to the Zimmermans' residence on Westwood Boulevard to arrest them. John was arrested wearing only his undershorts and a pair of glasses. Merrilee was wearing a housecoat and a half-slip and was carrying a brown leather purse. At the police station, matrons observed blood on Merrilee's half-slip and panties, so these were removed and retained as evidence.

Zimmerman was questioned at headquarters. After being advised of his rights, he said he would like to discuss the charges. He said he was a roofer and admitted that he had been in the neighborhood canvassing for leak-repair work. He admitted that he drove down alleys and, in some cases, entered back yards and even some houses, to look for leaky roofs. He said he had gone into a white house in which two small children were alone, but had left when he found out the parents were not home. He denied entering the Dean house and said he couldn't be sure he was in that exact area at all. When officers told him they had identified a fingerprint at the Dean house as his, he answered that there was no doubt that it was his print, but that he didn't know how it got there. He denied killing Brian and Vriana.

Zimmerman's wife waived her rights and told police she had been at the local public library around the time of the murders. Her story checked out and she was eventually released. The blood on her slip and panties was from her menstrual period.

In addition to the Deans' house and the house next door, at

least one other home in the neighborhood had been burglarized.
Both houses had been broken into in much the same way—
through a window broken by the burglar. Other people in the
neighborhood reported seeing a man answering Zimmerman's
description soliciting work in the neighborhood and "snooping
around" the afternoon of the murders.

While he was being held in the "lock-up," a temporary holding cell where everyone from murderers to traffic ticket scofflaws
are held, Zimmerman told fellow prisoners two different stories
about his involvement in the crimes of the previous day. In one
version, he had burglarized both the Dean house and the house
next door, but he denied having anything to do with the murders.
In the other version, he admitted to the burglary next door but
denied entering the Dean house for any purpose, claiming in
both cases that someone else must have committed the murders.
Zimmerman got in a fight with some of the other prisoners and
was moved to another cell.

In the late afternoon of Wednesday, April 19, 1978, only two
days after the murders, I was called in to examine John Zimmerman. Alone with him in a holding cell, I advised him of his rights,
that he didn't have to talk to me if he didn't want to, and that
anything he said could be used against him. I told him that I was
there to evaluate him psychiatrically. Zimmerman, a thin, weasely
man, agreed to the interview. He presented a calm, cooperative,
almost friendly demeanor.

We started talking about the afternoon of the murders.

ZIMMERMAN: I went back home and laid down and slept.
My wife woke me up about 2 o'clock or 2:30 or so. I do roofing
for a living and I was going to go out after the previous rain we'd
had and try to get some leak-repair work and make a little bit of
quick money that way and so I was out in Santa Monica canvassing around.

MARKMAN: Is that the way you have normally picked up
jobs like that before?

ZIMMERMAN: Yes. A lot of jobs. That's the way I get all
my side jobs. . . . I was more or less looking at people's roofs
finding built-up areas where there's lots of leaves, where the wa-

ter was dammed, and you know, create a leak in the house, broken ridges and things like that and curled-up wood shingles like that, and then I go and talk to people. And I did talk to a couple of people and I wrote down the number, I wrote down a little diagram of the places I talked to the people and the police say they can't find it anywhere or in the car or anything. They took me out today to try and find the place. Without my glasses, my vision is like I can't see from twenty feet what somebody else can see from a hundred.

MARKMAN: OK, so you're saying you stopped at two houses in that neighborhood?

ZIMMERMAN: Yeah.

MARKMAN: But not that particular house, the Dean house?

ZIMMERMAN: I have no idea about that house. I don't know where that house is in respect to anything.

MARKMAN: So how long were you in the neighborhood?

ZIMMERMAN: In the neighborhood, roughly about an hour and a half, something like that.

MARKMAN: So you were there at about the time this happened?

ZIMMERMAN: Yeah. Apparently.

MARKMAN: What time did you get back home? Did you go home after that?

ZIMMERMAN: No, I didn't. I had a job out in Inglewood that I've been trying to get at a coin shop. The guy's got a really bad leak up there and I was talking to him about it and I called my wife from over there.

MARKMAN: You went to Inglewood?

ZIMMERMAN: Yeah, and I called my wife from over there and told her that I was going to be a little bit late so that I'd be home about six-thirty or seven or something like that. So I went home from there.

MARKMAN: And you did see this guy in Inglewood?

ZIMMERMAN: Yes.

MARKMAN: What time did you get to Inglewood?

ZIMMERMAN: Oh, boy, I guess it was about four o'clock or so; four-thirty. I know I talked to him for quite a while.

MARKMAN: And did he give you the job?

ZIMMERMAN: Well, I, he, we, he was the guy that owns the place but he rents it from somebody across the street, so I was waiting to talk to the guy across the street but the guy never showed up, so I couldn't talk to him. That's why I waited around for as long as I did and then I left.

MARKMAN: When did you leave?

ZIMMERMAN: I left about six-thirty, I guess.

MARKMAN: So he can, this fellow, what's his name? Do you know?

ZIMMERMAN: Don.

MARKMAN: Don what?

ZIMMERMAN: I'm not sure what his last name is.

MARKMAN: But he can verify that you were there?

ZIMMERMAN: Yeah.

MARKMAN: And he can verify what you had on and everything, to the best that he can recollect?

ZIMMERMAN: Apparently, 'cause he had . . .

MARKMAN: What's the name of the Inglewood coin shop?

ZIMMERMAN: Don's Coin Shop. That's the name of the place.

MARKMAN: So you left at six-thirty and went home?

ZIMMERMAN: Um hum.

MARKMAN: And then I guess you stayed home the rest of the night?

ZIMMERMAN: Right. The next morning you know what happened.

MARKMAN: You got busted like at six o'clock.

ZIMMERMAN: Yeah. Shotguns at the door.

MARKMAN: Did you know about this murder?

ZIMMERMAN: No, I didn't.

MARKMAN: Did you watch TV that night or read the papers or listen to the radio?

ZIMMERMAN: I watched TV, yeah, but they didn't really say anything about it on TV. I don't think I watched any news program. I watch mostly movies and things. I watch the news once in awhile, not too often.

MARKMAN: Have you talked to an attorney yet?

ZIMMERMAN: Ah . . . I talked to . . . the public defender talked to me and he advised me not to talk to anybody without having him with me, you know.

MARKMAN: So why are you doing this?

ZIMMERMAN: Well, because I don't feel I have anything to hide. That's exactly it.

Unwittingly, in his story about the coin shop in Inglewood, Zimmerman had just told me something that would eventually help seal the case against him. He thought he was providing an alibi. In fact, he was doing just the opposite. I pressed on, mainly trying to gauge his mental status by observing his reaction when we talked about the crime and the circumstances of his arrest.

MARKMAN: OK, now there are a couple of things that undoubtedly are going to have to be explained away. I understand that they got a print that matches yours. How did that come?

ZIMMERMAN: I have no idea.

MARKMAN: Yeah, and also they got the license plate, that's obviously how they connected you up.

ZIMMERMAN: Yeah.

MARKMAN: The only thing you could say then about the fingerprint is that they're making a mistake?

ZIMMERMAN: Possibly. That's the only thing I could think of.

MARKMAN: It couldn't be that they're not making a mistake? I mean, if the assumption is that everybody has different fingerprints and they have a good print and they say the print is yours, they're making a mistake?

ZIMMERMAN: Yeah.

MARKMAN: What did you, how did you react when the police came? Was the place surrounded and things like that?

ZIMMERMAN: The whole place. My wife shook me and woke me up and said the police are outside and they're yelling and then I heard somebody yelling "You in the red house, come out with your hands up." And I put on my underwear and my glasses and walked outside and about seven, eight, or nine police standing around pointing shotguns at us yelling "Lay down on the ground, lay down on the grass, wherever you got to lay, get your ass down," so I don't argue when I see police with guns.

MARKMAN: Have you been busted before?

ZIMMERMAN: I have been arrested before.

MARKMAN: For what? As a juvenile and an adult?

ZIMMERMAN: As a juvenile, I was arrested once for, I broke a window in a car.

MARKMAN: That's malicious mischief.

ZIMMERMAN: Yeah, that was thrown out, I think, and then I had been arrested when I was in high school three or four times, something like that, for possession and driving under the influence of barbiturates. . . . I did one year of penitentiary time in Arizona.

MARKMAN: For what?

ZIMMERMAN: A burglary.

MARKMAN: This is as an adult now?

ZIMMERMAN: Yeah, that was in 1970.

MARKMAN: Any other arrests other than the one in Arizona? Any burglary arrests in California?

ZIMMERMAN: Yeah, I got one I am going on right now in Culver City. I guess it's been put out over here now.

MARKMAN: Did they find any of the supposed stuff, the contraband that was picked up there . . . from this house at your house? I mean, have they suggested that they found anything that was stolen from that place at all? Do you know what was taken?

ZIMMERMAN: No.

MARKMAN: Did they tell you?

ZIMMERMAN: No.

I was asking these questions to elicit and observe any emotional response on his part. There was none. The absent emotion was consistent with a man capable of butchering two teenage children.

MARKMAN: How long have you known this guy from Don's Coin Shop?

ZIMMERMAN: Oh, boy, about a month or so.

MARKMAN: Never knew him before that?

ZIMMERMAN: I'd gone into his shop once or twice a long time ago when I used to try and sell silver dollars and stuff like that.

MARKMAN: How are the police treating you?

ZIMMERMAN: Nice, if you don't mind being ignored.

MARKMAN: Being ignored?

ZIMMERMAN: Yeah. I mean I got pains 'cause I'm sick and they could care less, you know. But I guess that's their job.

MARKMAN: There's no way you could have been at this house and done this thing and not remembered it?

ZIMMERMAN: No. I never had a blackout like that in my life.

MARKMAN: Ever had a seizure?

ZIMMERMAN: No.

MARKMAN: Ever had a head injury?

ZIMMERMAN: No.

MARKMAN: Are you familiar with what happened to those two kids?

ZIMMERMAN: No.

MARKMAN: They didn't tell you at all?

ZIMMERMAN: They didn't tell me anything. I don't know anything about it. All I know is they got a fingerprint.

MARKMAN: You don't even know what they're holding you on?

ZIMMERMAN: I'm being booked for burglary and murder. That's all I know, that's it.

MARKMAN: I mean, you don't know anything about the facts or what allegedly happened or anything like that?

ZIMMERMAN: Uh-uh.

MARKMAN: When was the last time you had sexual intercourse with your wife?

ZIMMERMAN: Oh, Monday night.

MARKMAN: That was, um, that would have been the seventeenth.

ZIMMERMAN: Uh-huh.

MARKMAN: Ever cheat on her?

ZIMMERMAN: No, I got no reason to.

MARKMAN: No reason. You get along all right with her?

ZIMMERMAN: Yeah. We have little spats now and then but you know that's to be expected by living together?

MARKMAN: How often do you have sex together?

ZIMMERMAN: Well, since we've been on methadone we have it maybe two or three times a week something like that and it dulls the effects a little bit.

MARKMAN: So you aren't necessarily horny?

ZIMMERMAN: No.

MARKMAN: You ever forced a girl into sexual activity?

ZIMMERMAN: Uh-uh.

MARKMAN: How old were you when you first had sexual intercourse?

ZIMMERMAN: Fifteen.

MARKMAN: Ever had any gay experience?

ZIMMERMAN: No.

MARKMAN: Ever been a peeping tom?

ZIMMERMAN: Uh-uh.

MARKMAN: Ever been an exhibitionist?

ZIMMERMAN: I think I'm gonna be if these pants, you know they took me in my shorts and they gave me a size forty-four pants. They take me out everywhere and handcuff me behind my back and expect me to keep my pants up.

MARKMAN: Well, why don't they give you a belt?

ZIMMERMAN: They figure I might hang myself with it. They won't even let me have my glasses so I can see. The guy said you might file it down and cut your wrists with it, you know.

MARKMAN: Anything else you want to tell me, John? Anything you think I haven't covered that you want to tell me?

ZIMMERMAN: That's about it, I guess.

MARKMAN: Ever experience hallucinations? You know, hearing or seeing things that weren't there? Never felt people were out to get you?

ZIMMERMAN: No paranoia.

MARKMAN: Not even now?

ZIMMERMAN: No. There isn't any way I can get another cigarette, is there?

MARKMAN: I don't smoke or I'd give you one. We're almost through here. You were kind of in the wrong place at the wrong time.

ZIMMERMAN: Yeah.

MARKMAN: They didn't tell you who the victims were in this case? Male, female, you don't know anything?

ZIMMERMAN: I don't know nothing.

MARKMAN: I have a couple of questions that are really unrelated. How good are you at mathematics, things like that?

ZIMMERMAN: Pretty good.

I then proceeded to ask him some questions to gauge his fund of knowledge, intelligence, and general thinking abilities.

MARKMAN: How much is nine times eight?

ZIMMERMAN: Seventy-two.

MARKMAN: Who's the mayor of L.A.?

ZIMMERMAN: Bradley.

MARKMAN: Who's the first baseman for the L.A. Dodgers?

ZIMMERMAN: I don't know.

MARKMAN: You don't follow sports. What do you watch on TV?

ZIMMERMAN: Mostly comedy situation series like "Happy Days" and . . .

MARKMAN: Who are the stars of "Happy Days"?

ZIMMERMAN: Henry Winkler, Ron Howard. I watch shows like "M*A*S*H" with Alan Alda and, you know, mostly shows like that.

MARKMAN: If I said to you a table and a chair, what they have in common, I think the answer would be furniture. What are they? How about a pair of pants and a shirt?

ZIMMERMAN: Clothes.

MARKMAN: How about a bicycle and an airplane?

ZIMMERMAN: Transportation.

MARKMAN: How about a fly and a tree?

ZIMMERMAN: A fly and a tree? Places you live— No, I don't know that one.

MARKMAN: How about a match and the sun in the sky?

ZIMMERMAN: Fire and light.

MARKMAN: What does it mean when someone says you don't cry over spilled milk?

ZIMMERMAN: It means what's happened has happened and you make the best of it.

MARKMAN: How about: You can take a horse to water, but you can't make him drink it?

ZIMMERMAN: You try and show somebody the right way but they don't necessarily have to go along with it.

MARKMAN: How about: People in glass houses shouldn't throw stones?

ZIMMERMAN: That's people that do wrong things shouldn't go after people that are doing the same thing.

MARKMAN: How about: Mounted beggars race their steeds?

ZIMMERMAN: No. I never heard that one before.

MARKMAN: That's why I gave it to you.

ZIMMERMAN: Mounted beggars?

MARKMAN: Mounted beggars . . . race their steeds.

ZIMMERMAN: A person can get what he wants faster.

MARKMAN: That's not bad, that's pretty . . . I mean it doesn't have one single interpretation. But that's not bad. (Actually, I think the more traditional answer is that when a person gets something he never had before, he tends to abuse or overuse it.)

ZIMMERMAN: I'm glad to hear that. Does that mean I'm OK in the head?

MARKMAN: Pretty good, yes. Very few people get that one.

ZIMMERMAN: What's a fly and a tree?

MARKMAN: Life.

ZIMMERMAN: Life? OK.

MARKMAN: Agree?

ZIMMERMAN: Yeah.

MARKMAN: OK. All right.

ZIMMERMAN: Weird comparison, huh?

MARKMAN: Well, it's just . . .

ZIMMERMAN: Well, not weird, I mean it's a vast difference.

MARKMAN: Sure, but there's a vast difference between a bicycle and a plane, too.

ZIMMERMAN: There sure is.

If a person doesn't know what "Mounted beggars race their steeds" means, it may be an indication that there is something wrong with his thinking. Zimmerman didn't supply a suitable response because he wasn't intellectually resourceful. He got the earlier ones, but as they got harder, he had a tougher time. What I look for in the answers is a thought disorder. People with thought disorders will not be able to transpose these sayings into human experience. For example, if I say "Birds of a feather flock together," the person may say "Swallows fly with swallows," rather than explaining that people who think, act, or look alike are comfortable together.

The examples get progressively harder. In the similiarities, for example, a chair and a table are fairly easy to group together as furniture. A pair of pants and a shirt are obviously both items of clothing. Some people have trouble with the easy ones, though. I've had people say that both the chair and the table have legs. Or that an airplane and a bicycle both have wheels. Once, someone told me that a shirt has buttons and pants sometimes have buttons, too.

The ploy in these questions is that I'm asking for a broad connection, not a narrow one. I'm asking for inductive reasoning, not deductive. I'm not asking for minute details that these things might have in common, but for the general category that they both always fall within.

As for the fly and the tree, only a small percentage of people I ask are even in the ballpark. I've had people say that flies land on tree leaves, or even that a fly's wing looks like the pattern in leaves.

Shortly before I left, Zimmerman betrayed some curiosity.

ZIMMERMAN: Can you give me any idea about what you think?

MARKMAN: Well, I don't think you're crazy.

ZIMMERMAN: Good.

MARKMAN: I don't think you're . . .

ZIMMERMAN: You think I'm sadistic, or immoral, or . . .

MARKMAN: Ah, that you can't tell in one interview, whether—you know we're all capable . . . I've met some very docile people who blow their cool and I've evaluated hundreds of people who have committed very serious crimes. And there are very few people that if you sit down on a one-to-one basis with, they're not pleasant like you are now, pleasant, cooperative, friendly. But we're all human.

ZIMMERMAN: True.

MARKMAN: OK.

ZIMMERMAN: Do you have any pull outside so I can get my dough and get me out of here?

My conclusion was that Zimmerman was not insane. He demonstrated adequate intelligence and was not prone to a transient "flip-out" or lapse of consciousness. He was completely oriented and was not fantasizing. He was not psychotic. Zimmerman was a psychopath, or, in more up-to-date psychiatric terms, a sociopath, or antisocial personality. (All three terms are interchangeable.)

If you could crawl into Zimmerman's mind and examine the elements of his psyche, you would find one essential ingredient missing: a conscience. That is perhaps the most significant characteristic of a sociopath, because it allows full and often violent expression without significant hesitation, guilt, shame, or remorse. Sociopaths are unable to learn from experience or punishment, and they frequently get into trouble with the law. They often fancy themselves as antiheroes or rebels, but they are incapable of any true loyalty to a person or cause. Sociopaths are hedonistic, emotionally immature, selfish, impulsive, and devious. Their goals are often quite primitive, and usually are centered on power and pleasure. Sociopaths tend to consider other people only as objects to be exploited, avoided, or neutralized.

Successful sociopaths can make it big in business, politics, or sales, areas where they can manipulate others. Unsuccessful sociopaths bounce from trouble to trouble, arrest to arrest, jail cell to jail cell. In the extreme, they wind up committing crimes that are horrible, violent, and cruel. Although it is certainly a mental disorder, sociopathy does not reduce culpability for a crime. The sociopath knows right from wrong, and will commit the crime because his internal "policeman" is absent—but will not if there is an "external" policeman watching. When caught—even caught red-handed—a sociopath tends to shift the blame to others, to "circumstances," or offer rationalizations for the behavior. Or simply lie. A sociopath can look you in the eye and lie without blinking or registering any anxiety on a lie detector. So Zimmerman would know if he was lying. And apparently, he was doing plenty of that.

Even more important than my psychiatric evaluation, however, was the clue Zimmerman had given me about his going to the coin shop. He had told the police that he had gone to the

shop after he left Santa Monica, but he did not tell them that he
went to the shop to sell the things he had stolen from the Dean
house and other houses in the neighborhood. Zimmerman had
actually told police to call the coin shop as an alibi for where he
was at the time of the murders. From previous records, police
knew that the shop had taken stolen items in pawn from Zimmerman. But when the police first questioned the proprietor, he denied knowing Zimmerman, and the police didn't take it any further. As sometimes happens, an overburdened police department
simply failed to follow up on a lead which, in retrospect, appears
quite important.

I later urged the police to talk to the owner of the shop
again. They did. He was evasive and reluctant to get involved.
This time they impressed upon him the importance of telling
them what he knew. Under pressure, he cooperated. At the coin
shop, police found the silverware and other items stolen from the
Dean house. The owner identified Zimmerman as the person
who had sold him these things the afternoon of the murders.

Zimmerman also lied about the time. He said he was in Inglewood at the coin shop at four, four-thirty. The shop proprietor
testified that he was there between six-fifteen and six-thirty. Zimmerman was at the coin shop at almost the exact same time Jim
Dean was coming home to find his murdered children.

My interview with Zimmerman helped shatter his flimsy alibi. Before I got that information from him, the police had some
fingerprints and a person who saw him at the house and who took
down the license number on his Volkswagen. With that evidence,
they might be able to prove that Zimmerman was at the scene,
but not necessarily that he had committed the crimes. This new
information about the coin shop in Inglewood gave them solid
evidence. Without the knowledge about the stolen goods, the
case might have been more difficult to prove.

Apparently, Zimmerman thought he could use the meeting
at the coin shop as an alibi. He assumed the proprietor would lie
for him and hide the evidence that removed all doubt that Zimmerman had robbed the Dean home. Zimmerman thought he
was smart enough to fool everybody in the system. He was willing to take on anybody: police, prosecutor, psychiatrists—anybody. John Zimmerman, in true sociopathic fashion, believed he

could pretend to cooperate, appear to play the game by the rules, and beat the rap. He even expressed a willingness to take a lie detector (polygraph) test.

Let me explain about sociopaths. There are two kinds of people who can consistently muddle polygraph results: sociopaths and hysterics. Hysterics can answer the questions and not manifest anxiety during the test because their feelings are divorced from their thoughts. As a result, the physiological changes measured by the polygraph do not occur. There is no pulse elevation, no increase in blood pressure or respiration or galvanic skin response. The hysteric tends to put his or her head in the sand, to repress and deny reality.

Say a woman strangles her child and develops a hysterical reaction to the event. She's given a polygraph test. In such a test, the procedure is not to ask direct questions, such as, Did you strangle your child?—but to be rather indirect about it: Have you ever felt like killing a child? The hysteric will say, No—and the polygraph will not register as much as a blip. Why not? Because she has lost the connection between her actions and feelings. She will not feel the anxiety associated with the question, so the question will not evoke any of the physiological changes that go along with anxiety.

The sociopath can also distort lie detector results, but not for the same reason. The sociopath will likewise not register any signs of anxiety when the questions start to approach the crime. But whereas the hysteric has buried the anxiety, the sociopath has no anxiety in the first place. The hysteric feels and knows that the crime is wrong, and so reacts by disconnecting from the feelings associated with the knowledge. The sociopath expresses no anxiety because there is none. As far as the sociopath is concerned, he knows he did it—and responds by saying, So what? Both the hysteric and the sociopath have defective superegos, but at opposite ends of the spectrum. Where the former's is too harsh, the latter's ranges from too lenient to nonexistent.

This is the kind of mind that butchered the Dean children. The only thing that could have stopped John Zimmerman would have been the immediate prospect of getting caught or being, himself, hurt in some way. He felt no guilt or remorse whatever for his crimes, and no pity for his victims. Did he feel anything at all? While he tortured and murdered Brian and Vriana, he most likely felt an exhilarating sense of power. For those horrible moments, John Zimmerman felt a rush of godlike control over his victims. After that, he felt less guilt than a person who cheats on a diet. Zimmerman was able to discuss the crime and lie without flinching. In fact, he tried to manipulate me to get him out of jail or get his money back for him, the very money that helped incriminate him.

Zimmerman was tried and found guilty of two counts of first-degree murder. The prosecutor tried to get the death penalty, but because the jury was undecided, had to settle for life imprisonment without possibility of parole. Zimmerman appealed the decision, but the sentence was upheld.

In the Zimmerman case, information I provided helped lock up a dangerous sociopath. Remember, however, that I had been brought into the case by the prosecutor. Had I been brought in by the *defense,* everything Zimmerman told me during my evaluation would have been "in confidence." It would have been "fruit of the forbidden tree," so *I would not have been able to tell the prosecutor a word of it!* When I am brought into a case by the defense, everything I learn during my interview is confidential information, as between any doctor and patient. I do not even testify in court at all unless I'm first called to do so by the defense, or the privilege is waived.

In any criminal trial, everything discovered by the defense is confidential. The defense can use the information or keep it secret. Only the prosecutor is legally and ethically bound to reveal everything known before the trial. The defense, however, can conceal any and all secrets. For a long time, only defendants who could afford to shop around for favorable psychiatric evaluations could take advantage of this rule as it pertains to psychiatric testimony. A wealthy defendant could keep hiring psychiatrists until he found one whose evaluation suited his defense. Any unfavorable psychiatric evaluation could be kept out of court by simply not calling the psychiatrist to testify. A poor defendant did not have this luxury and was provided only one psychiatrist by the court. In many cases that evaluation was not confidential. This practice continued until someone pointed out that it amounted to unequal protection under the law. So the rule was changed to allow poor defendants to have the right to a confidential, inviolate psychiatric evaluation.

In contrast to the Zimmerman case, the Tripiccio case demonstrates what happens when I'm called in by the defense in a criminal matter. The rules that I function by, as you will see, are totally different.

I was called into the Tripiccio case by the defense. While under the influence of drugs, Tripiccio had killed his grandfather. The defense wanted me to evaluate the young man to determine his state of mind at the time of the murder. The defense attorney was hoping my evaluation would allow him to argue for a reduced charge, from second-degree murder to manslaughter. Recall that first-degree murder involves malice, deliberation, and premeditation. Second-degree murder involves only malice, but not premeditation or deliberation. To reduce a second-degree murder charge down to manslaughter, I would have to find that his state of mind was such that he lacked the capacity for malice.

I examined Tripiccio, went back to the attorney and said, "According to my evaluation, his mental state doesn't exclude malice." I was unable to say that mental limitations reduced his culpability from murder to manslaughter. It could have been second-degree murder. As a result, the defense attorney, Alan Oberstein, didn't want to use me at the trial at all, which was his right. Normally, then, I would not even show up on the day of the trial.

But this trial was different. The prosecutor subpoenaed me. I had to appear, and I had to take the witness stand when I was called. But once I was there, I claimed "privilege," the legal equivalent of confidentiality. In other words, I stated that the information I obtained in my evaluation didn't belong to me but to my patient. Therefore, unless he released the information, which could be self-incriminating, I couldn't reveal any of it. It was "fruit of the forbidden tree."

The judge, who was something of a courtroom tyrant (and, by the way, the same judge who, after Dontanville's second trial, scolded the jury for bringing in a not guilty verdict) ordered me to testify, despite the privilege.

"But there's case law that says I don't have to," I replied.

The judge insisted, and threatened to throw me in jail for contempt of court if I didn't testify.

If I did testify, I would be breaking privilege—but because I'd be doing it under order of a judge in court, I would be under legal protection. Some professionals will advise not to testify, even under those circumstances. Some will say it makes no difference, since with the law the way it was, the case was going to be reversed anyway if the judge forced me to do something against the existing law.

I then told the judge that I didn't have my records of the evaluation with me. They were at my office.

The judge said he would call a recess until one-thirty. I was to get the files and be back by then or be thrown in jail for contempt of court.

It was eleven-thirty in the morning. I had additional work to do over lunch, and there was no way I could pick up the files and get back in time. So I called my wife and asked her to retrieve the files and meet me outside the courthouse at one-fifteen to give them to me.

I was supposed to meet her at the corner of Temple and Spring in downtown Los Angeles. She was on time—but I was held up. As she was waiting for me, with our newborn son in the car, she saw a friend of mine, attorney David Guthman, walking by with another man. She called to him, told him she was supposed to meet me to give me some papers, and said, "I've got to run, are you going to see Ron?"

My friend David said he wasn't. But the man he was walking with said he was going to see me. So my wife gave the Tripiccio files to David, who gave them to the other man . . . who was also an attorney. He was Alan Oberstein, Tripiccio's defense attorney.

I got to the corner minutes later. My wife wasn't there, so I ran back into the courthouse and up to the courtroom to tell the judge that my wife hadn't shown up with the files yet. On the way, I ran past Alan Oberstein, who remarked, "Ron, I saw your wife."

"What do you mean you saw my wife?"

"I was with Dave Guthman, and we ran into her, and she gave me the report."

I asked him to give me the report.

He refused. "I don't have to," he said.

"Alan, you've got to give me the report. It's my report!"

"No, I don't have to." In a lawyer kind of way he was right. He got the report legitimately, not through any fraud or subterfuge.

Court reconvened, with me on the witness stand. The judge asked me if I retrieved the file.

I said, "Yes and no."

The judge asked me to explain.

I explained that I'd asked my wife to bring it down for me, but that she had given it to Alan Oberstein, whom she saw walking with a friend of ours. Mr. Oberstein had refused to hand it over to me.

The prosecuting attorney went into a tirade, alleging "This is a conspiracy!" and accusing me of withholding evidence and obstructing justice. I reluctantly realized that I was now in the company of Richard Nixon and the Watergate conspirators.

So the judge said to the prosecutor: "Ask Dr. Markman to ask the defense attorney for the report."

The prosecutor looked at me and said, "Dr. Markman, will you please ask Mr. Oberstein for the report?"

I looked at the judge and asked, "Is that a question?"

"Yes," he said.

"How am I supposed to answer it?"

"Follow the request," he replied sternly.

I said, "Mr. Oberstein, will you give me the report?"

Mr. Oberstein said, "No."

The judge excused me from the witness stand, but not before he said he was withholding his decision whether or not to hold me in contempt for conspiring to obstruct justice.

Days later the jury came back with a conviction: guilty of first-degree murder. The judge was said to have blanched. He had made an incorrect ruling despite controlling case law. In order to reach the ends, he was mangling the means. On appeal, the decision was reversed on the grounds of prosecutorial misconduct. Inasmuch as justices rarely reprimand their own, the judge's questionable decisions were not raised in the opinion.

If you look for this case in the law journals you won't find it.

In a masterful ploy used to hide the perversions of the system, the decision, though written, was not published in the case law journals. It exists only in the bowels of the records at the courthouse in Los Angeles.

CHAPTER 4

COLD-BLOODED

HEAT OF PASSION

Most people think of courtroom psychiatrists as helping criminals get by with less blame and punishment. That public perception is not only sometimes correct, but it's also shared by attorneys, judges, and juries. One night I was at my son's high school for an open house program when an attorney friend came up to me: "Ron, you're going to have to be a little more lenient in your reports," he said.

"What do you mean?" I asked him.

"Because the death penalty is back in," he explained, "we're going to have to use psychiatrists more and more to protect our clients."

My friend was not joking. In a jovial, friendly way, he was revealing his exact intentions, and the intentions of most other criminal defense attorneys. They know that psychiatric testimony can be used to lower the heat on their clients, and they have no qualms about using it to the fullest extent, even if it means abusing the medical information and further corrupting the justice system that allows it so much influence—influence that has spread way beyond the relatively simple issues of competency to stand trial and sanity at the time of the crime. Although psychiatrists were once limited to testifying about these two limited issues, the past four decades have seen them invade the very heart of the proceedings. Now psychiatrists supply information that not only helps determine a defendant's sanity, but also helps the court decide *what level of crime has actually been committed.*

Psychiatrists didn't ask for this power; it was thrust upon them by the appeals courts, egged on by ambitious attorneys.

In order to understand why and how this came about, it's necessary to understand something about the legal term "diminished capacity." The issue arises automatically when a crime can fall into various degrees of seriousness depending on the state of mind of the defendant.

The law says that a crime requires two things: an act and a criminal state of mind, or intent. In other words, you not only have to *do* something "bad," but you also must have a "bad" intent. This distinction is necessary to determine how serious a crime has actually been committed and how severe the punishment should be. The law recognizes that there is a difference between shooting someone accidentally while cleaning your gun, and planning the killing, lying in wait, aiming, and shooting the victim in the back. One is accidental and potentially not punishable at all. The other is murder, and potentially punishable by death.

Our society has a long history of making these distinctions, and they have become fairly sophisticated, as well as complicated. In order for a killing to be first-degree murder, the defendant must demonstrate three mental elements in addition to killing: he must premeditate, deliberate and harbor malice. If he doesn't premeditate and deliberate, but does harbor malice, then it's second-degree murder. If there is no malice, but merely an intent to kill, then the killing is voluntary manslaughter. If none of the elements are present, but there is reckless disregard for human life, then the killing is involuntary manslaughter. Any other homicide would be excusable or accidental.

As these definitions evolved in the courts, the distinctions were made according to the evidence at hand, even though they involve something that happens in the mind of the defendant. The questions were answered from the known details of the case. Did the killer's actions indicate that he premeditated and deliberated? Did his actions indicate that he harbored malice? Did his actions indicate that he intended to kill? The judge and jury drew their conclusions based on whether it *looked as though he did* from what facts were plainly evident. If there were disagreements, they argued over what the defendant's *actions* said about his state of mind, not over what a psychiatrist said. Psychiatrists were not even allowed to testify during this part of a trial. In California and many other states, the psychiatrists were not allowed in the courtroom until the issues of the degree of crime and guilt had already been decided.

But all that started to change after the Second World War, with the introduction of diminished capacity. In California, the Wells case, in 1949, involved a man serving a life sentence who threw a heavy pot at a prison guard. The law said that when a life prisoner intentionally attacked a prison guard, the crime was punishable by death. At the trial, psychiatric testimony was offered that Wells did not have the mental capacity to act intentionally because his mind was in a state of fear and tension. The trial court refused to allow the psychiatric testimony. The appeals court disagreed, and said that it was perfectly acceptable for a psychiatrist to testify as to whether a defendant had the mental capacity to form the required state of mind to commit a crime.

This decision was a big crack in the dam, and amounted to an invitation by the appeals court to have attorneys bring in psychiatrists in droves to shove aside the facts at hand about the case and substitute their own version of the defendant's state of mind. No longer was it just a matter of deciding whether or not a killer had, *in his actions,* premeditated, deliberated, harbored malice, or intended to kill. Now a psychiatrist could come in and testify as to whether the killer *had the mental capacity* to premeditate, deliberate, harbor malice, or intent to kill.

Obviously, the potential for complicating the system was enormous. The entire range of psychiatric knowledge that had developed since the middle of the nineteenth century could now be applied—not at two relatively limited points at the beginning and end of a trial—but at four or five critical junctures at the heart of the proceedings. At the very least, it gave every defense attorney two passes at the same brass ring. If the attorney couldn't successfully argue, for example, that his client did not *in fact* harbor malice, then he could bring in a psychiatrist who would say that the defendant *lacked the mental capacity* to harbor malice.

The dam was cracked, but it didn't burst quite yet. Over the next decade and a half, more and more psychiatrists trickled into the courtroom. Several more appeals courts' decisions eventually helped to open the floodgates and inundate the system with psychiatric testimony.

A second landmark case came in 1959. An appeals court reversed the second-degree murder conviction of a man named Gorshen by saying that a mental abnormality not severe enough to bring about a verdict of "not guilty by reason of insanity" could still be used as a defense. Short of letting him off totally, the court said his diminished mental capacity could reduce his responsibility by lowering the sophistication of his state of mind.

Now the dam was completely gone. Additional landmark cases widened the chasm still further, and made it increasingly difficult to prove that a killer's state of mind was sophisticated enough to sustain murder charges. In 1964, for example, in the Wolff case, the California Supreme Court reduced a first-degree murder conviction to second-degree murder on the basis of psychiatric testimony that was, apparently, ignored by the jury. The case involved a teenage boy who got it into his head that he would like to have sex with some girls at his high school. But he knew he could never do it at home because his mother wouldn't allow it. So he figured the best way to do it was to have an orgy where the girls lived. He went over there and, instead of knocking at the door, climbed up on the roof and tried to go down the chimney. He got stuck and the fire department had to be called to get him out. After that, he figured the only place he could have his orgy was at home. But what to do about his mother? One day he went after her with an ax—and killed her.

At his trial there was plenty of psychiatric testimony that said he was mentally disturbed, psychotic. But the jury looked at the facts of the case and decided that he did, in fact, deliberate and premeditate, so they convicted him of first-degree murder and gave him a life sentence. The California Supreme Court disagreed, and reduced the conviction to second-degree murder. On what basis? On their judgment that though it was obvious that the boy premeditated and deliberated, owing to his mental disturbance he could not do so at a "meaningful and mature" level. In effect, what they did for the defendant was to reduce a sentence of nine to life to a sentence of five to life, with the possibility of parole within three rather than seven years.

But what the court did to the criminal-justice system was to create an enormous loophole through which hundreds of killers escaped murder charges.

Another devastating, yet more sinister, effect was that attorneys started planning their defenses not only for the juries, but also for the appellate process. They started bringing in psychiatrist after psychiatrist to give expert opinions on the diminished capacity of the defendant's state of mind. The prosecuting attorneys countered with psychiatrists of their own. As a result, many trials became battles among psychiatrists and other experts. Juries, as might be expected, were often not sophisticated enough to understand the expert testimony. But the attorneys weren't playing for the juries—they were playing to the appeals courts, building a record for a potential appeal, where they knew the judges would relish the challenge of sorting out the complicated medical opinions and making their own decisions, the jury be damned.

Not a single solitary guideline for diminished capacity was created by a legislature passing a law. It was all court-created. No wonder trial judges, not to mention juries, grew suspicious and disdainful of psychiatrists. They knew that the psychiatrists were there to plant seeds that could eventually confound the system and overturn their decisions.

In 1976, for example, the California Supreme Court went so far as to rule that a person without a preexisting mental illness could, for all intents and purposes, be provoked into a diminished mental state that would reduce responsibility for a crime. In the Berry case, a woman taunted her husband by teasing him sexually while she openly carried on an affair with another man. Finally, the husband no longer could stand the torment of simultaneous sexual advances mixed with infidelity and demands for a divorce. He choked his wife with a telephone wire. Despite the fact that a psychiatrist testified that the man had been acting in the "heat of passion" and an "uncontrollable rage" because of the extreme provocation, the jury convicted him of first-degree murder.

The California Supreme Court reduced the charge to voluntary manslaughter. Although they drew a distinction between "heat of passion" and "diminished capacity," they had, in effect, established that even in the absence of heat of passion a reasonable man could be pushed into a mental state that would negate the malice requirements for murder. This was an important case, because it proposed that even though a killer was acting in what appeared to be cold blood—by premeditating, deliberating—if he lacked the necessary malice aforethought it diminished his capacity and his responsibility to a level of manslaughter.

Although I am generally critical of the liberties taken by the California Supreme Court, I was involved in a case that was, to me, a classic example of what I termed "cold-blooded heat of passion."

As the eldest grandchild, Kevin Green, whose name has been changed to protect his identity, was the "crown prince" of his upper-middle-class Bay Area family. His parents encouraged their three sons to do well in school and plan useful careers. The Greens had high expectations for Kevin and his younger brothers, Sean and Tim. Kevin planned a career in law, following in the footsteps of his father, who was a successful attorney and real estate investor. Kevin's mother provided a good example, too. She had recently returned to school and obtained her master's degree in literature at nearby San Jose State, the same university at which Kevin planned to begin his college career in the fall of 1985.

Their oldest son had never disappointed them. Kevin had always done well in school: he had always been in the "gifted" classes, he had a solid B+ average in high school, and was looking forward to an equally successful college career. He was a high achiever not only in school, but also in his extracurricular activities. When he was only thirteen, he became the youngest state-certified soccer referee and regularly volunteered his services. When his neighborhood flooded, he tirelessly helped others save property and reduce the damage. Kevin was interested in police work, too, and took a class taught by one of the local sheriff's deputies. He looked up to the deputy and thought seriously of becoming a member of the "police reserves." To do that, he knew he'd have to keep his record clean, but that was not a problem. Kevin had never gotten as much as a traffic ticket.

Kevin also took pride in keeping his 1979 Mustang in perfect mechanical condition and cosmetically dazzling. In fact, he was able to turn his fascination with cars into a profitable neighborhood automobile detailing business. He had two teenage employees who would pick up the customer's car and drive it to his house for washing, waxing, and fine detailing work. Out of the $100 the customer paid for this service, Kevin gave his employees $30 and kept $70.

Kevin also worked hard at his part-time job as a pizza delivery boy. He sometimes earned as much as $60 in one night, and often referred to himself as "the best delivery guy in the world." From these enterprises, and despite the great sums of money he lavished on his automobile, Kevin managed to save $3,000 by the end of his senior year in high school.

But to his parents, Kevin always seemed to be a somewhat lonely boy. When the Greens had lived in Belmont, until he was nine years old, he did have a number of close friends. But when the family moved to Los Altos Hills, several miles farther south on the peninsula, there were fewer children his own age in the neighborhood, and his former friends lived too far away for him to see regularly. He still had outside activities: for a while he was a member of the 4H Club and raised chickens. Yet Kevin seemed to become more isolated as he grew into adolescence.

Although he was always a very popular young man, by his own admission Kevin was not very open to developing friendships: "When I think about it, more people wanted to be friends with me than I wanted. I was in the gifted classes and didn't have anything in common with kids who weren't in those classes. Besides, I was real overweight. By fifteen, I weighed about 240 pounds and was really miserable about my weight."

Although the family remained close-knit, Kevin did not participate in family activities as often as his parents might have wished. When he was home, he seemed to come out of his room only for meals. His mother and father tried to reach out and make contact with him, but he did not respond. Instead, he spent long hours in his room with his computer.

Kevin had discovered computers at the age of thirteen. Before long, he was a real "hacker," with an array of computer hardware and the know-how to put it to imaginative and entertaining use. Kevin's parents didn't feel this was very strange, since they were living right in the middle of California's Santa Clara Valley, the so-called Silicon Valley. To them, Kevin's obsession with his computers was just part of his isolation. They had no way of knowing how wrong they were. For Kevin Green had a secret life—and his computer was not only a window into that life, but a door, as well.

One of the first pieces of peripheral hardware Kevin obtained for his computer was a modem, which enables a computer to tie in with other computers over telephone lines. Kevin could then communicate not only with any other individual who had a similar machine, but also with entire networks of computer operators—sort of like a computer "party line," in which people exchange messages directly or through an electronic bulletin board. Most of these computer bulletin boards tend to organize around a single shared interest. There are, for example, computer bulletin boards made up for people who all own the same brand of computer, who share the same interest in electronics or short-wave radio, and even computer bulletin boards for shoppers.

The bulletin board Kevin discovered and was most drawn to was the Gay Bulletin Board.

Kevin had been sexually attracted to other boys as long as he could remember. When he still lived in Belmont, he had engaged in sex play with a friend who had slept over. When he was twelve he went on a school trip to Washington, D.C., where he and his roommate found themselves "messing around" one night. Each boy blamed the other for what happened, and they almost got into a fight over the incident. Later, there were more incidents like this, in which Kevin and a friend would engage in sex play and then end their friendship in a storm of guilt and anger.

Throughout his early teenage years, Kevin's sexual fantasies always involved his male friends. Often, he rejected male friends because he felt too attracted to them. "I was afraid to get close to them," he said. These feelings contributed to Kevin's sense of isolation and self-doubt.

But the computer, and the Gay Bulletin Board, opened up a new world for Kevin Green. "On that earliest bulletin board," he remembered, "they were all adults and mostly into various types of S&M, so I didn't call back until I was about sixteen. By then, there were hundreds of gay bulletin boards, so I spent a lot of time contacting people through them."

Kevin also made a seemingly three-dimensional display on

his computer screen that read: YOU ARE A FAGGOT. At times he would flash the message at himself.

At first, his contacts with gay men were limited to his computer. Although he did make several good friends, Kevin had no actual meetings. One night he drove to the Castro District, a part of San Francisco with a high concentration of gays, and parked along the street. With his doors locked, watching the gay men walk by, Kevin was excited and frightened at the same time. Afterwards, he continued to just park outside the gay clubs and watch the people go in and out. When he finally got up enough courage to enter one of the clubs, he was immediately accepted.

When he was seventeen, Kevin made a date with an older friend he'd met through the computer bulletin board. They met once and engaged in fellatio and mutual masturbation. But the older man wanted to use drugs, so Kevin never saw him again. On another occasion, when his parents went away for a weekend, he returned to the Castro District and met another older man. They got together six or seven times, according to Kevin. "We really liked each other, but I told him never to call my house. I was so worried about it and afraid my parents would find out. He wanted me to go to the Gay Pride Parade with him, but I was afraid I'd get on television or run into someone I knew."

More than anything, Kevin feared that his parents would find out he was a homosexual, and he intended to keep it a secret from them forever. He knew he would even get married and have children in order to hide the truth from them. Kevin did have sex with a girl once, at sixteen. He enjoyed the experience but had no feelings for the girl. He continued to date girls, however, so that his family would not suspect that he was gay.

Although Kevin loved his father and wanted to emulate him in his choice of the law as a career, he also felt uncomfortable or embarrassed around him. "Dad was a lady-killer when he was younger. He and his girlfriend were labeled the best-looking couple in his yearbook." Kevin thought his father was a handsome man and his mother an extremely beautiful woman. "My parents always seemed like the perfect heterosexual couple, and I knew exactly how they would react if they knew about me.

"I knew I could never tell my parents that I was gay," Kevin said. "I remember what my dad once said when he was reading an article about AIDS: 'The faggots are getting what they deserve,' he said."

The young man also remembered the time a gay cousin was about to pay a visit to the family. Sean, Kevin's brother, quipped: "I'm gonna put a Band-Aid on my butt."

Kevin was so afraid his family would find out he was gay that he planned an elaborate and expensive masquerade to obtain a date for his high school senior prom. He had been thinking about the problem since the tenth grade. The execution of the plan began early in his senior year, with his determination to lose weight. With characteristic intensity, he plunged into a crash diet. During a six-month period that year, Kevin lost more than 75 pounds and got his weight down to 150. His waist went from thirty-eight to twenty-eight, and he liked himself for the first time in his life. He bought new clothes, and everyone at school—even teachers—noticed and remarked about the improvement.

Getting a girl to go to the prom with him was not that difficult, especially since he let it be known that he was renting a limousine for the evening. Kevin took the girl home early, pleading that he couldn't afford to keep the limo out very late. "I was relieved that I had to take her home early, so that I wouldn't have to do anything sexual with her. The important thing was that I had the photos to prove that I had a date."

The celebration Kevin was really looking forward to was planned for the night of his graduation from high school. His parents' beach house in Half Moon Bay was to be the scene of a small party for Kevin and his closest friends. He didn't know that there were to be uninvited guests at that party—his brother Sean and Sean's friend Roger Anderson.

Kevin and Sean shared their friend Roger Anderson. Kevin had gotten Roger a job at the pizza parlor where he worked and had washed Roger's car several times without charging him. Roger was a fanatic about guns. He had his own gun collection, and worked at a shooting range and gun shop. Roger had made it possible for the three boys each to purchase his very own "stun gun," which disables its victim with forty-seven thousand volts of electricity. At times, Kevin was afraid of Roger, and he felt he had good reason to be. "Roger was always armed. He always carried at least a dagger. Roger and Sean saw themselves as 'soldiers of fortune' and hung out at a survival store." As a matter of fact, Roger's habit of carrying a dagger got him fired from the job delivering pizzas.

Kevin knew that Roger lived in a violent fantasy world, where gays were "bad guys." One day Kevin saw Roger chasing another student across the parking lot, waving a heavy flashlight menacingly and yelling "Faggot!" When Kevin caught up with him, Roger said, "I'm going to beat the shit out of Rudy, because he's gay!"

Nevertheless, Kevin and Roger were friends. Kevin felt sorry for Roger because the boy came from a broken home. It was Kevin's impression that there were considerable family difficulties. In contrast, Kevin prided himself on the stability of his own family.

To help maintain that stability, whenever Kevin called his gay friends he was always sure to check that no one in the house was listening to his conversation on another telephone. It did not occur to him that his brother Sean might actually tap his phone. But the younger boy had done just that: Over a one-month period, Sean had not only tapped the phone and overheard several of Kevin's private conversations, but he had also tape-recorded them—and played them back for Roger Anderson.

Although Kevin told his brother Sean that he was taking a girl to the beach house and he didn't want Sean to come because the girl would be embarrassed, Sean and Roger knew better. Sean Green had overheard his brother making plans for the party. He alerted Roger Anderson, and the two "soldiers of fortune," outraged that Kevin was secretly gay, planned a "commando raid" on the beach house.

Kevin was graduated from high school on June 20, 1985. His parents held a small party for relatives at their house, and his grandparents were the last to leave, at around 9 P.M. Kevin then left to pick up his friends for the party at the family's beach house. Bill, Kevin's gay friend, brought along another boy, Reuben, and his lesbian girlfriend to the house in Half Moon Bay. The beer flowed freely at the party, and before too long all four of the young people were drunk. When Reuben and his girlfriend passed out, Bill and Kevin went off to another room to make out, unaware that they were being observed from outside.

Sean and Roger had snuck up on the house and observed the goings on inside for quite some time. Sean was carrying an electric stun gun, and Roger wielded a police flashlight weighted with lead so it could also be used as a weapon. When Sean and Roger first looked in the window of the beach house, they saw Kevin, two other boys, and a girl sitting on the couch watching TV. Roger and Sean watched them for more than an hour. Then they saw Kevin kiss the boy next to him, Bill, a tall boy with blond hair cut in a "Mohawk." Then Kevin and Bill went into one of the bedrooms. Roger and Sean went around to that window, but they couldn't see because it was dark and the curtains were drawn. The room was silent. Sean and Roger decided to make their move.

All of a sudden the languid calm inside the house was shattered as Sean and Roger burst in yelling, "Faggot! We're going to kill you!" They rushed toward the bedroom and flashed the light through the open door. Kevin came out naked from the waist up and immediately tried to defend himself and subdue the younger boys, who tackled him. Roger attacked Kevin with the flashlight and swung it into his face. Immediately, Kevin's nose gushed blood. Then Sean advanced on his brother with the stun gun. When Kevin grabbed at the gun, it went off and burned his hand.

Bill came out of the bedroom and, after a scuffle, the two older boys were able to subdue Roger and Sean, despite Kevin's wounds. During and after the scuffle, Sean yelled, "I can hold this over your head now!" at his brother, and warned that more of their friends were on their way over with a shotgun. Sean also said that he and Roger had taken photographs of Kevin and Bill making out, and that he had tape-recorded their telephone conversations.

At that point the boys started fighting again. Reuben was awakened by the sounds of the scuffle and went to Kevin's and Bill's aid. Kevin and his friends were again able to overpower Roger and Sean and take away their weapons. Sean admitted that the tapes he had made of Kevin's conversations were outside in his car. Kevin took Sean's wallet and car keys and all the boys walked outside. Once outside, Sean broke free and bolted toward a nearby convenience store, yelling, "Call the police! Call the police!" When he got there, Sean called the police and told them that his brother and another man were holding Roger Anderson in the beach house against his will.

When the police arrived, only Sean and Roger were there. Kevin and his friends had left. The police made no report of the incident. Sean went back to the store and called his father to come pick them up, since Kevin had taken his car keys.

An hour later Mr. Green arrived at the beach house. Roger Anderson told him that he and Sean had walked in and found Kevin and the other boy together "with their pants down."

Later that morning, Kevin left his friends at the motel where they had spent the night, and went home. His father was waiting for him. "We have to talk," Mark Green said to his oldest son. In the kitchen, he confronted Kevin. "Sean and Roger tell me you're a homosexual. Is this true?"

Kevin was terrified. "Of course not," he said. "That's ridiculous."

Then Kevin saw his father put his head in his hands and start to cry. "I'm so glad you're not gay, Kevin. It was killing me. We agonized over this all night. I pictured you in bath houses and bars. I thought I'd lost my son."

Kevin's father continued to sob for several minutes. Then his mother came in. The boy again denied he was gay, and now his mother started crying, too.

Then Kevin asked to speak with Sean, alone.

Kevin begged his brother to take back his story "in order to keep the family together." At first Sean refused, but he finally agreed to change his story. He went in and told his mother and father that he had lied. When he finished recanting his earlier story, his parents started crying again. They also said they were angry with Sean for telling such a hurtful story, which had caused them so much pain.

Witnessing all this, Kevin's worst fears were confirmed. "I was never so nervous in my life," he later said. "I was nauseous. Their reaction just confirmed everything I had been afraid of for so long. I was scared to death."

Kevin left to pick up his friends at the motel and drive them home. When he got back, the nightmare started all over again. While Kevin was gone, his father had talked to Roger Anderson. Anderson had insisted that he and Sean were telling the truth the first time: Kevin was a homosexual. Of that Anderson was certain. Now Kevin came home to find that his father once again believed he was homosexual. This time, instead of crying, his father "began acting like a lawyer. Dad seemed to think that the others had seduced me. He demanded that I give him names and phone numbers of the others."

Kevin resisted these demands and got into an argument with his mother and father. He told them he had not been seduced and refused to reveal any names or phone numbers. Finally, his father issued an ultimatum. He demanded the names and numbers one last time, and then said, "If you don't do that, you can leave."

The young man went up to his room and locked the door behind him. Then he started stuffing his belongings into plastic trash bags. He took special care to preserve photographs and his high school diploma, which he had received just a few days earlier. In a symbolic gesture, he turned all his trophies around to face the wall. Then he attached his prom photo to a piece of paper and drew arrows pointing at the smiling couple. He wrote "boy" next to the arrow that pointed at him, and "girl" next to the arrow that pointed at his date.

Kevin then spent the rest of the day and night recording his favorite records on cassette tapes. "I knew I was never coming back," he recalls. At 2 A.M. he slipped out of the house while his parents slept. He carried his belongings out in the trash bags and spent the rest of the night in his car, sleeping fitfully.

By the next morning, Sunday, Kevin had a plan. He would earn money by delivering pizzas, a job that had always allowed him to make a lot of money. After all, he was the "best delivery guy in the world." But he figured he would need his own truck to really make this job pay. So he went to a dealer and bought a small pickup truck, which cost $3,000. Kevin paid $800 down, so he now had $2,200 left in his bank account.

Aside from his extreme emotional distress—he cried frequently—Kevin's most serious problem was moving two cars around. He spent another night in his car, this time behind the pizza parlor where he was now once again employed delivering pizzas.

On Monday, when Kevin once answered the phone at the pizza parlor, it was his mother looking for him. He immediately felt "discovered" again, and knew he could not remain there for long. He was thrown into a deep, confused depression. All of his anger and terror returned. "I just couldn't stand to think that my Mom and Dad thought I was gay. I felt like nothing in front of them—just dirt. I couldn't stand to look them in the eyes. I knew the reason was Sean and Roger."

Kevin was plagued by persistent thoughts of suicide, as well as revenge. He went to a gun shop, but they refused to sell him a gun because he was under age. "I wanted to shoot up their cars to get back at them. I felt they had wrecked my whole life. I wanted a gun, both to kill myself and to shoot up their cars."

He got his gun. On June 24, he went to the same rifle range where Roger Anderson had once worked and discovered an Uzi semiautomatic rifle. The gun shop at the rifle range wouldn't sell him the gun, but he managed to find a sporting goods store that would sell him an Uzi. The clerk told him he couldn't sell him a handgun—since he was under age—but the Uzi was classified as a rifle, so he could legally sell him one. All he would have to do was order it, pay for it, and wait a couple of days. The clerk even threw in a few extra clips of ammunition. Kevin paid for the Uzi with his mother's credit card, which she had lent him the previous week to make some purchases for her.

Once again, Kevin spent the night on the back streets of the Santa Clara Valley, within a few miles of his home, sleeping in his car. On Tuesday, he put spotlights on his truck, to better equip it for delivering pizzas. Then he installed $400 worth of stereo equipment. On Wednesday, he picked up the Uzi he had ordered two days before.

Thursday, Kevin decided it was time for action. He said his plan was to use the gun to humiliate Roger and Sean for "totally ruining my life." He was going to destroy their cars with the gun and then kill himself. Thoughts of suicide grew stronger. But, he thought, "If I had to kill myself, Sean and Roger were going to go with me."

But Kevin also had thoughts of trying to get his old life back. He could not accept his exile, and he decided he would try to "put everything back right." The only way he could do that would be to persuade Roger Anderson to take back his original story, the way Sean had.

On Thursday night, Kevin drove over to the condominium complex where Roger Anderson lived, a cluster of townhomes set near the freeway among the rolling hills. The hills were brown and dry—a real tinderbox. Similar hills in the area, and in Southern California, were ablaze with the season's first brush fires. About 300 miles away, the entire town of Ojai was in the path of an advancing fire and had to be evacuated. Dozens of homeowners in the affluent, semirural community were abandoning, and losing to the flames, their half-million-dollar homes. Santa Clara Valley residents were beginning to be concerned that a similar conflagration could engulf and destroy the affluent tranquillity of their homes.

Kevin couldn't find Roger's car because he was unable to remember exactly which condo belonged to the Andersons. So he drove to his family's house to shoot up Sean's car—but it was not to be seen. Kevin considered shooting out the guest house windows. He decided against it and drove back to Roger's condominium complex, parked in the visitors' space, and spent another night in his car. The distant fires lit the sky with an eerie orange glow.

Kevin awoke at 6 A.M., drove out of the space, parked near the driveway leading to the street, and waited.

At around ten forty-five, Roger Anderson told his mother he was going over to the Green house and that if he was not back by eleven-thirty to "come and get me." Apparently Roger had been receiving several calls from Sean, who was still trying to get his friend to recant his story about Kevin.

When Kevin saw Roger's maroon Toyota coming down the driveway, he started his car and blocked the road. Roger stopped his car and got out. Kevin knew that Roger was always armed, that he carried at least one jungle knife, so as he got out of his car, he took the Uzi with him. When Roger got out of his car, Kevin could see that he did have a dagger in his belt. He also carried a "butterfly knife"—which cuts on both edges—in his back pocket.

Kevin recalls that all he wanted to do was ask Roger to recant his story. If Roger refused, there was always the Uzi with which Kevin could shoot up the other boy's car. He asked Roger to talk to him "for five minutes to settle this whole thing." He pointed the gun away from Roger and toward the car while they argued about "why Roger did what he did."

"Why'd you do all this?" Kevin asked Roger. "Get in my car so we can talk about it." He motioned Roger toward his car with the gun barrel.

Roger was adamant and angry. He was wearing a T-shirt that read "Mountain Shooting Range." "I'm not getting in your car," Roger shouted. "I don't talk to faggots!"

Kevin asked Roger to take back his story so that he could have his old life back. Roger, at one point, tried to get the gun away from Kevin by grabbing at the barrel, but the older boy pulled back and pushed him away with his free hand. Roger shouted at him, "I don't make deals with faggots!"

Then Kevin warned him not to do that because he didn't want to hurt him by accident. Kevin again motioned Roger into his Mustang with the gun. Roger refused. "I'm not going to get into your car, you fucking faggot!"

Kevin raised the rifle at Roger and fired. He was surprised when the first bullet came out and hit Roger. He pulled the trigger again . . . and again . . . and several more times. The Uzi is known for its ability to fire off several rounds with blinding speed. In an instant, Kevin fired more than ten shots into Roger Anderson's body.

Kevin was shaking and his mouth went completely dry. He couldn't believe what had happened. Roger was lying before him in a pool of blood. Kevin looked at him for a moment, hoping that Roger would move, but he didn't. Kevin realized at that moment that he couldn't go shoot up Sean's car because of what he might do if he got near Sean with the gun.

Kevin got back in his car and roared away.

There were several witnesses. A man was driving by when he saw Kevin's dark red Mustang speeding away from where the Toyota was parked by the traffic island. He saw Anderson's body on the island. Thinking that the Mustang had hit the boy lying on the ground, the witness took off after the Mustang. The Mustang entered the freeway and the witness followed him, driving south, toward the more densely populated center of the Santa Clara Valley. A few miles down the road the Mustang pulled off the freeway and rocketed off. After chasing the Mustang for a mile or so,

the witness lost him around Page Mill Road—less than a mile
from Kevin's home. However, before he lost the Mustang, he got
close enough to see the license number. He wrote it in the dust
on his dashboard, then returned to the scene of the killing.

Meanwhile, a witness who saw the entire violent drama
raced to the nearby fire station and told the firemen. They were
the first on the scene after the witnesses. Soon thereafter the police arrived and roped off the area. A yellow plastic cover had
been thrown over Roger Anderson's body. The firemen had
drawn white circles around the spent shell casings scattered on
the ground, and had put a rock behind the right front tire of the
Toyota to keep it from rolling. The police copied the license
number scrawled in the dust on the witness's dashboard.

Roger Anderson's mother had heard the short POP–POP–
POP bursts from the Uzi several minutes after her son had left,
but had not given them much thought. When a police officer
came to tell her that her son had been killed, she broke down and
asked that her boyfriend be allowed to identify the body.

During his high-speed flight from the scene, Kevin ran into a
curb and wrecked his right front wheel. He changed the tire right
away and then drove to a tire store and bought a replacement.
Then he called home. His brother Sean answered, and Kevin told
him, "Something happened. I'll never see you again."

Then Kevin got back in the car and drove back to the freeway. First he headed east toward Sacramento, but thought better
of it after driving several miles, and turned south on Interstate 5,
a four-lane freeway that settles down into a near-perfect straight
line as it stretches south of Sacramento and the Bay Area through
more than two hundred miles of the relentlessly flat farmland of
the San Joaquin Valley, before it climbs over the mountains ring-
ing Los Angeles.

At three-thirty that afternoon, the police set up road blocks
and sealed off the neighborhood around the Greens' house in Los
Altos Hills. A SWAT team surrounded the house and shot seventy
canisters of tear gas through the windows.

No one was home.

Fifteen minutes later, Mr. and Mrs. Green approached the
roadblock in their BMW. Mr. Green was told by the police that
no one was being allowed into the area because of the possibility

that a murder suspect was in the neighborhood. Mr. Green got out of his car and insisted that he and his wife be allowed to go to their house. He was once again told by the officer that a "containment" had been set up because the police believed a murderer was hiding out in the neighborhood. When the police found out who they were, the Greens were arrested.

At 9:10 P.M., Kevin called the sheriff's office and asked to talk to the deputy who had been his instructor for the course in police work that he had taken just a few months before. The deputy was one person who apparently had a great impact on Kevin, so much so that the boy had planned on joining the police reserves as soon as he was old enough. Despite the fact that this man had just a few weeks earlier served as a kind of father to the boy, Kevin felt so distant from his own life that he asked the deputy if he remembered him.

The deputy said that, of course, he remembered him, and then tried to establish a bond of trust with Kevin. Early in the conversation his tone varied from one of fatherly concern and closeness to one of gravity in contemplation not only of what had already happened but also of what might happen if Kevin did not give himself up.

For as long as Kevin had the weapon, the deputy stressed, every police officer in California would be looking for him, and if they saw him, would approach with guns drawn, "and the first cop that sees you on the street and you make a funny move, it's gonna be over."

The deputy asked Kevin if he thought he could trust him, and tried to get Kevin to give himself up. He wanted to meet Kevin "face-to-face," but Kevin told him he was "a thousand miles away." Throughout the conversation, the deputy tried to get Kevin to "come on down" or meet him somewhere. He said he would stay with Kevin as he was taken into custody and visit him in jail.

Failing at that strategy, the deputy stalled in order to keep Kevin on the line as long as possible in hopes the call could be traced. He was unaware that Kevin had "patched" the call through an intricate network of telephone–computer connections —all performed from a phone booth in Southern California.

Though Kevin and the deputy talked for almost an hour, the police were unable to trace the call.

Before the end of the conversation, Kevin not only sent messages of love and remorse to his family, but also tearfully gave away all of his belongings to his brothers. In final reply to the deputy's persistent plea that he give himself up, Kevin said he had to drive around for a while and think it over. The deputy advised him that an "all-points bulletin" for him had gone out and that "you're not gonna have the time to think it over that way."

But Kevin did have the time. Several weeks, in fact.

After ending the call, Kevin spent the night in a motel in Agoura, a Los Angeles suburb. The next day, June 29, Kevin called some friends he had met through his computer bulletin board and invited them to have dinner with him at his motel. While at dinner, he told them he was going to settle in the area. One of his friends offered him a place to stay at her house in Fullerton, a town in nearby Orange County. Kevin accepted the offer and stayed at his friend's for the next three weeks.

Despite the deputy's warnings about the "dragnet," Kevin was never apprehended. He did not particularly try to elude police. In fact, he would sometimes try to get them to chase him, hoping they might recognize his license plate and "take care of this thing in the field," as the deputy had warned they would.

During his life as a fugitive Kevin fell into severe bouts of depression. He knew the police were looking for him, and that because he was armed and considered dangerous they would have anxious trigger fingers. "I didn't want to be killed, but at the same time, I did want to be killed. All I wanted to do was go home, but if I couldn't do that, I just wanted to die."

Nevertheless, Kevin went just about anywhere he wanted to go and did anything he wanted to do. Though he drove a bright red car that stood out in any crowd—a car for which every policeman in the state had a detailed description, including the license number—he was never caught. In fact, Kevin brazenly succeeded in penetrating the police dragnet around his family's house. One night he actually drove right up to the home in Los Altos Hills, let himself in, and while everyone in the house was asleep, managed to make off with his own stereo, TV, and computer.

When Kevin returned to northern California, he also spent

some time in San Francisco with friends, then drove north all the way to Oregon. Realizing that using his mother's credit card might allow police to track him down, Kevin traveled far enough away from his regular haunts to obliterate the trail before abandoning the card.

Despite his success at eluding capture, Kevin was still plagued by depression and suicidal thoughts. On July 13, the head nurse at a private Los Altos Hills psychiatric hospital reported to the police that she had received a phone call at 4:30 P.M. The caller had asked her if she had read about the Los Altos Hills High School student who had been shot, and then told her, "I'm the one who shot him." He went on to say, "I know there were four or five people there when I shot him and that someone followed me when I left, but I don't care. I did society a favor by shooting him." Then Kevin told the nurse that he had a "pretty mean-looking, wicked, lethal weapon" and sixty rounds of ammunition.

The nurse asked Kevin if he wanted to turn himself in. No, he answered, and explained that he had talked to an attorney and knew how much time he would have to spend in jail if he were caught. Then Kevin said that his problems were the fault of his family and the victim, Roger Anderson.

The nurse asked Kevin if he wanted to talk to one of the doctors at the hospital. Kevin said he didn't know what he wanted to do. The nurse gave him a doctor's telephone number in the event he wanted to talk about it further. She then tried to get him to tell her where he was staying. Kevin asked the nurse if she was now going to call the police. The nurse said she didn't think she would.

Every now and then Kevin would take the Uzi and fire the unloaded gun at himself—practice for when he would presumably have the courage to do it when it was loaded. He was growing weary of his flight, but he didn't know where else to go. Besides, his beloved Mustang was showing signs of giving up. Kevin knew the signs of bad trouble in the engine. The oil pressure was dropping and the main bearing in the crankshaft, the very heart of the motor, was not long for this world.

Meanwhile, the police obtained a search warrant that enabled them to look at a list of phone calls charged to his parents' home phone number. Some of these calls were made to phones in Southern California. Kevin had been talking to his parents. The police followed these leads and located a woman in Fullerton who admitted that Kevin had been living at her residence since July 1. On July 19, she said Kevin had left in the morning and was expected back that evening. Police kept watch on the house. Kevin returned to the house and saw the police in time to get away without being detected. The next day he called the police and told them he knew the house was being watched and would not return again. He told the police he was going back to the Bay Area.

By the time Kevin got back to Los Altos Hills, the oil pressure in the Ford was down to zero. The crankshaft main bearing was shot. Kevin roamed his old haunts in the Santa Clara Valley. He went into a favorite ice cream shop, then to a trendy Mexican restaurant with sawdust on the floor and festive outdoor tables. But now the festive atmosphere of the place mocked him. Kevin knew he "couldn't be gay in Los Altos Hills." Kevin's plan was to find a lonely back street somewhere in the Valley and shoot himself.

But he couldn't bring himself to load the Uzi and fire it one last time. Kevin called his attorney, his psychiatrist, and his mother and father. He wanted to give himself up.

Kevin arrived at his psychiatrist's office the night of July 22, just before midnight. He handed over the Uzi. The doctor and the attorney took him to the local hospital, where he was admitted into the psychiatric ward and given routine tests to determine if there were any drugs in his system. The tests showed that the only drug Kevin had taken was caffeine.

Kevin's attorney contacted the police, who arrived at the hospital at 2 A.M. The attorney told the police that the Uzi was safely secured at his office and that Kevin's car was at the doctor's office. The police arrested Kevin on the charge of murder and then drove to the attorney's office to retrieve the Uzi and the ammunition. At 4 A.M. on July 23 they took Kevin from the hospital and drove him to jail.

The mental status report on Kevin's discharge papers included the following: "Patient was alert, oriented, cooperative, highly anxious, over-controlled, at times fighting tears and fatigue. . . . He was very, very ambivalent over his future, mildly to moderately suicidal when facing the reality of his future, but in contact with reality. During the patient's stay in the hospital, the patient's father was present, was consulted by the undersigned [psychiatrist], and in addition, his two attorneys were also present and arranged personally for the transfer of custody to the homicide detectives. The patient was in the hospital for a total of three hours. The patient was discharged with instructions to the sheriffs to communicate to the custody officials that suicidal precautions should be observed. The transporting homicide detectives informed us of their intention to have the patient housed in a special unit of the jail. He was discharged in fair condition, stable and calm."

I examined Kevin Green on December 17, 1985, almost six months after the killing of Roger Anderson. Kevin told me that while he was a fugitive he had thought about suicide on several occasions and called the Suicide Prevention Center for help. Many times during that month he had put the unloaded Uzi to his head and squeezed the trigger. "I couldn't shoot myself," he told me. Kevin cried when he talked about Roger Anderson.

It was clear to me that Kevin had been unable to deal with the intense stress of being exposed as gay to his parents, and then being rejected by them. Because of the enforced alienation from his home and family, his ability to think and act were severely impaired. I don't believe he was capable of the kind of "malice aforethought" that the law normally requires for a murder conviction. I believe Kevin acted within an ongoing "heat of passion," which severely diminished his mental capacity.

Legally, if a person kills while in the heat of passion, even if there is the intent to kill, it's not murder but manslaughter. However, courts have generally held that heat of passion must be instantaneous or, at least, within a certain short length of time after the incident that provokes the passion. But in Kevin Green's case, there was not one provocative event, but a continuing series. It was one spark, then another, then another, then another. I testified that Kevin was acting in a continuous heat of passion.

The argument against my testimony was standard: it couldn't have been heat of passion because Kevin did not actually lose control. His behavior, after all, was "in control" enough to get a job, buy a truck, purchase a weapon, and take target practice.

Yet Kevin was clearly in a depraved state. His life was in shambles. At 6 P.M. on June 20 he was a high school graduate with a 3.3 grade-point average, on his way to college and a law career. Within twenty-four hours he was a pizza delivery boy exiled from his family. He didn't shower regularly or sleep in a bed the entire week. He was an outcast from the life that he loved.

"Everything I had built up, my car, my reputation, were all gone," Kevin said. "Before this happened, it was the most happy time in my life. I was in the right spot—just graduated from high school and had been accepted at college, lost some weight so I could put on my nice clothes, and found some gay people. It was all shattered right there."

Kevin had a strong need to at least appear to conform and contribute to the rest of society, especially as it was represented by his family's environment in Los Altos Hills. He was convinced that he could not be openly gay and still live in Los Altos Hills, and yet he felt that was the only place he could live. Although Kevin felt his parents were "terrific," he inwardly knew that they would totally reject him if they found out he was gay. When they did, in fact, do just what his worst nightmare said they would, he was suddenly plunged into a personal hell. His world and his life were crumbling. His worst nightmare was coming true.

As far as Kevin was concerned, the events of that week were a threat to his life. He felt he was being attacked. And when he fought back for self-preservation, Roger Anderson—at the moment of their confrontation—became the focus of all of Kevin's anguish, of all his embittered resistance, of all the fighting back he had never done. Roger was, in those tragic, fatal moments, no longer just Roger—he was Sean, he was Kevin's father and mother, he was all the forces of society that Kevin felt aligned against him, hurting him, forcing him into hiding, telling him "I don't talk to faggots!" and trying to destroy him.

Kevin said, "I had built an image of myself, and after Sean and Roger blew my cover, it was all gone. It was like my life was over, ruined."

For his part, Sean admitted to the police that he and Roger had gone to the beach house because they both shared a "deep prejudice against homosexuals." Their intention was to catch Kevin with another male and humiliate him, and "have something to hold over his head."

The sheriff's deputy that Kevin had called the night of the murder never came to see him as he promised he would. Kevin told me he "understood."

Kevin eventually reconciled with his mother and father. When I spoke with him last, around the time of his trial, he told me that his father had sent Sean to Europe, "to get him away from all this."

"Imagine that," Kevin said, with a smile tinged with amazement and bitterness, "imagine that."

Kevin was kept in jail awaiting his trial. When he came to the courtroom, he wore one of his own suits, yet it looked pathetically large on him, he had lost so much weight in jail. This put a crimp in the defense attorney's strategy to make the defendant look as much like the "all-American boy" as possible. Kevin testified that he had never intended to kill Roger, but he did admit to having fantasies about killing him and Sean. He said that if he had really planned to kill Roger, he wouldn't have done it in broad daylight, at a time and place when there would be witnesses.

In Kevin's sorry condition, however, it was all the more difficult for him to win the sympathy of the jury, which was undoubtedly aghast at the weapon used in the killing.

Furthermore, one of the disadvantages of our jury system is that it is often impossible to get a true "jury of one's peers." Justice is not, after all, blind to human prejudices. A gay man shooting a "macho" man will quite often have a rougher time of it that a macho man killing a gay man or a woman. As far as most juries would be concerned, the "all-American boy" was the one who lay in a pool of blood on the traffic island in the middle of that Silicon Valley road.

In July 1986, despite my testimony and that of other mental health professionals that Kevin acted within a heat of passion, he was found guilty of second-degree murder and given a sentence of fifteen years to life in prison. He should be eligible for parole around 1995.

The perverse irony of the way the criminal-justice system works stands out in the stark contrast between the Kevin Green case and the Dan White case, which occurred a few years earlier, at the high point of the "diminished capacity" flood. The fact that Kevin Green was severely punished while Dan White was not shows just how perverse the system can be.

Dan White had resigned his seat on the City Council of San Francisco, but then he changed his mind and decided he wanted it back. The mayor of San Francisco, George Moscone, a political opponent and the person empowered to appoint a successor, told him it was too late for him to get it back. Carrying a gun, White broke into San Francisco City Hall through a window. He knew that if he tried to go through the front door, the metal detectors would go off and the guards would take away his gun. Once inside the building, he went to the mayor's office and begged to have his seat on the City Council returned to him. Moscone once again said it was impossible, so White pulled the gun and shot Moscone dead. Then he shot and killed Councilman Harvey Milk, who was a homosexual councilman, and a political opponent.

Dan White was charged with two counts of first-degree murder, but the prosecutor wasn't able to sustain the charges. The defense brought in psychiatric testimony that said that White had diminished capacity because he had been depressed, eating a poor, high-sugar diet, and that his mental state had deteriorated significantly, to the point where he no longer had the capacity for malice. It became known as the "Twinkie Defense." And it worked. White was eventually convicted of manslaughter.

As the testimony began to evolve, I saw the manslaughter conviction coming and predicted it. Although I never examined Dan White, from what I heard it sounded like there were grounds for the medical conclusions rendered. Don't misunderstand me. Based on the act alone, he should have been convicted of first-degree murder. But remember, a crime also requires a necessary state of mind. And psychiatrists who examined Dan White did report that his depression impacted on his capacity to premeditate, deliberate, and harbor malice. As I've said many times, I'm often distressed at what the criminal-justice system does with psychiatric testimony.

Plenty of other people were also shocked. White had gunned down two of San Francisco's most able and beloved politicians. And he spent only a few years in prison.

Why did Dan White get off so easily while Kevin Green did not? On the surface, their scenarios parallel each other. Part of the reason may lie in social prejudices and politics. Dan White shot a homosexual, while Kevin Green was a homosexual. If the system worked the way it should, it really would not matter who killed whom. Similar crimes would carry similar penalties. But that's not the way the system works. It's not simply a matter of the way juries carry their prejudices into the courtroom, either. Psychiatrists, judges, and attorneys do it, too.

Another reason was that by the time Green shot Roger Anderson, the people of California had decided they'd had enough cold-blooded heat of passion. Proposition 8, which became known as the Victim's Bill of Rights, abolished a decade and a half's worth of court-created diminished-capacity loopholes. Diminished capacity was still a viable defense, and, to be sure, there was still a big market for courtroom psychiatrists. But, you might say, as the floodwaters receded before the public will, Kevin Green was simply carried away with the tide.

Dan White was resettled, with a new identity, in Los Angeles. However, not long after his release, he committed suicide, succumbing to a more powerful internal tide.

C H A P T E R

5

Justice delayed, justice denied?

One of the oldest legal maxims says that "justice delayed is justice denied." Many times, the system makes a mockery of the law's guarantee of a speedy trial, and all too often the quality of justice decreases as the length of time increases between the crime and the final judgment. Delays result from many factors, including the built-in sluggishness of the system, the enormous volume of cases that must wait their turn for trial, the length of time taken up by various hearings, motions, and appeals, and, finally, the delaying tactics of defense attorneys, who know that the longer they keep their client "innocent until proven guilty," the more favorable will be the final result. I'm awaiting the day when a defense attorney, after filing every appeal and delaying motion imaginable, will finally seek the dismissal of charges with the excuse that the long delay has inflicted "cruel and unusual punishment" on his client, or, better yet, has deprived him of due process.

The story of Louis and Laura Schindler is an ironic tale of justice delayed. I'll leave it up to the reader to decide whether or not justice was ultimately denied.

Louis Schindler was born in New York City on May 11, 1922, the son of a merchant who imported and sold "raw" furs, or animal skins to be used in making coats and other articles of clothing. After graduation from high school, Lou's father took him into the family business. But World War II broke out and, after two years of working with his father, Lou went into the Army Air Corps. He served as a radio operator in B-29s and saw action in the Pacific. He was honorably discharged in 1946, after four years of military service.

The family fur business was waiting for Lou when he returned from the war. Soon, however, his father, brothers, and sister moved to California and left him in charge of the company. Years later, when Lou was earning far more money, he would look back on these less pressured, less harried years in New York and reminisce that these were happier times. Nevertheless, in 1952, he left New York and followed his family to California.

Lou did extremely well in California. He started his own wholesale carpet business, which flourished. But by 1956 the pressures of his new life and business were starting to take their toll, and he started making regular visits to a psychiatrist. Uppermost on his mind was his marriage, which took place in 1942, during the uncertain early years of the war. Now, fourteen years later, the marriage, which had produced two daughters, was showing signs of strain. Lou's wife was dissatisfied with the role of housewife. She started taking college extension classes and ultimately had an affair with another student. She and Lou separated, but because of her interest in psychology, she suggested they seek marital counseling. The couple began seeing separate therapists, reconciled, and even attended some college classes together. Lou took classes in literature, political science, and economics.

To his therapist, Lou presented the picture of a very anxious man extremely disturbed about his relationship with his wife. Aware of his lack of emotional control, Lou pleaded that he wanted to keep his marriage together but felt that it was impossible. Indeed, five years into their attempted reconciliation, he and his wife were divorced. The official explanation was that they had grown far apart in their goals so, amicably, they decided to split up for good rather than perpetuate their unhappiness.

Convinced that married life was best, despite this failure, Lou wasted little time in pursuing another woman. He dated only women who, he felt, were "prospective marriage material." Less than a year after his divorce, in his own words, "the day after my fortieth birthday I met June and immediately fell in love with

her." June was a beautiful, charming, thirtyish about-to-be divor-
cée. But her fourth marriage could not take place until her third
one was officially terminated. She told Lou that would not happen
for several months yet. June also told him, to Lou's frustration,
that she wanted to date other men.

Lou responded by pursuing her even more intensely. He
finally won her over, and on December 19, 1963, June and Lou
were married.

The marriage began on a positive note as June expressed her
desire to have a child. Her three previous marriages had been
barren. But before long, Lou's second marriage sailed into even
stormier waters than his first. Though at first he had admired
June's devotion to her parents, he soon grew to feel that his in-
laws were interfering in his marriage. "I found that my mother-
in-law was overriding all my decisions with my wife." For example, June and Lou had begun to build a new house closer to her
family's residence. But while Lou was paying for the construction,
he felt left out of all the decisions regarding design, cost, and
furnishings of the house. June and her parents seemed to be completely in charge.

June's parents didn't feel much better about Lou. They described him as a jealous, possessive person with a "nasty, vile
temper." They admitted, however, that he could "turn on charm
like flicking on a light switch." Lou was unjustly jealous of June,
they felt, because she had always been faithful to her husbands—
and was still friends with all of them. She was, after all, a very
popular, well-liked person.

Lou described June, somewhat wistfully, as a "woman who
had some fine qualities about her. A very beautiful girl. And
kind. And I was very much in love with her . . . inextricably in
love with her." The problem was, however, that he "couldn't
control any of the money. I had very little to say about how the
household was run. She exhibited an extreme temper on a number of occasions and we just couldn't get along."

When the marriage began to flounder, Lou went back to the
same psychiatrist who had counseled him during the breakup of
his first marriage. This time the doctor noticed that Lou was even
more agitated and distressed than before. He complained of
problems that had begun in the earliest days of their marriage.

June just seemed to need to call the shots wherever they went, whatever they did. According to Lou, "She was a person who was driven and wanted every excitement that life had to offer. She just ran through life that way." He wanted to spend more time at home, rather than going out "more than I cared to," and spending "more money than I could afford." There was never any rest for Lou and his bride. "How many restaurants, how many night-clubs can you take in?" he once asked. But Lou loved June and so he "conceded mostly to her whims and wishes. I let her win every battle."

Though Lou was very happy with June in many ways and generally felt proud of her, he bristled at her domineering personality and her quick temper. There was also an increasingly icy distance developing between them. When he came home from work, he complained, June never asked him how his day had been, although she was always ready with a list of her own concerns. Their sex life was not one of the happier areas of their marriage. Lou complained that it "deteriorated to a very low ebb. She denied my advances."

As their marriage quickly drifted closer and closer to the rocks, one argument led to another, and finally, in 1964, after less than a year of marriage, divorce proceedings were begun.

During an especially stormy period in the proceedings, Lou angrily told his in-laws that if he couldn't have June, he would fix it so no one could.

But before matters progressed much further, the couple reconciled. Lou professed his love for June, and confessed that perhaps he had been unfair in his objections and that he had placed money above their happiness. Once love rather than economics controlled Lou's purse strings, he and June went on a three-and-a-half-year spending spree that left a trail of over $215,000 in receipts. They built their dream house on Mulholland Drive in North Hollywood, furnished it lavishly, and went on expensive vacations to Europe, Canada, and Mexico. The couple shared many happy, and expensive, moments. In April 1966 June bore a daughter, Kimberly.

But 1966 also brought less-blessed events into the Schindlers' lives. Lou's business partner had been objecting all along to the large amounts of money Lou was withdrawing from the com-

pany's accounts. Then a building slump dealt a serious blow to
their business. During the fall of 1966 and early months of 1967,
their volume dropped to about half of what it had been in previous years. Adding to the financial strain was the fact that the
general slump in building meant that Lou's customers were having trouble paying their bills. So some of the accounts receivable
from the previous good months' business were not forthcoming.
Furthermore, the possibility was increasing that Lou could lose
more than $100,000 in real estate investments that threatened to
go sour.

When Lou explained what was going on and said that they
should try to economize, June told him not to bring his business
problems home. As the business problems and pressures grew
worse and Lou again asked June to economize, she answered by
threatening him with divorce. He threatened her right back.
When she confronted Lou with her desire to get a divorce, he
backed down from his threats and suggested marriage counseling.
However, June did not respond to his suggestion. Finally, after
being advised by her attorney that it was to her advantage to
strike first, June Schindler filed for divorce.

Lou did not find out that the divorce papers had already been
filed until his bank notified him that his accounts were all under
legal restraint. Suddenly, he was facing another divorce, and this
one wasn't promising to be anywhere near as amicable as the first
one. June was asking for $2,250 a month in alimony.

What kind of man went into court to face his soon-to-be ex-
wife and her attorney in a hearing to begin divorce proceedings
and determine temporary support and living arrangements?

Lou Schindler, forty-four years old at the time, was short
(five-feet-seven), stocky (160 pounds), and athletic, though he
smoked a pack of cigarettes a day. His favorite forms of recre-
ation were tennis, handball, and sailing on his twenty-nine-foot
sailboat. As a businessman, he always paid his bills on time and
prided himself on his fair and honest dealings. Lou bragged that
his customers had confidence in him, and that he had never once
been sued in a business deal.

Lou's friends knew him as a dedicated father to his daughters
from his first marriage. One friend wrote: "In the seven years I
have known Mr. Schindler he has been a model of good moral

character. His integrity and honesty is [sic] beyond any question whatsoever. I have found him to be a devoted father to his two daughters by his previous marriage. I know that every Wednesday no matter how important his business or how busy his schedule, he set aside that evening for the sole purpose of taking his daughters out to dinner for a pleasant social evening. He also took them for at least a two-week vacation every year, provided them with schooling, and took care of their financial and personal needs. I know he went far above and beyond the things he was required to do under the divorce settlement.''

Judging from the early sparring and his wife's enormous demands, there was little indication that Lou's second divorce and June's fourth would proceed amicably. However, both parties presented themselves peacefully in court. June's attorney did not ask for a restraining order, although he did ask that Lou be ordered to pay more than $800 in bills June had run up in the week since filing for divorce. Neither husband nor wife asked for the eviction of the other from the family home.

The judge denied the request for Lou to pay June's $800 in bills, and, instead, ordered Lou to pay $50 a week for food and household expenses, and to pay the maid's salary. Then—a move that many judges make in what I believe to be blissfully negligent optimism—the judge allowed them both to live in the same house. After all, they had been getting along, sleeping in separate bedrooms, without incident for weeks.

As the couple left the courtroom with their respective attorneys, Lou mentioned that it was not his desire to win a lawsuit against June. In an attempt to settle the matter, he offered her the house and $1,250 a month alimony and child support for the first year, decreasing to $1,000 the second year and to $750 the third. Lou said, "I really didn't want the divorce, but thought after we got the financial matter out of the way there would be a better chance for possible reconciliation later, which had happened between us before.''

But Lou's offer was turned down, and the estranged husband and wife settled into their bizarre living arrangement. The seeming amicability of the initial hearing soon gave way to something more closely resembling a pair of scorpions dancing around each other, trying to keep out of each other's stinging distance while waiting for the right time to move in and strike. For one thing, June's apparent willingness to share the house with Lou was little more than a strategic smoke screen. She was apparently advised that the best way to get Lou out of the house and make him the villain in their divorce proceedings was to provoke him into some kind of violent attack on her. Then she would go to court and ask for a restraining order forcing Lou out of the house.

Lou's attorney advised him of the danger he was in, and told him to avoid confrontations with June at all costs. He was told to leave the house before June got up and to come home as late as possible—and not to abandon the house under any circumstances, despite the fact that June would certainly try to make his life there miserable.

Sure enough, June mounted a campaign to separate him from his temper and his house at the same time. Several times through February and March 1967 she demanded that Lou leave the house. He replied that he did not want to leave either his home or his baby daughter, Kimberly. Inwardly, he felt that if he could remain in the house there was a chance the marriage could somehow be saved. But June held no such delusions, and within a few weeks, neither did Lou. He complained to his attorney that she and the maid were conspiring by hiding and denying him food, and refusing to clean his room. June picked arguments with him whenever she saw him. "The minute I'd walk in, she'd start yelling and screaming. If I did something, I was doing it wrong. If I didn't do it, I was wrong."

On two occasions, Lou found the harassment intolerable and asked his attorney if there wasn't some way he could move out and still preserve his rights. The attorney told him there wasn't, so Lou dug in deeper and readied himself for battle.

Suspecting that June was having an affair, Lou hired a private detective to follow her. The detective was unable to supply any evidence of infidelity. A business associate suggested that Lou should "bug" the house. So he bought an electronic listening device, a microphone-transmitter that could be monitored through the radio in his car, and planted the device in June's bedroom.

On Wednesday, April 5, 1967, June called her attorney and told him that a handgun they had usually kept in the closet was no longer there. Lou had bought the .32 caliber French automatic in Arizona and shot it off in the desert a couple of times to try it out. The gun held six bullets in the clip and one in the chamber. Lou had kept the gun in a drawer in a nightstand by the bed, but had removed it to the hall closet when baby Kimberly began to explore the house.

June also called her mother with the same message: She was afraid Lou was going to kill her.

On Thursday, April 6, as Lou left to go sailing with a friend, he turned on the listening device and heard a conversation in which June told a friend that Lou had stolen the laundry. He also overheard her tell his friend Bill, "I hope he drowns and winds up at the bottom with his boat."

On Sunday morning, April 9, Lou went to his brother's office to study for a navigational course he was taking. He called a few friends to try to find someone who would go sailing with him, and then went to the yacht club.

Meanwhile, June had made arrangements to have a pot-luck dinner with friends at the house. She had cooked some chicken and each of her guests was to bring some food. At five-thirty, just before her guests were scheduled to arrive, Lou came home and noticed that June was in the middle of preparing for visitors. When her friends started arriving, Lou greeted them. Shortly thereafter, he left to go bowling with his friend Bill.

Bill and Lou bowled until almost 9 P.M. and then came home. June's friends were still at the house. Lou ushered Bill into the living room. They had a drink and then saw some leftover chicken on a plate on the counter between the kitchen and living room. Lou offered the chicken to Bill, and reached for a piece himself. June saw him reaching for the chicken, grabbed his arm, and told him he couldn't have any of that chicken because it had been brought by one of her guests.

Lou told June not to get physical, proceeded to eat the chicken, and then left the house with Bill.

As they drove away, Lou decided to tune in to the listening device. One of June's friends said, "It must be terrible living like that."

June replied, "The only way I can get him kicked out is an act of violence, but he wouldn't do that."

Then June and her friends started talking about men, especially men they had dated. When Lou heard June talk about men who had been her lovers, he grew despondent. He and Bill thought they recognized the name of one of the men, and decided to drive to his home and confront him. When they arrived at the man's house, they learned that the man was now divorced. His former wife said she doubted that he had ever had an affair with June. Lou and Bill left.

By now it was ten-thirty and the two friends called it a night.

When Lou got home, he heard June and Inger, the maid, in the maid's room. Inger had apparently just returned from her weekend off. First Lou went to June's bedroom and removed the listening device. Then he went to the kitchen and poured himself a glass of milk. While he was drinking it, he could hear June and Inger conspiring on how they were going to get him out of the house. The young Swedish woman Lou and June had brought over from Europe apparently had taken sides. Lou had been thinking about firing her for some time, and now decided it was time to even the sides. He walked over to the doorway of Inger's room. She and June were sitting on the floor. Lou told Inger to leave: "I think it's foolish for you to continue here under these circumstances." She would have no trouble finding another job, he said, so he gave her two weeks' notice as of that moment.

Inger angrily told Lou to get out of her room.

Lou replied that she had no right to talk to him that way. "How dare you! This is my house!"

June got up and charged at Lou, shouting, "Get out of this house!"

Lou backed up into the kitchen, but June kept after him, yelling. The argument became louder and hotter. Lou tried to retreat into his bedroom, but June kept yelling at his heels, so he ducked into the guest bathroom and slammed the door in her face. Once safely inside, he went to the sink and threw cold water on his face to try to cool his temper, remembering his attorney's warnings.

Reaching for a towel to dry his hands and face, Lou found only the monogrammed towels they had bought in happier times.

Both he and June were avoiding these towels, so to dry his hands and face he would have to leave the safety of the bathroom to get a towel in the kitchen. June apparently was not laying siege to the bathroom, so Lou left his sanctuary and headed for the kitchen. There, he found June sitting on a high chair at the counter, talking on the phone. "Hi, Ceil, the big mouth is home now. I had to call you and give you a big laugh. The big mouth just walked in and told me that he met you outside the house and that you told him I was in love with another man."

The way Lou remembered it, he reached into the cabinet under the counter and took out a towel. When he looked at June again, she was still talking on the phone, but in her other hand she held a gun, aimed at him.

Lou remembered lunging at June to get the gun, grabbing her wrist and slamming it down on the counter to dislodge the gun. The dog started barking, and a shot or two went off. June's friend Ceil, on the other end of the phone line, heard the shots and also heard June cry out, "Help! I need help!" Then the line went dead and Ceil called the police.

At that point, Lou's memory went dead, too.

But Inger, the maid, had been listening to the little drama being played out just a few yards from her door, and she was soon drawn right into the action.

From her room, Inger heard what sounded to her like a dog's leash striking against something. She came out of her room and walked to the kitchen, where she found Lou standing at the high chair aiming a gun at June, who was now standing five or ten feet away and looking very upset. No one said a word. The phone was on the floor.

Inger ran back to her room. Then she heard that loud snapping sound again—one, two, three, four, five times the dog's leash cracked—and Inger realized it was the gun going off.

Suddenly, June came staggering into Inger's room. There was blood all over her face and arms and clothes, and her hair was an awful mess. June reached down for Inger's telephone and tried to call the police, but the phone wouldn't work. The extension in the kitchen was still off the hook.

Then June told Inger to go next door to the fire station and call the police from there. The two women ran out of the room, and the house, together. Inger took the lead, as June quickly fell behind. Inger ran down the road to the fire station, about 150 feet away. June made it to the end of her lawn and then fell face down into a flower bed at the curb.

Inger rang the doorbell at the fire station. A captain answered the door, and the maid told him that June had been shot and to please come. The fire captain and Inger headed for the Schindler home, and heard June's last cry for help from the flower bed. The fire captain saw that June was bleeding from several wounds and that she was still breathing.

Meanwhile, Lou Schindler was waking up from a nightmare. It was dark all around him. He thought he was at Bear Mountain and he was a teenager again, on a biking trip. He was riding a child's bicycle . . . he saw a hill . . . and a stream . . . a split rail fence . . . and the lights from the houses around him. His feet, socks, shoes, and lower trouser legs were wet and he had bad cramps in his legs from pumping the bicycle more than two miles to the dead-end of this residential street off Mulholland Drive. "I didn't know if it was real or unreal," he later said. "I tried to collect myself. I saw these lights in the houses and it reinforced the thought that it was a dream. As I looked at the surroundings I realized I wasn't a teenager. It's hard to describe the feeling. I finally realized where I actually was and remembered fighting . . . and the shots that had gone off . . . and became extremely alarmed."

Lou suddenly dropped the bike, climbed over the fence, and ran across the yard. "I was frightened. I wanted to get to a phone booth." He half ran, half walked down the hill to busy Ventura Boulevard and found a phone booth at a gas station. First he called his house and heard a busy signal. Then he called his brother and told him about the fight and the memory of shots being fired. Lou asked his brother to come and get him. His brother said he would be right there, and told Lou to call his attorney right away.

Lou's brother came and picked him up. A short time later, Lou and one of his attorney's young assistants waited in front of a West Los Angeles restaurant for his attorney to drive in from

Malibu. Lou still wasn't sure what had actually happened at his house that night. When he saw his attorney's car pull into the restaurant parking lot, Lou went to greet him. His attorney, a man named Jerry, stepped out of the car and said, "I just heard on the radio . . . she was fatally shot."

The fireman had called an ambulance, but by the time it arrived June had stopped breathing. At 11:07 P.M. she was pronounced dead by the ambulance personnel. June died of multiple gunshot wounds that caused massive internal bleeding. She had been shot five times: in the right front chest, in the right shoulder penetrating to the chest, in the right side of the back, in the left side of the neck, and in the left side of the cheek. Her right lung and larynx had been penetrated by bullets. She also had bruises on her right hand and cuts on her fingers, injuries consistent with a struggle with Lou for the gun. However, whether Lou or June had the gun first could not be determined. Two bullets were found in the wall.

When he heard the news that his wife was dead, Lou ran into the men's room of the restaurant and screamed. "I became nauseous," he later said. The other men took him out of the restaurant and into his attorney's car. On the way out to Malibu, "I kept sobbing and couldn't believe it and begged him to tell me it wasn't so." Lou was so distraught that he tried to jump out of the car on the freeway. His attorney grabbed him and held him in the car. Lou was getting so upset that he begged his attorney to "take my finger and push the bullet back."

Once they arrived at the house in Malibu, Lou was given a sedative by his attorney's wife, who was a nurse. After spending the night there, at ten-forty-five the next morning he went with his attorney to the North Hollywood Station of the Los Angeles Police and surrendered.

Three days later, Lou Schindler was out on bail. He had been examined by a physician who expressed concern that he might become suicidally depressed, withdrawn, and perhaps even psychotic, but who felt that otherwise he would not present a

danger to himself or others. Lou immediately made an appointment with his own psychiatrist. At the first of many visits over the
next six months, he told him what had happened and pleaded
with the doctor to explain how and why he could have done such
a thing. In search of the answer to this question, Lou was seen by
his psychiatrist three times a week while waiting for his trial to
begin.

In criminal cases it is not unusual for friends and family of the
concerned parties to write letters of support or condemnation to
the judge, prosecutor, and probation officials, in hopes of affecting the outcome of the trial. However, in the Schindler case, well
over one hundred letters were written testifying to Lou's superior
character, morality, and overall goodness. Letters were written by
friends, relatives, business associates, attorneys, officials of charitable organizations, and a Superior Court judge who had known
Lou for twenty-seven years. Even the father of the eight-year-old
boy who found the murder weapon wrote a letter of support. The
letters pleaded for mercy on behalf of Lou, on behalf of his children, and even on behalf of the community itself, all of whom
would suffer if this "good and productive" citizen were removed
from their midst.

One friend, who had known Lou for eighteen years, wrote:
"I still find it difficult to believe what happened. Lou has always
been of high moral character and honest in all business dealings, a
very concerned family man. We were guests together at many
social functions and charity fund-raising affairs. He always gave
fully of himself and his money for worthwhile charitable purposes, quite often in a quiet, unobtrusive, anonymous way."

Some of the letters not only praised Lou, but criticized June
—stopping just short of saying that she got everything she deserved. One such letter, from an attorney, said: "I know that he
did everything to make the marriage work. . . . I saw how she
attempted to undermine his self-confidence and provoke him to
action so that she would have grounds for divorce. As old friends
we accepted his second marriage and wished him only happiness.
June resented all the friends that he had before his marriage to
her. Louis was a very happy man when his baby Kimberly was

born. . . . He had high hopes that by having a child, this would result in a happy marriage. Unfortunately, June's character would not permit this. She had been married three times before. None of her prior husbands were wealthy. Where Louis wanted love and companionship, June required and demanded substantial expenditures from him for homes, furniture, clothing, and other possessions to demonstrate his love for her. To the fullest extent of his ability, he gave her everything she desired. This was not enough. . . . Louis believed that to June he was just a meal ticket. . . . Based upon my observation of June and Louis in the several times I was with them together, and also upon conversations with Louis when June refused to be with my wife and myself, it is my belief that she was deliberately trying to provoke him. I never observed Louis give her such provocation. When I learned of June's death, I could not believe that he was capable of such an act. During the years I have known him he was always gentle and considerate. Even on occasions when June embarrassed him by her language, or even more so by her nonappearance at a social event to which she had accepted our invitation, he never assailed or condemned her but always attempted to excuse her actions."

Lou's psychiatrist, who could be said to have known him in a different capacity than his friends did, explained Lou's actions this way: "At the time Lou Schindler shot his wife, he did not have the mental capacity to premeditate or deliberate an intent to kill his wife. He did not have the mental capacity to conceive of the specific intent to kill his wife. His acts at that time were inconsistent with planned activity. . . ." With these words, the doctor was saying that Lou was not guilty of first-degree murder, since first-degree murder requires the mental capacity to premeditate and deliberate. He then went on to relieve his patient of the responsibility for second-degree murder as well, by saying that, "because of mental illness and defect he was emotionally incapable of preventing and was not conscious of the impulsive acts which resulted in his wife's death. This mental illness and defect prevented Louis Schindler from acting with malice aforethought, and he was unable at that time to comprehend his duty to govern his actions in accordance with law." According to his psychiatrist, Lou Schindler was, at most, guilty of involuntary manslaughter, since voluntary manslaughter requires the intent to kill, and the doctor's report had erased that from his mind.

But the doctor went even further than that. By saying that Lou suffered an "acute dissociative reaction," and that he was "very mentally ill at the time," his doctor was rendering an analysis that could completely relieve Lou of responsibility. He was describing legal unconsciousness, a "complete defense" for criminal activity, in that it totally extinguishes culpability. "I feel that he's a very sick man, was very sick, and still is, mentally. I would say that he had an acute psychotic reaction, a total temporary break from reality. He was unaware of what he was doing at the time. He did the shooting while he was completely unaware of what he was doing. He not only couldn't remember what happened, but he regressed back to an earlier age. This fits in with a person who suffered a psychic trauma and was reacting unconsciously and not knowing what he was doing. His ability to commit violence is totally outside of his usual behavior pattern. He had a great love for his wife. Why would he go ahead and destroy someone who meant so much to him? It had to be unconscious." Because unconsciousness is a total legal defense for any crime, including homicide, the doctor's report attempted to free Lou Schindler from any responsibility at all.

Because I never had the opportunity to examine Lou Schindler, I cannot say whether his doctor was correct in his diagnosis or whether he was simply adding his professional expertise to the chorus of support for Lou. The doctor also called Lou a "paranoid personality," which, if true, means that Lou had a tendency to misinterpret reality in such a way that he felt threatened. This tendency, plus his hot temper, might help explain the ever-escalating tension and hostility once the divorce proceedings were begun.

Lou also confessed to his psychiatrist that he "wondered what kind of person he was," and "whether this could ever happen again." The answer to the first question is that Lou Schindler —his doctor's calling him "acutely mentally ill" notwithstanding —was not very different from most of us. I'm certain that all of the letters written on his behalf were sincere and mostly true, insofar as the authors knew the man.

The answer to the second question is that it certainly could happen again, despite the fact that Lou's brother said that he was a gentle, jovial, tolerant man and that "it wouldn't happen again in a million years."

But while Lou and his psychiatrist were asking whether it could happen again, the criminal justice system had to deal with the immediate offense. On June 19, 1967, Lou pleaded not guilty to murder charges. Normally, once a plea has been entered, the trial is supposed to begin within sixty days. Lou's trial did not. There were numerous delays and postponements, most of them coming from Lou and his attorneys. The trial was postponed because of his attorney's surgery, because of his psychiatrist's illness, and because his attorneys were needed in other trials. With all the delays, the trial did not begin until October 1967, six months after the killing.

On November 3, 1967, the jury brought in a verdict of guilty to second-degree murder. Lou was sentenced to state prison. While his case was being appealed, he began serving his sentence at Chino State prison, generally regarded as a minimum security facility. Ironically, his cell mate was a former assistant district attorney who had murdered his wife and her lover and devised an elaborate scheme to evade suspicion: he drove at breakneck speed to Las Vegas, and stopped along the way to make sure he was noticed by asking service station attendants the time and directions, so he could claim that he was there when his wife was killed. The scheme didn't work. He was convicted, though he claims to this day that he is innocent.

The accuracy of the evaluations given by Lou's psychiatrist may be reflected in what he said about Lou's prison experience: "In prison, Lou was so ridden with guilt for his grave offense against his own moral code that he thought seriously of suicide, and it was on the basis of this that he received so much treatment there."

While in prison—and presumably contemplating suicide— Lou also found the spirit, time, and energy to put his forceful, driving, athletic personality to good use by becoming handball champion and playing shortstop on the baseball team.

Lou also served as inmate assistant to the prison psychologist. In his capacity as chief clerk, he conducted all the standardized psychological tests on the other inmates. The senior psychologist was Lou's therapist as well as his prison employer. Popular among the other inmates, Lou was elected chairman of the Advisory Board. The prison chaplain chose him as his clerk.

In August 1969, after serving twenty months, Lou was eligible for parole. But just a few days before his parole hearing, his conviction was reversed on appeal. The appeals court said that the judge had incorrectly instructed the jury as to the requirements for second-degree murder. A second trial was scheduled and Lou was released on bond. He was a free man again.

With a new trial scheduled, the letter-writing campaign began again. The probation officer and the court received another enormous batch of letters from friends, relatives, and business associates—including the attorneys and the Superior Court judge —in support of Lou Schindler. He also received favorable reports from all the psychiatrists and psychologists who saw him during his stay in prison, including the chaplain, who said that he had seen a lot of Lou at Chino and that he had never been so impressed with anyone. According to the chaplain, Lou was very sincere, kind, and sensitive to the feelings of others.

Lou's brother also wrote a letter, in which he said, "Lou has already paid and been punished for his 'alleged' offense. I say 'alleged' because knowing him as I do I am convinced that it was an involuntary act. I saw him almost daily for one month prior thereto in his torment, emotionally disturbed and upset by the pending divorce and mental conflict from the constant harassments of his wife as well as his serious business problems at the time."

Meanwhile, various motions by Lou's attorneys to dismiss, continue, and postpone held up the second trial until March 1970, seven months after the reversal of his conviction. Once it began, the trial took three weeks. Essentially the same evidence and facts were reviewed. On April 13, 1970, the jury found Lou guilty of voluntary manslaughter, which would normally require a much shorter term in custody.

Before he was sentenced, Lou wrote a letter to the judge in which he said, "My gratitude is boundless for those dedicated people at the Department of Corrections who during my twenty months of incarceration at Chino after two months in county jail had recognized the utter despair I felt for having taken the life of my wife. My conscience was shocked by the act. With compassion and understanding they had, in therapeutic sessions, made me come to the realization that such things can happen in human relationships. I feel reconstructed today, though I shall always carry the sense of the tragedy that occurred."

Lou went on to tell the judge about his relationship with his daughter. Custody of Kimberly had been granted to her maternal grandparents while Lou was in prison. However, when he was released on bond, Kimberly spent weekends with Lou at his brother's home: "It is now three years since the time of the tragedy. The time that I was on bail had permitted me to spend each weekend with my baby Kimberly, so that a fond relationship has developed between us. As I write this she is asleep in her bedroom, having just been put to bed after a kiss and a hug to me, and after her having said her prayers for her father, grandparents, sisters, uncle and aunt, and our dog. I feel a deep regret that her mother is not there to help put her to sleep each night. I vow to you and God that I shall endeavor to do my very best for her as the circumstances allow."

In his letter, Lou was obviously trying to impress upon the judge that he had been punished enough and that more harm might be done if he went back to prison. This, plus his appeal to the judge's sentimental side, apparently worked. Lou was once again sentenced to state prison, this time for the statutory period of six months to fifteen years. But the execution of the sentence was stayed by the judge and Lou was released on his own recognizance pending the outcome of his second appeal.

So another round of letter-writing and legal delays began.

But notwithstanding his personal psychiatrist's official characterization of him as a person who was severely mentally ill, Lou did not waste any time while awaiting the decision of the second appeal. In fact, not only did he take up where he left off in business and yachting, but in other areas as well. Lou and his brother went to court to wrest custody of Kimberly from her grandparents. However, custody could not be granted to Lou until his case was resolved, so his brother became Kimberly's guardian. And finally, Lou resumed his love life. During the winter of 1970–71, he met Laura.

Laura and her twin brother Jack were born February 27, 1927, in New York City. Their father was sales manager of a dressmaking firm, and their mother was a model. When she and her brother were four years old, their parents placed them in a boarding school while they traveled. Laura and Jack lived with several different foster families during the next two years. In 1933, Laura and Jack moved back with their parents and the family moved to San Francisco. Nine years later, they moved to Los Angeles.

Laura's father was aggressive and overbearing, though her mother was depressed and dependent. She described her father as "independent, very outgoing, hyper, strict, and impatient," and said he was more in charge of her and her brother than her mother was. Spankings were not uncommon.

Laura grew up to be a rather smallish young woman, prone to underweight even for her height. Emotionally, she tended to be like her mother: quiet, withdrawn, a stay-at-home much of the time. Her mother had grown up with a "very rough and exacting stepfather." Laura followed her mother's example in love, too. Over the years, she got into relationships with men who were similarly abusive. At the same time, she suffered from depression and lack of self-esteem. At age sixteen, she quit school. Though she went back years later, she never got her high school diploma.

In 1950, Laura was married to a man named Frederick, who was gentle and shy. The marriage lasted less than two years. Laura said the marriage broke up because "It was my fault. . . . I was young and foolish and he was really wonderful. I was immature. I felt life was passing me by. I divorced him. We had no children and I just didn't want to be married anymore."

In 1954, while looking for a job, Laura met William, a man who was hiring staff for a trade show. She worked for him briefly and they became platonic friends.

In 1955, Laura married a man named David. According to Laura, this marriage failed because David was "manic-depressive," and behaved chaotically. Furthermore, David was an actor and didn't want to be married. He was hyperactive, strongly opinionated, and prone to emotional outbursts. After less than a year of marriage, he divorced Laura.

In 1959, Laura married husband number three, Harold, who could not hold a job and depended on her for financial support. This marriage lasted barely two years. Laura found out that Harold was bisexual and accused him of being "morally bankrupt." Harold had also been arrested for armed robbery when he was a teenager and spent time in prison. Apparently, he had not mended his ways. Not only was he still stealing, but he was also cheating on Laura.

During the early 1960s, Laura worked as a receptionist at Hollywood West Memorial Hospital. She worked the late shift— 3 P.M. to 11 P.M. After her third marriage failed, she saw a psychiatrist to help her deal with the problems she had developed during this relationship and others. But despite any therapy she might have received, Laura remained a potential victim. On the night of April 1, 1963, as she was leaving work, she was attacked in the parking lot, knocked to the ground, and dragged into a storage shed. Laura struggled to defend herself and escape from her attacker, but she was stabbed in the wrist and abdomen, and then raped. Her ankle was broken during the struggle. She reported the attack to the police, but the attacker was never caught.

During the remaining years of the 1960s, Laura remained single. She worked as a receptionist at another hospital until June 20, 1971, when she married Lou Schindler.

Laura had met him during the winter. To her he was "charming, ambitious, and very intelligent." Of course, there was this little matter of his having shot and killed his previous wife. Lou told her all about it on their very first date: The killing had been an accident. Lou told her the gun went off accidentally. Laura did not find out until after they were married that he had "accidentally" fired at least five shots at June, hitting her three times in the front of her body and twice in the back as she turned to run away from him.

Lou's second appeal was still pending when he met, courted, and married Laura. In early 1972, the second conviction was also reversed on technicalities. A third trial was scheduled.

But the third trial never took place. The rules of the game say that once a conviction has been reversed on appeal, the accused cannot be retried for a more severe crime than the previous conviction. Since Lou had been convicted of voluntary man-

slaughter at his second trial, he could no longer be charged with
first- or second-degree murder—only manslaughter. In light of
the meager stakes, in April 1972 Lou's attorneys and the prosecutor worked out a plea bargain. Lou pleaded guilty to involuntary
manslaughter, another notch lower on the homicide scale. Since
he had already served almost as much time as he would normally
receive for an involuntary manslaughter conviction, his sentence
was thirty days' probation. Lou Schindler was a free man—once
and for all.

The new couple settled down to married life, free at last of
the threat of another trial. Lou regained total custody of his
daughter, and Kimberly came to live with him and Laura.
Though he had lived quite modestly when they first met, soon
after they were married they bought a new home. They were a
complete, happy family.

Sort of. Laura soon came to think of her husband as a "Jekyll
and Hyde" kind of man. To her, he could be very charming and
disarmingly sweet—"and then when the door was closed, it was a
whole different story." She never knew when he might "go off."
More and more she saw Lou as overbearing, aggressive, and
prone to violent outbursts. "My heart was pounding all the time,"
she said. "Everything that was wrong was my fault. Nothing I did
was right. I became passive and withdrawn. I didn't want to rock
the boat. He gave orders—no 'thank yous' or 'pleases.' It built up
and up over the years."

Lou constantly talked about June's killing. This frightened
Laura and Kimberly, as if he were threatening them. Apparently,
he enjoyed having this effect on Laura. At times he would sneak
up behind her and do or say something scary. "What frightened
me about Lou was that he enjoyed frightening me." Laura always
felt threatened. She constantly thought of leaving—but also kept
hoping things would get better. So she stayed. She still loved her
husband, and as time went on she became more and more attached to Kimberly.

After about a year of marriage, Laura decided to leave her
husband. She spent the night with her sister-in-law, in whom she
had come to confide. For some time, Laura had enlisted the aid of
her sister-in-law in an effort to try to understand her husband.
The next day she went to Kimberly's school to tell her where she

was. Six-year-old Kimberly got upset and begged Laura to take her away with her. Laura was torn. "I'm very family-oriented," she said, "and very fond of Kim." Though she never discussed divorce with Lou, she did consult an attorney. But she never went beyond that stage. "I just never wanted a divorce," she said. Laura knew that Lou would never allow her to see Kimberly if they were divorced. So she took Kimberly home and "tried to be the best mother and wife I knew how."

Despite the fact that Lou could be an explosive tyrant who tended to blame others for his frustrations, he was a good provider and a successful businessman. Lou's carpet business was thriving once again. In 1974, Laura went to work for him doing general office work. But she had to leave the job after a few months because the pressure made her ill.

As Laura grew more passive, gentle, depressed, and fearful, Lou became more domineering, explosive, paranoid, and irrationally hostile. Although his physical abuse never went beyond pushing, his verbal and emotional abuse could be intense. As their marriage wore on into the mid-1970s, Laura became more severely depressed and withdrawn and suffered from anorexic weight loss. Not only did she grow ever more afraid of her husband, but she also grew more nervous. She had increasing trouble sleeping, perhaps with good reason. Lou sometimes slept with a knife under his pillow for fear that he might be attacked by anti-Semitic groups in the middle of the night.

And then there were the times when, to Laura, it seemed as though he was actually boasting about killing June and "getting away with it." Laura was afraid to even discuss the prospect of a divorce, since he had killed June during their divorce proceedings.

The picture of Lou Schindler that Laura carried in her mind was not a pretty one. She said he "hated the system" and was abrasive and explosive not only with her and Kimberly, but also in his friendships and business relationships. Lou was also apparently estranged from his two adult daughters from his first marriage. He had not seen them in over seven years. He could be vindictive, too, especially toward June's parents. As soon as he obtained custody of Kimberly, he immediately restricted their right to visit her. He also held the restriction of these rights over his daughter's head.

For her part, Kimberly corroborated Laura's view. The daughter felt that her father bragged and made light of her mother's death. He also criticized and demeaned June's relatives, who rarely said anything negative about him. Kimberly said that her father behaved "like an angel" socially and among relatives. But at home it was a different story. "His temperament flared up all of a sudden," she said. "He just became a whole other person. He would yell and scream and he was just impossible." Kimberly, too, was afraid of her father. "He was intimidating and he always yelled and ranted. And he was always yelling and blaming other people for things that were totally his fault."

Kimberly said that Laura never resisted Lou. "He would just go on and on and she would just sit there and say nothing." Kimberly felt that her father "liked to make people sad."

Laura knew Kimberly was troubled about her father, and so counseled the child to try to be patient and understand and respect him. She considered Kimberly "as much my own as if she had come from my own body." Laura knew she was losing face with Kimberly by not standing up to Lou. But she also knew that June had stood up to him—and "look what happened to her."

So Laura became more and more withdrawn. Little by little she gave up arguing with Lou. She felt she was always "on a powder keg." She suspected that he manipulated her because she allowed him to, but she didn't know what to do about it. A friend said that Laura was "just not the kind of person who really complains. She didn't want to burden anyone with her problems, but I knew she was unhappy."

To call Laura unhappy is a gross understatement. By 1978, she had lost more than twenty-five pounds. She went from a size ten dress to a size three. Since 1971 she had suffered from a chronic cough. In 1973 she was diagnosed as diabetic. In 1974 she had a hysterectomy. She was so nervous most of the time that she couldn't eat. Tranquilizers became a regular part of her life. As soon as she woke up in the morning she would take one. When she heard Lou's car in the driveway, she would take another. "My heart would start pounding something fierce when he came into the house," she said. Laura was regularly consuming up to ten tranquilizers per day.

In 1976, with Lou's support, Laura sought professional help. She was seen by a psychologist who later went on to become a radio celebrity. After three sessions, Laura was told she couldn't help herself unless she left her husband.

Next, Laura tried to get her husband to join her in counseling. Lou said he didn't need any help and suggested that she see his psychiatrist, the same man who had treated him during his previous troubles. In the doctor's opinion, Laura was "so depressed and seemed so despondent that I was afraid that she might harm herself. She had a very strong conscience, which would tend to make her feel responsible for helping others. She felt very concerned about the welfare of Mr. Schindler's daughter and very concerned about the welfare of her own parents, and she was a sensitive person who would tend to have her self-esteem lowered or feel guilty fairly regularly."

After eight visits with this doctor, Lou insisted that Laura stop seeing him. "He didn't seem to be helping me. I was getting worse and so was my husband."

Despite their psychological difficulties, the Schindler marriage prospered materially. In 1976, Lou paid cash for a brand new Rolls-Royce and a brand new Toyota. But material possessions were little consolation. As a matter of fact, they even became part of the problem. Lou's sailboat, for example, was not the scene of happy family outings. Instead, as Laura complained, "We always did whatever he wanted to every weekend. He had a boat, and Kim would get seasick. And I'm not the sailor type. It was a sailboat and we were forced to do things we didn't want to. . . ."

On the evening of March 6, 1978, Lou and Laura had a dinner engagement with Lou's brother and sister, their respective spouses, and another couple who were celebrating their anniversary. They all met at the Schindler home, and then went to Yamato's Restaurant for an early dinner. Twelve-year-old Kimberly went along. At around 8 P.M. the group returned to the Schindler home, where they socialized for a little over an hour. Laura had asked them to stay awhile. She felt uneasy, vaguely scared. Lou had been acting a bit erratic lately. About a month before he had pushed her against a wall during one of their arguments, right in front of Kimberly.

But so far the dinner party and the get-together at the Schindler home were perfectly normal and without incident. Lou's brother and his wife were the last to leave, at around nine-fifteen. Before the family retired for the night, Laura set up Kimberly's breakfast for the next morning.

When Laura came into her bedroom, Lou was already there, sitting up in bed, dressed in his pajamas. Laura sat down in a chair next to the bed. Suddenly, though neither said a word, she sensed Lou was in a surly mood. He turned to Laura "with a maniacal look on his face" and said in a low voice that was almost a whisper, "What happened to June is going to happen to you. I know what I have to do."

The next thing Laura knew . . . she was in jail.

At 11:20 P.M. that night, the police had responded to what is known as an "ambulance-shooting" call. Laura greeted the first police officer at the door and pointed to the rear bedroom and said, "He is in there." The officer went to the bedroom and saw Lou Schindler lying in bed with the covers pulled up to his neck. No signs of life were evident to the officer. Nor could he see any sign of blood.

Returning to the living room, the officer asked Laura what had happened.

"I shot him," she said.

Kimberly came into the living room, along with a neighbor, Sheila, and her son, Paul. Sheila was a family friend who knew all the stories about both Lou's and Laura's previous marriages—and how they ended. Paul was Kimberly's friend.

Kimberly had been in bed asleep when her stepmother came in, woke her up, and cried, "I think I've done a terrible thing. I think I shot your father." Even though there was a phone in Kimberly's room, the two went to the kitchen phone, which had a sticker with the police and ambulance phone numbers on it. First they called the police, then the ambulance, then Sheila. Then Kimberly phoned her uncle, June's brother.

Sheila advised Laura not to say anything more to the police.

Laura and Kimberly were both taken to the West Los Angeles Police Station. The authorities tested Laura's and Kimberly's hands to determine if either or both had fired a gun. Kimberly's hands were clean. Just as she was about to be taken into protective custody, her uncle (June's brother) came and took her home. Kimberly was now an orphan, both her parents the victims of homicide within eleven years of each other. She went back to live with her maternal grandparents.

When the ambulance and the coroner arrived at the Schindler home, they examined Lou and found a small entry wound at the back of his head. The weapon Laura had used was a .25-caliber automatic, blue steel pistol, which she had bought for protection many years before she met Lou. Normally, the gun was kept in Laura's clothes closet—loaded.

The next day, Laura was released on bail. She moved out of the house she and Lou had bought for over $200,000 after their marriage, and moved in with her parents, where she remained for the next fifteen months.

Laura felt tremendous guilt for killing her husband. "It all has the quality of being unreal. It's so untrue it doesn't seem real. I would do anything to undo it." She also said that "It must have been an accumulation of everything. I couldn't handle it. I must have short-circuited." For taking a human life, "the most precious thing in the world," Laura said she was prepared to be punished.

Her defense attorney was not quite so eager for her to be punished, however. Laura hired the same man who, as an assistant district attorney, had prosecuted Lou Schindler three times for June's killing. Now in private practice, he went to work defending Laura.

Laura's defense was based on the fact that she did not remember going to get the gun or firing it at her husband as he lay in bed. "I'm devastated that I could be capable of such an act," she said. "It is totally against my nature. I can't sleep. I'm going through a very bad period of terrible guilt and upset."

I was called in to examine Laura in March 1979, almost one year to the day after she killed her husband. My job was to determine two things: whether she was legally sane at the time of the killing, and whether she had the mental capacity to form the specific intent to kill her husband, to premeditate and deliberate, or to harbor malice.

Laura was a small woman. She weighed only seventy-eight pounds on the day she shot her husband. In the year since his death, she had regained most of her lost weight, and then some. But she was still of small stature. She wore her hair long and spoke in a soft monotone. I reviewed the results of standard psychological tests Laura had taken. They reinforced what I could tell from examining Laura myself, that she was a very passive, dependent person who had a tough time dealing independently with problems. Such people do tend to repress, or push back, their anger until they wind up feeling depressed, sad, alone, and helpless.

The other doctors who had examined Laura said she was so incapacitated by her fear and depression that she was unable in her mind to form the intent to kill. She had lost control of her behavior because she was in a "state of panic," and in "mortal terror for her life." One doctor said that immediately prior to killing Lou, she was "at the end of her rope," and that when he intimated a threat that she would wind up like his previous wife, she "exploded in an angry crescendo of years of pent-up frustration, fear, and despair." In other words, she was not in emotional control, and was acting in the heat of passion. If this could be sustained in court, it would mean she was guilty of, at most, voluntary manslaughter.

But I did not see heat of passion as a viable explanation for Laura's actions. She simply was not given to wide and potentially violent mood swings.

During our session together, Laura told me that she and Lou had not talked about their problems that evening. There had been no argument or abuse. It was impossible for me to see her action as an explosive outburst, since she was not an explosive person and there really was not enough going on that night to provoke a violent, aggressive act from such a normally passive person. There may have been enough confusion and fear in her mind to impair her ability to reflect upon the gravity of the act, thus erasing the mental capacity required for first-degree murder. But there was not enough to melt away her ability to harbor malice, a necessary ingredient for second-degree murder.

Nor was she legally insane at the time she shot him. There simply was not enough mental impairment to blind her to how wrong the act was. In other words, she may have been at wits' end and had not really known what to do, given her personality, but she still knew it was wrong to kill her husband. She wasn't out of control. After all, she was able to properly inform others of the act immediately thereafter.

Laura may have been experiencing extreme fear of her husband, and killing him was certainly inconsistent with her personality, but there simply was no evidence of a legally significant mental breakdown. She was able to form the intent to kill and to harbor malice. In short, though I felt tremendous sympathy for her and her plight, I felt she was mentally capable of committing second-degree murder.

The jury apparently agreed, because on March 16, 1979, after deliberating for twenty-two hours, they brought in a verdict of guilty to second-degree murder.

Laura was sent to Frontera (women's facility) for evaluation and to await sentencing. While she was there, she received a letter from William, the man she had befriended back in 1954. Over the years their friendship would, from time to time, pick up and drop off. Now it was evidently on the upswing. During the seventy-seven days Laura was at Frontera, she and William corresponded. In one of her letters she asked him if she could go to work for him when she was released. William wrote back that she would have a job waiting for her.

When Laura left Frontera, William offered her a job at his advertising business. First, she had to undergo surgery to repair the bones in her foot, which had separated. She believed that this problem had been caused by malnutrition when her weight had fallen so dramatically. Once healed from her surgery, she was able to take advantage of William's offer. At first, she performed general office duties, such as opening mail, sorting orders, collecting unpaid bills. Before long, she and William started dating.

Meanwhile, the same letter-writing machinery that had gone into action years earlier during Lou Schindler's trials, once again cranked into action. Letter after letter was addressed to the judge and probation officer preparing a sentencing recommendation for the court. The letters were similar to the ones that had been sent a decade earlier. There was an avalanche of letters praising Lou and condemning his wife. The only difference was that this time Lou was the victim, so rather than plead for leniency, the letters cried out for the killer's blood. Lou's brothers and sister, who heard that Laura's psychological evaluation from Frontera was in favor of leniency, wrote a scathing letter condemning not only Laura but the criminal justice system as well: "Their evaluation is based on self-serving declarations, calculated conduct the defendant would naturally put on while at Frontera, exercising her wiles, cunning, and histrionic abilities to influence bleeding hearts. She fooled our brother at the cost of his life. They have only seen one side of the coin—her version. Unfortunately the victim is dead and can't be heard from."

This time, however, not only were there letters from relatives, friends, and associates of Lou Schindler, but also letters praising Laura from people who knew her. A social worker and child and family counselor who had known Laura for several years wrote about her, "As a friend I have found her to be kind, considerate, concerned, and very gentle. I have noticed that these qualities are characteristic of her relationship not only with me but with all people. I trust Laura's honesty and integrity."

The probation report to the judge, which is routinely completed to apprise the judge of all the facts to help him pass sentence, called attention to the contradictions and ironies in Laura's situation. While acknowledging that her marriage was difficult, the report also noted that "before his death the victim made the defendant the major beneficiary of his rather substantial estate, as well as appointing her the guardian of his minor child." The report also acknowledged that the offense was "situational" and not likely to happen again, and that Laura would normally be a good candidate for probation. However, the report concluded that since Laura knew what she was doing, had used a firearm, and had killed the victim while he was asleep, probation should be denied and a prison sentence imposed.

In September 1979, although Laura received much sympathy not only from the probation report but also from the judge, she was sentenced to seven years in state prison. For a second-degree murder conviction, that would be considered quite lenient. With good behavior, the length of confinement could be reduced to fewer than four years.

Laura's attorney appealed, and she was released on bond.

Meanwhile, Laura's friendship with William had blossomed into romance. They were married in November 1979.

Laura said about her fifth husband, "Bill is a good, down-to-earth, hard-working, gentle man. He always loved me. He was steady and dependable. And I loved him very much for these wonderful traits. He's quite shy."

Several months later, the appeals court reversed Laura's conviction. At her trial, the prosecution had used Laura's jailhouse interview to counter her defense claim of diminished capacity. Laura was interviewed by a police officer several hours after she had been advised of her constitutional rights. That was not a problem, since she was once again asked if she understood her rights. However, the policeman also heard Laura ask a friend to get a specific attorney for her—the man who had prosecuted her husband. The prosecution made the valid point that Laura had the mental capacity and clarity of mind to not only understand her rights, but also to ask for a specific attorney.

Her attorney moved for a mistrial on the basis that the court could not use Laura's exercising of her rights against her to support the contention that she acted with a sound mind. By doing so, her right to counsel was impaired. His motion for mistrial was denied during the trial. He appealed the conviction on the same basis, and the appeals court agreed with him. Laura's asking for a specific attorney, and thereby demonstrating what could be interpreted as clear thinking, could not be used as evidence against her.

A second trial was scheduled, but the same kinds of delays that kept postponing Lou Schindler's trials delayed Laura's. In September 1982, after Laura's trial had once again been delayed, Lou's brother wrote, "When is justice finally to be done? Is she waiting for the witnesses to die or be worn down?" Lou's other brother and his sister wrote to the presiding judge: "It is an outrage and a crying shame that the ends of justice can be so easily thwarted by the machinations of a criminal defendant with the connivance and delaying tactics of an attorney. . . . It seems all a clever criminal has to do is . . . engage a very busy lawyer, and thus keep from being brought to trial indefinitely. . . . Justice delayed is justice denied.''

Apparently, the irony of his statements was lost on the judge.

In December 1982 Laura's second trial ended in a hung jury. A third trial was scheduled. More delays. And in June 1983 the charges against Laura were reduced to voluntary manslaughter.

The barrage of letters continued. Now they attacked Laura for, as Lou's brother wrote, "living the good life . . . while my brother lies moldering in his grave." They accused her of pillaging Lou's estate, after he was "murdered . . . while he was asleep in his own bed. She crept up on him and cold-bloodedly shot his brains out five years ago. She committed this crime strictly for financial gain. The money she got from him, his Rolls-Royce, boat, home in Beverly Hills, the Cadillac, all the proceeds from same she is enjoying now. She planned this for a long time just for material gain," wrote Lou's sister. "Is this justice that the poor go to jail and the rich murderers get a good lawyer? She must be punished for her crime of taking a life. The Bible says 'Thou shalt not kill.' "

Actually, Laura did not "plunder" the estate at all. Despite the Schindler family's allegations that she was living the high life, there was no evidence that she was living at any more than a modest, middle-class level. She and her new husband had a second mortgage on their house, and they both had to work very hard to keep the business afloat. They often worked well into the evenings and on weekends.

Lou's estate was substantial—over $1.6 million. Laura's community property share of that estate was over $800,000. She gave more than half of her share to Lou's children. Approximately three quarters of what remained went to her attorneys. The rest was put in trust. After all her legal fees were paid, Laura was left with about $30,000. An objective investigator for the court came to the conclusion that Laura did not profit from the death of her husband.

In addition to the letters from Lou's family, Laura's family and friends wrote letters on her behalf. Her parents, both in their late seventies, pleaded with the judge to allow them to have their daughter with them for their few remaining years.

Laura's twin brother, Jack, wrote that "Laura is essentially a gentle person, more often than not dominated by those around her. . . . Laura has been profoundly shaken and remorseful about her act. No sentence imposed can possibly punish her greater than the punishment she carries within her mind and soul."

A good friend of Laura's wrote, "I have an old sick mother and Laura is always calling her and making her feel better. My mother adores her. . . . She lives a very quiet life with Bill and works very hard with him. . . . I have been to their modest home many times. No matter what her problems have been, and we know they have been considerable, she always asks about the other person's problems and tries to help."

Many people who had known Lou before Laura also came forward and testified for her. A business associate of Laura's new husband wrote: "Laura is a very warm, sensitive, caring, gentle, genteel, loving, considerate and fine person. These qualities are also demonstrated by her love not only for people but for all animals as well. We have a Doberman who immediately took to Laura and Bill. Our dog would seat himself next to Laura and put his head on her lap."

Laura pleaded guilty to the charge of voluntary manslaughter. Sentencing was scheduled for September 1983—five and a half years after the crime.

In a letter she wrote to the judge, Laura said, "Five years ago after seven years of an increasingly nightmarish life I did the most horrible act I can imagine. I shot and killed my husband, Louis Schindler. . . . In spite of Lou's personality and the problems we had, I blame only myself for what happened. It has taken me years of consultation with psychologists and psychiatrists to understand how I could have remained in such a terrible situation. . . . No amount of understanding makes it easier to live with the feeling of guilt and remorse that I feel. I loved Lou Schindler once and I loved his family and daughter. I grieve for all of them. I wish I could end the pain for his daughter, who I orphaned, for his family, and for my own dear parents who have suffered with me during these past five years. . . . There is no prison as strong or harsh as the prison of the mind. I don't want to go to jail, but I am ready to accept whatever happens. What I really want more than anything is something no one else can give me. I want to be forgiven. I'm doing better. I still have fears and apprehensions about my fate. But I am very comfortable with my husband. I have had a few phone calls at 4 A.M. that implied some threatening things. . . . I am now working. My life is largely uneventful. . . ."

In September 1983 the California Department of Corrections evaluation recommended that Laura be placed on probation in lieu of incarceration. The sentencing judge followed that recommendation.

Laura now walks with a limp, a result of the surgery she had on her feet and legs in 1979. She has tried her best to reestablish order and purpose in her life.

The Vampire
of Sacramento

Richard Chase's lifestyle could easily be described as eccentric. However, no one took sufficient notice of his strange behavior in time to avert the terror that plagued Sacramento in late 1977 and early 1978. Not his parents, not his doctors, not his psychiatrists, not his teachers, not police, and not the courts. Before it was over, there would be six people dead, including a twenty-two-month-old infant and a young pregnant woman, all victims of a predator known as the "Vampire of Sacramento."

According to his mother, Richard's delivery into the world on May 23, 1950, was normal. He achieved all the milestones of infancy and childhood at the usual ages. He walked by nine months, talked by fourteen months, and was "fully potty-trained" by the time he was two years old. However, he did continue to wet the bed occasionally until he was eight.

Richard's mother, father, and grandmother agreed that the best word to describe the boy's temperament during his early childhood was "passive." Though not overly affectionate or outgoing, he presented no disciplinary problems, but did like to play with matches. On at least one occasion, he actually set a fire. Richard's bed-wetting and fire-setting, when combined with his later cruelty to animals, comprise what, in my experience, is a triad of signs indicating that a person is highly dangerous. Nevertheless, Richard's family remembered him as a peaceful child.

Unfortunately, the same could not be said for his home. The

family situation became increasingly stormy during Richard's childhood. His father had problems with alcohol and his mother was tormented by suspicions that her husband was unfaithful to her and was trying to poison her. The household was beset by constant bickering, accusations, arguments, and tension.

The Chase family rented an apartment until 1953, when they moved into their first house. When family difficulties escalated around 1962, Richard's mother was seen by at least two different psychiatrists. Because of these marital problems the Chases slipped financially and lost the house in 1963, when Richard was in junior high school. It is difficult to say just how great an impact his parents' conflicts had on Richard's mental stability, but it certainly couldn't have helped. Indeed, he appears to have withdrawn into a world of mental chaos, controlled by fantasies of power and magical thinking.

Richard attended Mira Loma High School from 1964 until 1968. He managed to finish high school, though his grades were generally poor—mostly C's and D's with several F's. His sister, who was three years younger, recalls that her brother was selfish and inconsiderate of the rights of others. He tended to be a loner and had considerable difficulty forming relationships with young women. Though he went out on dates and had the opportunity to have sex on several occasions, he was impotent. Increasingly preoccupied and disturbed by this impotence, Richard got drunk at a friends' party one evening, broke down, and uncharacteristically divulged his problem for the first time. As a result, the traces of whatever minimal self-esteem he may have possessed were essentially destroyed.

During those high school years, Richard began to use alcohol, marijuana, and LSD—but would deny it when confronted by his father. Father and son would argue frequently. Richard was shiftless, lazy, slothful in his personal habits, sloppy in his dress, rebellious and defiant against his parents' values. His sister remembers him yelling at his mother, "You're controlling my mind, I want you to stop."

During his sophomore year of high school, Richard was arrested for possession of marijuana. He was subsequently ordered by the juvenile court to work on weekends. In his later high school years, as his drug abuse worsened, Richard came to experience periods of panic.

In 1968, Richard was admitted to American River College, which he attended until the spring of 1971, when he took a leave of absence. While at college he was a consistently low-C student, and a heavy user of drugs. He appeared to be constantly stoned and was always unkempt. When he became ill, he neglected to seek treatment, though he was seen briefly by a psychiatrist in 1969. Frequently, he would appear nude in the presence of strangers.

In February 1971 Richard moved in with some friends who were renting a house and arranged to share the rent. Once he moved in, however, he proceeded to board up his bedroom door, and then make a hole in the closet wall for exit and entry to his room. Then he bolted the closet door from inside the room. He said he did this so no one could sneak up on him. His housemates were not happy about the situation. Richard used so much marijuana that they believed he was dealing, although they had no hard evidence. He had also been seen one day waving a handgun out the window at someone who was coming up the driveway.

Richard didn't seem to care about keeping up his end of the house responsibilities. After three months, his housemates asked him to move out. When he refused, they moved out instead, forcing Richard to move back with his parents.

Richard's parents separated shortly after his twenty-second birthday in 1972, and were divorced six months later. Thereafter, Chase divided his time between them.

At around this time, he went on a solitary journey to Utah, where he was thrown in jail for a traffic violation. When he returned after two weeks, he claimed he was "quite ill" because the officers had "gassed" him while he was in jail. His father had to talk him out of trying to sue the Utah authorities.

Afterward Richard seemed to withdraw even further into a slovenly life-style. Seldom showering or shaving, he would lie in bed for hours. There were violent spells, too. On one occasion he broke one of the doors in the house. On another, during an argument with his mother, he hit her over the head with the telephone.

About this time Richard began obsessively worrying about

his health and, reversing his previous behavior, began seeking medical help for his imagined conditions. One night fire trucks and an ambulance pulled up to his mother's house. They were looking for the "heart patient" who had called in the emergency. Another day, after he shaved his head, allegedly, to see it change shape, he complained that the bones at the back of his head were coming through the skin.

While at his mother's house, Richard often acted as if he were hearing voices of invisible people. He would answer the voices, saying, "I'm not going to do that," and, "Stop bothering me."

In April 1973, while at a party at a friend's apartment, Richard tried to grab a young woman's breasts. He was ordered to leave, but he soon returned and had to be forcibly restrained. The police were called and, during the ensuing struggle, a .22-caliber revolver fell from his belt. He was arrested, but his father bailed him out of jail. Though there was no evidence of serious injury, Richard complained of head injuries and claimed to have been badly beaten by the police and other young men at the party. He was examined by physicians, but would not accept their conclusion that he was not seriously hurt.

From that point on friends and family noticed that Richard often complained of imagined illness. He carried his obsession to Los Angeles in May 1973, when he went to live with his grandmother, who operated and taught at a school for the retarded. Richard drove one of the buses for the school. Whenever he drove, however, he always took the back alleys rather than the main streets. Worse, he did not do the necessary maintenance work on the bus—he failed to check the gas, oil, and water. As a result, the bus often ran out of gas and was eventually ruined.

At home with his grandmother, he wasn't much better. He insisted on cooking for himself, yet he burned all the pots and pans. His grandmother also heard him talking to himself when he was alone in his room: "Are you a good boy?" he would ask himself. Then he would answer, "Yes, you're a good boy." Richard walked around the house with his head wrapped in cloth, and frequently stood on his head in a corner of the room. When his grandmother asked him why he was doing this, he told her his head hurt and he needed to get the blood to run down into it.

Finally, she could take no more of his behavior and put Richard on a plane back to Sacramento.

Richard continued to bounce back and forth between his father and mother. When he lived with his father, he occasionally helped with work around the house. They completely redid the floor in the kitchen and Richard helped place slats in the chain-link fence. Refusing to accept the fact that Richard was mentally ill, his father maintained that the boy's problems were the result of "misguided values and attitudes." He continued to pester his son to "shape up," get a job, and function normally.

Still, his father did bring him to several physicians in 1973. He saw a doctor for the stomach problems he often complained of, but walked out in the middle of the exam. He was also seen and evaluated psychiatrically, for the first time since 1969. A neurologist concluded that Richard "had a psychiatric disturbance of major proportions."

On the first day of December 1973, Richard walked into the emergency room of the American River Hospital in Sacramento. To the doctors, he had a wild look, and they described him as "filthy, disheveled, deteriorated, and foul-smelling." Their patient was extremely tense and wild-eyed as he nervously complained that he couldn't breathe and that his head was changing shape. From his descriptions of his symptoms, it was obvious to the doctors that this young man had some understanding of medical jargon, but he used the terms inaccurately. For example, he claimed to have had "cardiac arrest." If the emergency-room physicians needed any further evidence that this was a case for the Psychiatric Unit, Richard gave it to them when he complained that someone had stolen his pulmonary artery and his blood flow had stopped.

At the Psychiatric Unit, Richard's statements grew wilder and less coherent. The examining psychiatrist diagnosed him as a chronic paranoid schizophrenic—though he allowed for the possibility that the mental illness was caused by drug abuse. After two days in the hospital, Richard's mother showed up and made quite an impression on the doctors, who described her as "highly aggressive, hostile, and provocative . . . the so-called 'schizophrenogenic mother.'" She could not tolerate the thought of her son being in a mental ward, so, against the doctors' advice, she took him from the hospital.

Richard's father and mother disagree on how things went for the next two years. His mother claims that her son was frightened by the experience at the hospital and that she was then able to "work with him." She saw improvement in his eating habits and hygiene. His father recalls no such extended period of improvement.

In any case, whatever recovery may have existed, Richard's mother became convinced by late 1975 that her son was once again abusing drugs.

In the early months of 1976 Richard began another period of marked deterioration. He became convinced that he was the reincarnation of one of the Younger Brothers, bank robbers who rode with Jesse James. He did strange things: talked to himself, placed oranges next to his head "so the vitamin C would filter through to his brain," threw food, used foul language around his mother and sister, destroyed furniture, and had fits in which he chased people out of the house. He was unable to live very long with either parent, and was generally destructive, hostile, and uncontrollable.

While living with his mother, Richard went on welfare so he would have more spending money. He and his mother frequently argued about this and other matters, and quite often, Richard's father was called in to calm the storm at his ex-wife's house. One day in early 1976, while his mother was eating in her bedroom, Richard walked by and asked her for some food. She told him to use his own money to get some. Angered, Richard entered the room. When his mother stood up he slapped her, knocking her to the floor.

The arguments between mother and son continued, and became so violent that Richard knocked a huge hole in the wall of the house. He then became so enraged that his mother and sister fled the house and summoned the father. This time, before he drove over to his ex-wife's house, Richard's father tried calming his son over the telephone. In the middle of the conversation, Richard tore the entire telephone off the wall, wires and all, and the line suddenly went dead.

That incident prompted Richard's parents to find a small

apartment for their son and move him into it as soon as possible. They continued to deny their son's need for treatment, however. Now on welfare, Richard kept his new living quarters—and himself—reasonably clean, for a while. Eventually, however, both became filthy.

It was apparently about that time that Richard started drinking blood. He initially bought rabbits—presumably to cook and eat. But he didn't always cook them. More often than not, he simply killed and disemboweled them, and ate the meat and viscera raw. Preoccupied with blood and convinced that he needed fresh blood to survive, Richard also drank the rabbits' blood. He experimented with various ways of preparing and consuming them, and on occasion, he blended the blood and viscera together. On April 26, 1976, his father visited him and found him very ill. Richard was shaking and complaining of blood poisoning. He told his father he had eaten a "bad rabbit." Actually, unbeknown to his father, Richard had injected himself with rabbit blood.

This fact was discovered later at Sacramento Community Hospital, where his father took him. Richard began by saying only that he had been poisoned by a rabbit he had eaten. Then the story grew more and more bizarre: the rabbit, he said, had battery acid in its stomach, which, when he ate it, started burning through his stomach. Richard was transferred to a psychiatric unit. There, he was once again diagnosed as suffering from paranoid schizophrenia. His doctor decided he was a "danger to others" and requested that the young man be held for seventy-two hours and sent to the special Psychiatric Unit at American River Hospital as soon as possible.

At American River Hospital it was determined that Richard had killed the rabbit, drunk some of its blood, and injected some into his own body. Though he was basically reluctant to confide in his doctors, he finally admitted he needed to drink blood because his heart was weak and his body was "falling apart."

Once again, the doctors diagnosed him as a paranoid schizophrenic, acute—which meant that the disease, which can go into remission, was now flaring up. Indeed, Richard was withdrawn, suspicious, and uncooperative. Refusing to acknowledge why he was in the hospital, he insisted that he was suffering only from food poisoning. When hospital authorities would not give in to his constant demands to be released, Richard successfully escaped from the hospital on May 18, 1976, and showed up at his mother's home.

This time his mother and father cooperated long enough to return Richard to the hospital. Once there, however, he became even more withdrawn than before. His doctors described him as "almost nonverbal," and noted that he refused to exercise or attend group therapy sessions. From time to time, his condition would change. There were days when he was merely delusional, when he believed that his body was falling apart because his circulatory system was not working. Then there were days when he was unpredictably aggressive, hostile, and threatening. Richard again blamed the beating he received at the party many years earlier for his present problems, and asked doctors to supply him with enough evidence to sue his attackers. Neurological exams were carried out to determine if there was a specific organic problem. None was found.

On May 19 Richard was transferred from American River Hospital to an extended-care mental hospital. He resisted the transfer, and, upon arrival at the new hospital, continued to insist that he was there solely because of food poisoning.

Despite his initial resistance, however, Richard seemed to settle in to the routine at this facility. He gradually became more cooperative and even participated in the hospital's regular activities. Still, he was short-tempered and, the staff noted, he always refused lunch. He still spent a lot of time lurking quietly in the halls and staring silently at people.

One day two dead birds were found outside Richard's room. Their heads had been broken off. The housekeeper spotted Richard in the vicinity, but she could not see what he was doing. When he came back into the building, he had blood all over him.

Richard denied having anything to do with the dead birds. When asked why he was such a bloody mess, he said he had cut himself shaving. From time to time, the staff continued to find mutilated birds outside his room. No one fully investigated this behavior.

One day the nurse in charge during the swing shift found Richard's notebook. She opened it and read entries cataloging animals (rabbit, cat, bird) in terms of the taste and consistency of their blood—whether it was sweet, thick, and so forth. She recalled that she had often seen Richard sneaking around the yard . . . as if he were stalking something. She noticed that he seemed to be more active when the moon was full. Another day, an aide overheard Richard tell an orderly that he drank the blood of the birds he killed. When one of the nurses at the hospital asked Richard why he killed the birds, he answered that it was because he "didn't want to die." When it was Richard's turn to have a blood sample taken for a medical test, he struggled violently and had to be restrained and told exactly why the sample had to be taken before he would relax.

Though there were setbacks, Richard seemed to gradually improve over the weeks he was at the hospital. The antipsychotic medication and hospital treatment were producing positive results. By July, he seemed to enjoy volleyball games and other group activities. He socialized more and took part in all scheduled events. He even admitted that he had drowned the rabbits and then drunk their blood.

By mid-August, though he wanted to go home, he was also running for president of the resident council. He was still withdrawn from time to time, but the staff noted that he could sometimes function at a high level, and was better at keeping his room clean. As far as developing any insight into his mental illness, however, Richard had made no progress.

Still, he was able to go on group trips and on furloughs with his parents. In mid-September, the staff noted that no mutilated birds had been found for "some time now," and Richard had not requested any blood to drink. His general appearance improved, and though he was still essentially a loner, Richard made friends with another patient.

At the end of September, he was discharged from the mental hospital. The diagnosis was unchanged: paranoid schizophrenia, and the prognosis remained "guarded." His doctors felt that the hospital could not help him improve further but that continued medication was required. His parents, furthermore, wanted him out of the hospital, and were willing to take care of him.

At the time of his discharge his doctors felt he was not dangerous.

Once out of the hospital, his parents set him up in another apartment. They paid his bills, brought him groceries, and monitored him from time to time. His mother initially took charge of making sure he took his medications. The drugs helped Richard get by, but his mother felt they were only to make him "easy to handle" and rendered him "like a zombie all day." So she took it upon herself to wean her son from them. By January 1977, Richard was taking none of the drugs his doctors had prescribed—drugs which they assumed he would continue taking when he was discharged from the mental hospital.

Not only was Richard off his prescribed medications, but he also received no continuous follow-up care. He was not seen regularly by a psychiatrist or any other professional.

But he did make new friends. Richard had a habit of hanging out at a local bowling alley. He would stay out all night, come home at dawn, and sleep well into the afternoon. His mother described him as a "night person." On occasion he would bring home some of his friends from the bowling alley, and they would sleep over at his apartment.

With neither regular psychiatric treatment nor medication, Richard began to slip again. He frequently complained that his mother was controlling his mind and he wanted her to stop. One day he accused his mother and sister of trying to poison him with dish soap. Shortly thereafter, his mother found the milk at her house had been contaminated with dish-washing soap—apparently by her son.

Richard's preoccupation with his body developed into full-blown somatic delusions. He was convinced that his organs were moving around inside, that his heart was getting smaller because of lack of blood, that his stomach was rotting away. He felt that if he shot and killed animals and ate their viscera and drank their blood he could save himself. To this end, he often mixed the internal organs of cats and dogs in a blender—sometimes with cola—and drank it as if it were a cocktail. On a rare visit to his psychiatrist's office, Richard presented himself, head shaved, on one particularly busy day. He merely told the nurse he wanted blood—and then left before the doctor could see him.

As Richard continued to deteriorate, his apartment became dirtier and dirtier. Whenever his father would visit he would

bring groceries and, inevitably, comment about the filthy condition of the apartment. Father and son continued to argue, and
finally, Richard's father stopped coming. His mother was also
unhappy about the condition of the apartment, and by the spring
of 1977, Richard simply would not allow either of his parents
inside it. They continued to bring groceries for their son, but they
never entered his home.

When Richard had been committed to the mental hospital,
his parents had, through the court, become conservators of his
estate and his person. Because of his mental disability, he received Social Security checks, which his parents cashed for him
and used toward his rent and other expenses. In April 1977,
Richard was tiring of the arrangement and wanted to be fully
responsible for himself once again. Furthermore, he wanted to
take a trip.

Richard's psychiatrist advised against terminating the conservatorship, but, since the young man was insistent, his parents let it
expire automatically. He was now on his own. He could cash his
own checks and spend his own money—which he did. Though his
father tried to get him to stay in Sacramento and get a job, Richard's mother helped him plan his trip. In June 1977 she gave her
son $1,450, which she had saved from his Social Security benefits,
and drove him to the bus station. Richard bought a ticket for
Washington, got on a bus, and was gone.

Almost three weeks later he returned, driving a 1966 Ford
Ranchero wagon which he had bought for $800 from a man in
Steamboat Springs, Colorado. The half-car, half-pickup truck was
gray with a black stripe. In the back was a Florida license plate. In
the front, a plate stating I'D RATHER BE FLYING.

With his parents' help, he moved into a new apartment. His
father occasionally brought groceries, while his mother checked
his mail and paid his rent and bills. Though she lived nearby and
tried to visit him often, Richard would not let her into the apartment and always kept her outside as he spoke to her with the
door half open.

But the new car and the new apartment didn't add up to a
new life for Richard. He still behaved in a bizarre fashion. He
was reclusive, and seemed to come out only at night. He stayed

inside the apartment, usually sleeping, all day, and then cruised the dark streets of Sacramento until dawn.

Linda, Richard's neighbor, often was witness to his strange behavior. She often heard loud noises coming from his apartment, and frequently observed him walking around with his mouth hanging open, shuffling as he walked and dragging one foot. On occasion when Linda would greet him, he did not reply. But one evening he did enter her apartment—uninvited. When he saw that she had two male friends for company, he left immediately without saying a word.

It was around then that Richard started carrying a shotgun around the apartment complex. The other tenants reported him to the manager, who advised him to cover the weapon when he carried it around. From then on, residents observed Richard carrying "something wrapped in a blanket," which they assumed was the shotgun. One can only surmise as to why this issue was not pursued further. Were the neighbors paralyzed by fear or simply disinterested?

Then the weird episodes with animals began. A tenant reported to the manager that she saw a large black dog in Richard's apartment. Linda saw him carry a cat and two dogs into his apartment, but she never hear the animals or saw any sign of them ever again. On several occasions she observed him carrying large boxes in and out of his place.

Richard's parents noticed his strange behavior around animals, too. His mother owned a cat, a small white dog, and a German shepherd. Both dogs disappeared from his mother's home that summer, first the small one, and the large dog a few weeks later. His parents suspected that their son had kidnapped the animals, but when they confronted him, he denied it, just as he had denied his drug use. But they felt otherwise. They had seen him abuse the larger of the two dogs several times just before it disappeared. Richard would squeeze the dog's feet and make it yelp. His mother noted that he seemed to enjoy watching the dog suffer.

One evening Richard's mother heard a knock on her door. She assumed it was her son so she didn't answer it. Suddenly, there was a loud bang outside. She opened the door and saw Richard holding up her black cat by the tail. The cat was bloody and obviously dead. Before her eyes, Richard threw it on the ground and thrust his hands into its bloody body. Then he brought his bloody hands up to his head and smeared the blood all over his neck. Then he smoked a cigarette and disappeared while his mother stood frozen in horror.

A short time later he reappeared and cleaned up the porch with some papers. His mother later discovered that he had buried the cat in her front yard.

On August 3, 1977, officers of the Bureau of Indian Affairs at the Pyramid Lake Reservation in Nevada found Richard's ranch wagon stuck in the sand by the lake. The inside of the truck was smeared with blood, and they found a .22-caliber rifle and a 30-30 rifle, both bloodstained. On the floor of the truck was a white plastic bucket with a large bloody liver in it, and some blood-soaked tennis shoes. The officers searched for the owner of the truck and, about a half-mile away, came upon Richard squatting nude, covered with blood. The officers approached and asked him his name and address, which he gave them. However, when they asked him where the blood came from, he told them it "seeped from my skin."

The federal officers arrested Richard and impounded the car. The following day, lab tests revealed that the liver had come from a cow. Richard was released when the U.S. Attorney declined to prosecute. This bizarre matter ended with no further follow-up.

Richard's father went to Nevada to retrieve his son. When asked what had happened, Richard explained that he had been rabbit hunting, had gotten blood on his body, and was about to wash the blood off in the lake when he was arrested. His father had known about the rifles (he thought the .22 was O.K. but felt Richard wasted his money buying a larger-caliber rifle without any real need for it) but he was not concerned that his son would represent any danger. He did let Richard know that he was upset with him, and that he thought it was a stupid thing to be arrested with a car that wasn't properly licensed.

For his part, Richard was angry because he had paid a towing charge and still couldn't get his truck back from the authorities. Nevada authorities wouldn't release the truck because Richard didn't have a registration—the vehicle still had a Florida plate. They were able to get a notarized receipt from the original owner in Colorado, but they still needed Florida documentation. Richard eventually got the proper papers and got his ranch wagon back. He was never able to retrieve the guns.

Richard's mother was fully aware that her son went on "campaigns," killing and eating animals. Often, she found straw mixed with blood in the bed of his truck. By this time, his entire family was aware of his delusion about requiring blood to survive. Meanwhile, more of his neighbors at the apartment complex noticed his strange behavior. He seldom returned greetings and was frequently seen wandering aimlessly around the grounds. Several more residents noticed him carrying various animals into his apartment—animals that were never seen again.

During the fall of 1977, Richard purchased and stole several dogs. He bought two from the S.P.C.A. for $15.90, one on October 1, and another on October 10. He also prowled around the neighborhood picking up strays and untended pets. One woman who happened to have a Saint Bernard had just left her driveway when she saw Richard drive up to her house. She drove back, approached him, and asked him what he wanted. He just stared at her, then left without saying a word. A week later she spotted a prowler on her property, whose identity was never verified.

Later in October, Richard went shopping for a black Labrador puppy and got two for the price of one by telling the owner he wanted to breed "all sorts of dogs." However, he then selected two pups without paying any attention to their sex.

In mid-November, Richard telephoned to torment a family whose dog he had apparently stolen. About ten days after the dog disappeared, the family put an ad in the newspaper. Richard called, spoke to the daughter, and gave a detailed description of the missing dog. The child became frightened and gave the phone to her father, telling him the caller sounded drunk or high, but Richard hung up.

Richard's mother owned a duplex with an empty lot next door. On several occasions, neighbors saw Richard in the lot at odd hours. Sometimes he would just stand and stare, but there were times when he was considerably more busy. One neighbor saw him digging there and assumed he was planting a garden. But nothing ever seemed to grow on the empty lot.

On December 2, Richard paid $69.99 cash, for a .22-caliber semiautomatic pistol. In answer to the question "Is purchaser a mental patient or on leave of absence from any mental hospital or has he ever been adjudicated by a court to be a danger to others as a result of a mental disorder or mental illness?" Richard answered, "No." He could not pick up the gun until December 18, however, as the law required a waiting period during which the purchaser's credentials were supposed to be verified.

On December 15, Richard bought the Sacramento *Union* with a front page article on the "Hillside Strangler." He saved the section of the newspaper with the article. Around that time, his father took him out to buy a Christmas present. Their first stop, however, was a barber shop where Richard got a haircut and had his beard trimmed. They went to a store where he picked out an orange ski jacket that his father bought for him. Richard was anxious to return to his apartment, so the father-son outing came to an end.

A few days later Richard went to the sporting goods store and picked up his pistol. Apparently, his psychiatric history had not been discovered. He also bought a box of bullets.

As Christmas drew near, Richard seemed preoccupied with the desire to spend the holiday at his mother's home. To this end, he cleaned himself up, and called his mother frequently to plead with her to invite him over for Christmas dinner. His mother, however, refused. Shortly before Christmas, Richard tried to force his way into his mother's home, but failed.

On December 22, Richard bought the Sacramento *Bee,* and kept the pages about singles' bars and articles about how people at those bars pick up dates. He also kept the want ads and circled the ads for free dogs.

And Richard practiced with the gun. Between December 18 and 26 he fired the gun at least fifty times, using up an entire box of ammunition. Things were taking a serious turn.

On Christmas Eve, Richard's father paid him a visit to give him some presents. But Richard seemed distant and unconcerned about the holiday. He appeared preoccupied, and refused to tell his father what his plans were.

The day after Christmas, Richard bought another box of bullets. On the evening of the twenty-seventh, he went cruising in his ranch wagon, fired from the street, and hit the windowless wall of a house. Later that evening, at around six-thirty, he fired into the kitchen window of another house. He could see people in the window as he fired, and one bullet did rip through the hair of a woman in the room, narrowly missing her head.

On December 29 Richard again went cruising with his gun stuffed under his orange jacket. Around 8:30 P.M., as he rode down a nearby street, he noticed a man walking across his yard, carrying groceries in from his car, which was parked in the driveway. Richard slowed down the car and pulled over. Without warning he fired two shots at the man. One shot missed and hit a tree. The other struck Ambrose Griffin in the chest. Then Richard sped away. Inside the Griffin home, family members thought they had heard a car backfire. Mr. Griffin's wife and daughter ran outside and found Mr. Griffin on the ground. Initially, they thought he had suffered a heart attack—until they saw the bullet wound in his chest. Mr. Griffin was taken to American River Hospital, where he died a short time later.

Police were baffled by the apparently random, motiveless shooting.

On January 5, Richard bought the Sacramento *Bee* with an editorial on the killing—which he kept. He bought the paper again the next day, this time saving a section with an article about a knifing murder.

On January 10 he bought three more boxes of bullets, most of which he used up practicing . . . or otherwise.

On January 11, when Linda was moving out, Richard cornered the young woman by the mailboxes and, the blank look on his face totally unmoving, demanded a cigarette. She gave him one and started walking away but he grabbed her shoulder and demanded more. So she gave him the whole pack and he let her go.

Around this time the manager again received a report that a large black dog was seen in Richard's apartment. When the manager checked it out he found no sign of a dog.

During the week of January 16, one of Richard's windows was broken from the inside. He denied responsibility but offered to pay for it if the landlord insisted. Also that week, he set two fires in nearby apartments because he felt the people there were persecuting him.

For most of the month of January, Richard's mother and father observed no particularly bizarre behavior on the part of their son. On January 21, he even went hiking and rock-hunting with his father. He seemed to enjoy himself and was in good spirits. On January 22, he visited his mother's house. His grandmother was there. Seeming in good spirits, he got $10 from her and asked her how her dog was.

Although aware of his bizarre concerns, his family apparently had no inkling that Richard was leading a secret life. Having killed once already, he was prepared to do it again. This time he would go further toward fulfilling his grisly desired.

On the morning of January 23, Richard again went out hunting for a victim. At ten-fifteen he walked into a back yard not too far from his apartment. The house he was approaching was one of two on the street with no cars in the driveway. But unbeknown to Richard, someone was home at this house. The lady of the house saw him try to force a door open, fail, and then walk toward some windows. At the kitchen window he came face to face with her, said, "Excuse me," and then proceeded to sit down on her patio. She called the police, but he got up and walked away before they arrived. There was no immediate follow-up.

Less than a half-hour later, at 10:40 A.M., Richard was caught in the act of burglarizing a house just a few doors down—the only other house on the street with no car in the driveway. The owner came home and surprised Richard, who escaped through a window, and chased after him until Richard hopped over a fence. When the man yelled for him to stop, Richard yelled back, "I'm only taking a short-cut." The man got in his car and drove around; at one point he saw the intruder in the vicinity of his apartment, but was unable to catch him.

Richard had escaped with $16 in cash. He had collected binoculars, a tape player, a dagger, and a stethoscope in a brown bag. Strangely he had not attempted to take watches, rings, or prescription drugs from the house. But he had urinated on an open drawer of clothes and defecated on a child's bed.

At around 11 A.M., Richard's father showed up at the apartment. Richard had asked him for some money to help him get through to the end of the month. His father agreed to provide it and had come over to drop it off. Richard did not act too strangely when he saw his father, just a bit nervous. He did not seem to want to talk, so his father left.

Richard had hardly begun. About eleven forty-five, he went to a nearby supermarket, taking with him his loaded gun and rubber gloves. He wore his orange jacket to better conceal the weapon and maintain his anonymity. He knew he couldn't wear the blue jacket, since he had been spotted wearing it at the scene of the burglary earlier that morning.

At the supermarket, Richard ran into a woman he had known several years earlier. To her he looked unkempt: his hands were dirty and there was a yellow crust around his lips. She didn't recognize him at first, and said, "Who are you?" when he approached her.

"Were you on the motorcycle when Kurt was killed?" Richard asked her. She was startled by this question about her boyfriend, who had been killed in a motorcycle accident almost ten years before. Thinking he looked strange and that he was probably on drugs, she made small talk for a minute and then walked away. But Richard kept after her. She got in line and Richard grabbed an orange drink and got in right behind her. She then paid for her groceries and walked out to the parking lot, with him in pursuit.

"Hey, wait!" he called. But she kept going. As she drove away, he grabbed at the door handles of her car. The failure of this encounter stoked his rage and sealed the fate of his next victim.

The young woman having escaped, Richard turned his attention to the houses across the small park just beyond the supermarket parking lot. A husband and wife who lived in one of the houses saw him walk across their porch. He was headed for a house two doors down, where he'd seen a young woman walking across her lawn. He entered through the front door, cocked his gun, and fired a bullet into the mailbox. Then he encountered twenty-two-year-old Theresa Wallin as she came through the front room carrying out a trash bag.

Theresa Wallin, who was three months pregnant, tried to

defend herself against the first two shots, by blocking them with her right arm. But the first bullet went through her hand and into the left side of her scalp. The second shot went through her right forearm, struck her left temple, and lodged in her neck. She fell, and Chase fired one more shot to the right side of her head. But the violation of Theresa Wallin wasn't over yet.

Richard dragged the dying woman into the master bedroom. He pushed her sweater and bra up out of the way, exposing her breasts, and then pulled down her pants, exposing her pubic region. Then he got a carving knife from the kitchen and went to work.

While she was still alive, but most likely unconscious, Richard cut her open from chest to umbilicus, then pulled out her spleen and loop after loop of her intestines, which he dropped to the floor. He stabbed her liver, cut her diaphragm, severed one lung, sliced her pancreas in two, cut out both kidneys and put them on the bed, and then stabbed her in the heart. Then he stabbed her through her left nipple and thrust the knife repeatedly through the same opening. He smeared her blood all over his face and hands and licked it off his rubber-gloved fingers. As he tasted her blood, he pulled her left leg out of her pants, spread her legs, and made blood smears all over her inner thighs. He dipped a yogurt container into her blood and drank it, then crumpled the cup and left it next to her body. Finally, he defecated and stuffed feces in her mouth.

Then he went to the kitchen, washed off the knife, and returned it to the rack, hiding it under a casserole dish. He left a small spot of blood on the edge of the knife handle, and a tiny, barely noticeable splatter of blood on one of the freshly washed dishes near the sink. Next, he went to the bathroom where he removed the bloody rubber gloves and washed the blood off his hands and face—but left smears of blood all over the sink.

Richard left by the back door, went through the yard and out the back gate, avoiding detection.

The next day, January 24, Richard was in a different neighborhood, looking for new victims. He bought the Sacramento *Bee,* with a long article about the killing on the first page. Theresa Wallin had been found by her husband. Richard kept the entire paper. That day he also canvassed the neighborhood, going from door to door asking for old magazines, newspapers, and books. He also called his mother's house and spoke to his grandmother, telling her he wanted to ask his mother about going on a picnic.

On January 25, Richard went back to a home at which, two months earlier, he had bought two black Labrador puppies. This time he didn't bother to buy a puppy, he just took a four-month-old, shot it in the head, and split open its stomach. He removed the dog's kidneys and drank the blood.

That night, around 11:30 P.M., Richard phoned his mother again and said he just wanted to talk. He said he was lying in bed watching TV, that nothing was wrong, and that he had been panning for gold and swimming that day with his girlfriend's dog. His mother told him he was acting silly, he couldn't have gone swimming, it was too cold. To his mother, Richard seemed in good spirits. They made small talk and then hung up.

The next day he went asking for magazines and old papers again. He bought the *Bee,* with an article about a robbery-shooting, plus another article on the Wallin killing.

On the morning of the twenty-seventh Richard went after human blood again. Not too long after 10 A.M., he parked his car at a shopping center next to a large concrete planter, partially blocking a traffic lane. He walked three doors down from where he parked, and entered the home of twenty-seven-year-old Evelyn Miroth. There in the hallway he encountered Evelyn and immediately pulled his pistol and shot her in the head.

But there were other people in the house. Evelyn's boyfriend, fifty-two-year-old Daniel Meredith, and her six-year-old son Jason heard the shooting and rose from their seats in the living room. Richard was ready for them. First he shot at Jason, and hit the child in the back of the neck. Jason fell and Richard shot him in the head, execution-style, to kill him. Then he fired at Meredith as the man came toward him. The bullet crashed through Meredith's head and brain and didn't stop until it hit the wall of the entryway. As he fell, Meredith stepped in Jason's blood. Then, as his victim lay dying, Richard shot him at close range in the head. This second bullet also went completely through Meredith's head and came to rest in a blood-soaked spot on the carpet. Richard then rolled the body over and removed Meredith's wallet and car keys.

Then Richard went to work on Evelyn. He dragged her into the bedroom, where he found a fourth person in the house: twenty-two-month-old David Ferreira, Evelyn's nephew, was sleeping in his playpen. Richard shot the infant in the head at close range. Then he dragged the body of six-year-old Jason into the bedroom.

Now he could focus his attention on Evelyn. He stripped off her clothes, then his own, put on his rubber gloves, and found two carving knives and a green plastic pail. Standing over her barefoot and naked, he cut her open with two slices across her abdomen. As she lay dying, he proceeded to mutilate her body in much the same way he had mutilated Theresa Wallin. Her intestines were not touched by the knife as he went about his work. He made superficial slices on her neck, almost as if he were trying to make up his mind whether to continue cutting. He partially cut one of her eyes out of its socket and left it protruding. He sodomized her, then stabbed at her rectum over and over again with the knife. Then he drained her blood into the pail.

Richard found a coffee cup and used it to drink Evelyn's blood out of the pail. Next, he turned his attention to the baby's body. Leaving bloody footprints all over the house, he carried the body to the bathroom and ran some water in the tub. Then he used a knife to open a hole in the infant's skull, spilling pieces of brain into the bloody water. As he worked on the baby's body, he contemplated what he was going to do with that of Meredith.

But then Richard was interrupted. There was someone at the front door. The neighbor had sent her six-year-old daughter to the Miroth home to play with Jason. The little girl waited for some response. . . . But none came, so she went home. Her mother called the house, but there was no answer.

Meanwhile, Richard slipped out of the house. He left behind his bloody socks and the bodies of Evelyn, Daniel, and Jason. He took the infant David's body with him.

Stealing Meredith's red Ford station wagon, he drove home and parked it in the lot of an apartment building next to his. Somehow, he managed to carry the infant's body into his apartment without being seen. Leaving the baby's body there, Richard then went back to retrieve his ranch wagon.

Once back at his apartment, he was now able to focus on the

body of David Ferreira. Starting at the back of the skull, he severed the child's head completely from the body. He attacked the chest and abdomen, breaking several ribs, opening the body and removing organs and blood. He also stabbed at the child's rectum and opened the head in several places. Richard drank the child's blood and removed and ate parts of the brain.

At 2:20 P.M. police officers discovered the massacre at the Miroth home. Meredith was found in the living room, face down, jacket pulled up, rear pocket exposed, car keys and wallet gone.

Evelyn Miroth's nude body was found on the bed in the front bedroom. Her abdomen had two distinct cuts, through which her internal organs protruded. The right eye was extended from its socket. On the floor near the body was a circular stain, caused by the bloody pail.

Jason's body was found, fully clothed, in the same bedroom.

In the playpen where David normally slept the police found a bloody pillow and a .22-caliber slug. In the bathtub they found bloody water, feces, and brain matter.

Unable to find the infant David, the police acted on the possibility that he was still alive, so they launched a massive man-hunt to find the kidnapper and the child. (They eventually deduced from the amount of the infant's blood at the scene that he could not have survived.)

On January 28, the next day, as Richard was reading the Sacramento *Bee,* whose lead article focused on the murders, the police were canvassing his neighborhood. A city-wide dragnet was launched to find the missing Ferreira baby. At 5 P.M., an officer knocked on Richard's door and got no response. The detective left.

An hour later, following up on a lead given to them by a neighbor who thought she heard a baby crying, three detectives were back at Richard's door. Once again, they got no response, even after identifying themselves. But they heard movement inside the apartment, so they didn't leave. While one of the detectives went to the manager's apartment to telephone Richard, the other two stayed behind, positioning themselves several feet apart, with the front door between them.

The door opened, and Richard stepped out, wearing the orange ski jacket and carrying a cardboard box. He saw one of the detectives, started to back into his door, but then turned and ran in the other direction. The detective stepped in his path and ordered him to stop. Richard threw the cardboard box at him, and bloody papers, rags, a green plastic bucket, a diaper pin from David Ferreira's diaper and pieces of the baby's brain spilled out. The detectives charged and were able to subdue and handcuff the suspect after a brief scuffle. They removed the automatic pistol from a shoulder holster underneath Richard's orange ski parka. The pistol was fully loaded, with the safety off. Then they found a pair of bloody rubber gloves and a box of .22-caliber bullets in Richard's pockets.

Detectives then entered the apartment to look for the missing infant. They were greeted by an overwhelming odor of putrefaction. And almost everything in the apartment—floor, walls, bed, clothing, bathtub, furniture—had bloodstains on it. They found fecal matter on the bedroom floor. Chase's bloodstained clothing was in disarray all over the bedroom, and boxes and other containers found in the kitchen and bathroom were all spattered with blood. There were bones in the bedroom and bathroom, too. Not finding the baby, the detectives returned to the police station with Richard, and got a search warrant to allow a more comprehensive investigation of the apartment.

"Let me go," he insisted as they took him away. "I've done nothing." He reached for his pocket three times and after the detectives put him in their patrol car, they took a wallet out of the pocket. It was Daniel Meredith's and contained his driver's license and credit cards.

As the detectives drove off with Richard, he remarked, "My apartment's a lot cleaner, isn't it? I didn't do anything in my apartment except kill a few dogs."

Later that evening, with a properly executed search warrant, the detectives re-entered Richard's apartment and found out for themselves just how clean it was. The pungent odor of decaying tissue remained. On the wall, they noted two pictures of internal human organs. They counted bullet holes in the living room ceiling.

In the bedroom, on the bed, they found bloodstained men's

clothing and a dinner plate with a piece of brain tissue swimming in fresh blood. Also on the bed were more pieces of the infant David's brain. On the floor were loose .22-caliber bullets, a bloodstained machete, and fecal material.

In the kitchen they found that the refrigerator shelves were arranged so that something large could fit. In the freezer they found a half-gallon container with organs—human or animal—in it. There was a large bloodstain on the kitchen floor and a blood-stained hatchet in a kitchen drawer. In the bathroom they found an amber cup caked with blood.

The detectives went through Richard's reading material and found books on totalitarianism, a book entitled *Psychic People,* gun magazines, psychology magazines, newspaper articles about violent deaths and Old West outlaws, and, finally, Richard's high school yearbooks.

At the police station, Richard was interrogated repeatedly that night and the following morning. Although he admitted that he had killed animals, eaten their viscera, and drunk their blood, he denied any knowledge of the murders, even when confronted with the incriminating evidence gathered so far by the detectives, including the contents of the very box that Richard threw at them as he tried to get away. He maintained that the blood and other material were the result of his having killed dogs, not people. He said he had found David Meredith's wallet in a parking lot.

Richard repeatedly denied any involvement in the crimes. "My parents didn't bring me up that way. I wouldn't do anything like that." His responses were bizarre and erratic.

He said he thought he was being framed, and that the officers had "the wrong guy." He said, "It wasn't me . . . No shit, I didn't do it," and "I honestly don't know anything about it. It must have been somebody else."

Richard said he saw a "blond guy" who "had on an orange coat" in the vicinity of the murders. Then he told the police, "Somebody's been coming in and out of my apartment."

The officers tried to get him to tell them where David Ferreira's body was, but he denied knowing anything about the child. Subsequent questioning provided few real answers amid a confused series of contradictory remarks and evasive comments.

When asked why he tried to flee from the officers, he said he "did not know who it was" at the door and thought it was the manager beating on his door to complain about the dogs.

When asked about his possession of Daniel Meredith's wallet, he said, "I didn't have that on me. You sure you got it out of my pocket?" A little later he said, "I bought it at a five-and-dime two or three months ago."

Richard now readily admitted killing dogs. He explained the bloodstains on his clothing by saying, "It's just animal blood, just blood from dogs. I just killed a dog, that's all." He said he killed one because the animal was sick and he could not take care of it, another because "it was a mean dog." At first, he denied "cutting up" the dogs, but later recanted and said he "used a machete on it." Richard said that the meat in his freezer was all dog meat, and that he had eaten dog meat.

The detectives asked him if he liked to eat organs, like liver, heart, and kidneys. Richard replied, "Well, yeah, I've eaten it."

Then the detectives accused him of eating his human victims. Chase replied, "You're crazy. . . . I haven't. I'm not mixed up in anything like that."

"You've been eating animals and people," they accused him.

"I have not," he replied.

"What would you do if you found a dead child?" they asked.

"Turn it right in . . . call the police."

"You wouldn't flush it down the toilet?"

"No way," Richard answered.

When the detectives asked him what he thought people would do with a kidnapped baby, Richard said, "Sell it."

"To whom?"

"Down the street, I guess."

The detectives asked him if he would eat a child he had kidnapped.

"No," he stammered, "I don't, I didn't never want to. Why would I?"

"Do you think it would be wrong if you ate people?"

"The Nazis ate a lot."

The detectives were silent for a moment.

"I didn't eat anybody," Richard continued. Then he denied "having a liking for blood."

The next morning, January 29, two psychiatrists were brought in by the district attorney's office. Richard, having been advised of his rights, at first refused to speak to them, but later agreed to the interviews. When he talked about his crimes, he betrayed no emotion, remorse, or feelings of guilt or sadness. Instead, he described the crimes in a concrete, detached manner.

In jail, Richard behaved much as he had in the mental hospital. He kept to himself, was suspicious and paranoid about his food, slept with the covers over his head, and had to be continually instructed to flush his toilet after using it. On one occasion, he spit at a prison officer and yelled, "You guys have been poisoning me! I want out of this jail, now!" Chase later confided to this same officer that he preferred kidney meat and would often mix kidneys with lung meat and cola in a blender.

Richard told parts of his grisly story to another inmate: "I had to do it. I have blood poisoning and I need blood. I thought about it for several weeks and decided I was tired of hunting and killing animals so I could drink their blood. I decided I would kill humans for their blood. . . . On the first one I was walking down a street near some houses. I was close to a store. I saw a lady out in front of one of the houses. I walked by and watched her. She went into the house. I followed her. The door was left unlocked. I pulled my gun and went in. As soon as I was inside I saw the lady. I shot her in the head. She fell to the floor. I took my knife and started to stab and cut her. I then drank some of her blood."

Then describing the killings at the Miroth home: "I was walking around just like before. I saw a lady in the house. I walked up to the house. The front door was unlocked. I took my gun out and opened the door. I walked in. I came across the lady. She started to scream. I shot her in the head. She fell down. A man came running from another room. He saw me and tried to run away. I shot him in the back of the head. I looked around and saw a boy, just standing there looking. This all happened so fast I just shot him too. I then heard a baby crying. I went to it. It was screaming and crying. I shot the baby because it was making too much noise. . . . I then carried the baby out with me. I took it home where I drank some of its blood. . . ."

The infant's remains were not discovered until two months later, on March 24. It was decomposed and partially mummified. Richard had disposed of the child's body by putting it in a cardboard box, with its clothes and the keys to Meredith's car, and dumping it over a fence in a vacant area between a church and a market.

During interviews with the assistant district attorney, Richard revealed many unknown facts about the depths of his madness. For example, when asked about the murder of Ambrose Griffin, he said that he believed that Germans lived in the Griffin house and that "threats were coming from that house."

Richard admitted that he bought "25 dogs." "I would read about the dogs in the paper. I would pick up the dogs and take them to my apartment. I hung a couple of dogs. I bought my gun and then I started shooting them."

When asked how he felt as he approached Theresa Wallin's house, Richard said, "Like I was starved." He then went on to describe what he did after he shot her: "I pulled her into the bedroom to get her out of sight. I got some blood out and drank it. I used a glass. I cut her organs open, moved her entrails to one side and I drank the blood with a glass."

About the Ferreira baby, Richard said, "After I got to my apartment I took the little boy out of the clothes hamper and sucked some blood out of him. It was dead. The police started knocking on my door and I got scared."

When asked where he put the baby's body, Richard maintained that he stashed it in a "silver garbage can with a lid on it."

Richard justified the killings by saying, "The whole neighborhood was a bunch of drug addicts and Nazis. Everybody who lived around there for a square mile, for ten square miles, knew what was going on."

Richard admitted that he also ate the dogs' brains, and that in addition to rabbits, dogs, cats, and birds, he also killed two cows.

Because everything in Richard's apartment was splattered with blood, the district attorney's office removed as evidence just about every article of furniture, clothing, carpeting, and personal belongings, including the occupant's notebook. There was no pattern to the entries. Few had any discernible relationship at all to the previous pages. On one page, he had written a famous quote from Edgar Allan Poe's "The Raven": "Quoth the raven, nevermore." And in German: *"Anführen die Rabe nie mehr."* Also, Richard compiled lists of words with their German counterparts, words such as "brain, eye, latent tendency, sex, God."

He also wrote: "I will end the world by flooding if I get killed. *Gott"*

On one page he made a crude drawing of the internal organs of the human body, with the major blood vessels. On another he compiled a list of people who were conspiring against him. On the list were such names as Hugh Hefner, Frank Sinatra, Raymond Burr, and Bill Cosby.

On another page he wrote "dracula . . . Sadist . . . Seethe."

When asked about his paranoid delusions, Richard replied, "There seems to be enough evidence that proves that I don't think I'm suffering from any delusions of persecution, but that I am really persecuted."

Throughout his questioning Richard insisted that his mother had poisoned him, and that caused his physical and mental problems. "I know it [that she poisoned me] because I can prove it by all the feelings, you know, the lack of circulation in my body."

When asked how he knew about his mother's plan against him, Richard said he heard the messages on the telephone:

Assistant District Attorney: Richard, you've been hearing voices, haven't you, in the past? You know, hearing things in your head, is that true?

CHASE: No.
A.D.A.: You never heard voices?
CHASE: What kind of voices?
A.D.A.: Messages. They can give you messages.
CHASE: On the telephone? I got messages on the telephone.
A.D.A.: How would you get them?
CHASE: I don't know . . . Somebody rang my phone and

told me some stuff. . . . That my mom's been poisoning me and I was going to die.

Richard's mother, when interviewed by the assistant district attorney, blamed her ex-husband for planting such accusations in her son's mind. She believed Richard's father had done so in retaliation for her having accused him of poisoning her years earlier.

Chase was also asked about his father's treatment of him as a child:

CHASE: He was easy to get along with and he never really punched me around, I guess, just tortured me, you know.

A.D.A.: How would he torture you?

CHASE: By watching me, you know. He didn't care if I was getting poisoned or not.

A.D.A.: He made you eat everything on your plate? Did that go on?

CHASE: Yeah, and half of it was liquid detergents and stuff.

When Richard's father was interviewed by the A.D.A. he broke down and said he felt responsible, that "If I had handled that better, it would have been different. . . ."

In June 1978, Richard's paranoia about his food persisted. He told the A.D.A. that he found "volatile acid" and "venereal disease" in his food, as a result of a conspiracy against him by the prison officials. Convinced that his body was deteriorating further, he insisted on an angiogram and further extensive physical examinations to ascertain and document his body's declining condition.

In prison, Richard told the assistant district attorney that "they couldn't give me capital punishment because of psychiatric problems."

During the interviews Richard's appearance was always filthy and sloppy. He would frequently blow his nose or spit on his shirt, or onto a piece of paper which he would then put in his pants pocket. He appeared to be always physically ill, walking or sitting with stooped shoulders. He seemed to not be able to walk in a straight line, but would wander unsteadily from place to place. He showed no emotion whatever in his voice, and spoke in a soft monotone. He expressed a belief that he was of Jewish ancestry, although this was not true and it became part of a larger paranoid delusion. Richard was convinced that most people he encountered were either Germans or members of the Mafia, and were persecuting him because of his religion.

The district attorney's contention was that the killings were the result of Richard Chase's sexual sadism, not his global mental disorder. Psychiatrists and psychologists who examined him were not in agreement as to his sanity at the time of the killings. Some theorized that he committed the crimes directly as a result of his mental disorder and was insane. Others, including the psychiatrists brought in by the prosecution, concluded that despite his disorder, he was sane under California law.

Because of this conflicting psychiatric testimony, the district attorney set about to demonstrate that Richard Chase built up to the killings and that the initial murder of Ambrose Griffin was not undertaken to obtain blood for sustenance but rather as a means of developing the nerve to kill the rest of his victims. However, the poor condition of the various bullets made it difficult to connect all three events. In the first place, the bullet that killed Griffin could not be matched with those fired at Chase's apartment. The bullets recovered at the Wallin and Miroth scenes were also too damaged to be matched to Richard's gun.

Fortunately, the investigators found a way to match all the bullets and conclusively demonstrate that Richard Chase's gun was used not only in the Wallin and Miroth killings, but also in the murder of Griffin. The key was a bullet that Chase had fired wildly at a house on December 27. The occupants of the house heard the shots but thought it was a car backfiring. Several days later, the owner went into his basement and saw that the paneling was warped in a strange way. He found the bullet and brought it to the police. The police were then able to match this bullet to those fired in Richard's apartment and to the bullet that killed

Griffin and the other victims. This evidence undoubtedly played a pivotal role in the ultimate jury verdict.

The grisly murders and the resultant media attention created such a furor in Sacramento that a change of venue was sought by the defense, and the trial was transferred to San Jose. The standard justification for such a move is based on the belief that if broad publicity and emotion accompany a crime it can be impossible to find an unbiased jury panel from the county of origin to hear the case. So the original prosecution and defense teams continue with the proceedings while a jury is chosen from the rolls of the receiving county. The assumption is that the distance from the immediate area of the crime will eliminate emotion from the deliberations and eventual verdict.

However, in this era of instant mass communication, the Richard Chase case was publicized throughout the entire country, not only the rest of the state. So the same knowledge of the case —and, perhaps, the same emotional impact—that was available to residents of Sacramento had made its way to California's other twenty-two million citizens.

The crucial issue was whether or not Richard Chase could be convicted of six counts of murder in the first degree. The heinousness of the killings called for a forceful response by society, and the prosecutor didn't want the "Vampire of Sacramento" to get away with these crimes on psychiatric grounds.

Ronald Tochterman, the Assistant District Attorney in charge of the case (and now a superior court judge) was a thorough, well-trained, meticulous prosecutor, who prepared himself for any conceivable roadblock the defense could create. However, his task was a formidable one. It was his burden to prove beyond a reasonable doubt all elements of the crimes, namely premeditation, deliberation, and malice aforethought. In addition, to overcome an insanity defense it was necessary to demonstrate that Chase lacked substantial ability to appreciate the wrongfulness of his acts and to conform his conduct to the requirement of law.

I was called in as a consultant to help the prosecution prepare for the issues that might arise in a psychiatric defense. I informed

Tochterman that in reviewing the case, it was clear that Richard Chase was suffering from a major, chronic psychiatric disorder of psychotic proportions, and that a persuasive case for an insanity defense existed. Some members of the prosecution team and some expert witnesses felt that Chase was malingering or exaggerating his psychiatric condition. To the contrary, the medical data depicted a highly disturbed individual, consumed by his delusions. Though acting intentionally, Chase was unable to control his passion for fresh tissue and blood. My conclusions differed from those of other prosecution-retained experts.*

It was my opinion that, with such an analysis, under California law as it then existed, a prosecutor would be hard-pressed to sustain anything greater than a manslaughter conviction. At the time, the broad definition of malice included "an ability to control and conform one's conduct to the requirement of law." I felt it would be nearly impossible to successfully argue that Richard Chase, consumed by his serious mental disorder and his insatiable, unnatural need for human blood, had this ability.

Tochterman felt otherwise, and went about presenting his view to the jury. He argued that Chase acted in a deliberate, premeditated way that was not "wild," haphazard, or out of control. As examples of premeditation, Tochterman pointed out that Chase practiced with his gun, that he cut the women's bodies in straight lines, and that the mutilations were sadistic and sexually deliberate. In addition, he noted to the jury, Chase apparently went trolling for victims. He went to the homes with a loaded gun and rubber gloves; he tried to get away and avoid detection; he deliberately, and with precision, killed his victims.

The prosecutor also postulated that there was a progression to Chase's behavior. First, he bought the gun, then he practiced.

* This predicament raises an important issue in the use of experts. If a psychiatrist—or any other expert, for that matter—is engaged by one side in any lawsuit, how compelled is he to render an opinion that supports the position of that side? Is he an adversarial consultant or must he retain his objectivity? On ethical considerations alone, the answer is clear. An impartial evaluation and opinion is called for, regardless of who pays the fee. However, in the real world of law, economic considerations rear their head. How often would an expert be rehired if his opinion did not support or reflect the goals of the side that retained him? Attorneys are not interested in objectivity, they are interested in prevailing, in winning. They are looking for expert testimony to bolster their legal arguments and are not desirous of paying fees for unknown opinions. As a result, many experts acquire reputations as prosecution- or defense-oriented psychiatrists. Indeed, I have overheard certain colleagues state that they will only assist either the defense or the prosecution regardless of the case at hand. This has led to the use of words such as "prostitute" and "whore" to mean "medical expert."

Next he shot someone from a distance. Finally, he was able to kill face-to-face. Therefore, Tochterman argued, the defendant exhibited behavior and thought processes that were intentional, premeditated, and deliberate.

All of this was, indeed, evidence of premeditation. But insanity does not preclude premeditation. Overlooked in the prosecution's case were the numerous descriptions of Richard Chase's state of mind, most of which indicated that he was easily one of the craziest people ever handled by the criminal justice system.

Surely, Chase did progress from one level to another. But that, again, does not mean he wasn't insane. His madness was progressing, too. He began by preying on animals. First, small animals like rabbits and birds, then bigger animals—dogs and cows. Then human beings. All to obtain what he considered life-sustaining blood.

Chase's crimes were despicable. The fact that he was insane does not detract from that.

Nor did it blunt the jury's response. The prosecution prevailed: Richard Chase was convicted of first-degree murder. In the sanity phase of his trial, both of the court-appointed psychiatrists found him sane and he was declared sane at the time of the murders. Finally, at the penalty phase of his trial, Richard was sentenced to death.

Chase was sent to death row at San Quentin State Prison. He had some difficulties with his medication, so he was temporarily sent to Vacaville State Hospital, but was eventually returned to death row. While in prison, he repeatedly asked for fresh blood, human or otherwise, to drink for sustenance. Naturally, these requests were denied. As might be expected, Richard had no friends on death row.

Meanwhile, his case was automatically appealed, as all death-sentence cases are.

There are three theories that attempt to explain what happened next. The first is that Chase became more and more depressed because he could not obtain fresh blood to drink. Certainly, Chase did appear to grow more and more depressed the longer he remained on death row.

The second theory is that Chase simply became more and more despondent as Christmas Eve approached. It had become a significant date for him because of his mother's refusal to allow him to spend the previous holiday in her home.

The third theory is that Chase wasn't really depressed at all, and that he merely wanted to cure himself but felt that his illness was so severe that he needed a super-large dose of his medication to get well. So when he was given his daily medications, he surreptitiously hid them, saving them up.

Whichever theory is correct, on Christmas Eve 1979, Richard Chase mystified his doctors one final time. The Vampire of Sacramento, who in all of his psychiatric interviews had never betrayed any suicidal thinking, died of an overdose of his medication.

The crimes committed by Richard Chase reflect the depths to which human beings can sink in thought and behavior. The horrendous brutality suggests that he was motivated by subhuman forces. Is psychosis a prerequisite for such actions? No. Brutality is not the exclusive domain of the psychotic. Most psychotics are not dangerous, and most dangerous people are not psychotic.

Richard Chase was both psychotic and dangerous and, more important, the evidence was there for a long time. His bed-wetting, animal cruelty, and fire-setting were the earliest signs of future danger. Adding his blatantly psychotic thinking and behavior, the scenario for the disaster-to-come was long in place. Why, then, weren't our institutions able to prevent Richard Chase's crimes? Why didn't his family respond to the clues with which he littered their lives? Were they acting protectively, or blindly? Were his teachers and peers indifferent to his behavior? Were psychiatrists and other examining professionals careless or inattentive to his constant manifestations of madness? Did they underreact, or assume that his condition was limited in scope? Did the police and courts fail in their vigilance? And what about other relatives, friends, and neighbors who witnessed his peculiar behavior?

One way of looking at it is that Richard Chase cried out for control most of his life. Unfortunately, our institutions are geared to act only in an emergency, after a catastrophe has occurred.

Prevention is not our strong suit, especially when it competes with civil rights and concepts of fairness. Richard Chase was certainly treated fairly from start to finish. But can we say the same for his victims?

CHAPTER 7

HEARTS
UNBLAMABLE:
WHY ROMAN
POLANSKI
MAY NEVER COME
BACK
—AND THE
MANSON FAMILY WILL

The ironies of the criminal justice system, and life, sometimes create incredibly bizarre situations. The saga of Roman Polanski and the Manson Family is such a case. I was drawn into the irony because I not only examined some members of the "Family" that murdered Polanski's pregnant wife, Sharon Tate, and at least six other people, but years later I also examined Polanski himself when he was charged with a sex crime.

Not only did my testimony almost set one of the Manson Family free and come close to sharply reducing the charges against another, but the inevitable clumsiness of the system eventually saved all of them, including Charles Manson, from death row. Now, it looks as though at least two of them may be released on parole. Meanwhile, though his crime was minor when compared to the Manson murders, Polanski may never be able to legally return to this country without facing a prison sentence. Though I know he would like to return, I also know the dark memories and terrible fears that keep him away.

Roman Polanski was born in Paris in 1933. He was his parents' only child, although his mother had a daughter from a previous marriage. His parents were Polish immigrants who had met in Paris. The family's worsening financial situation forced them to leave Paris and return to Poland on the eve of World War II. At the end of the summer, in 1939, Roman started school in Cracow —one week before the invasion of Poland by German troops.

The Polanski family fled to Warsaw, believing the city would remain safe from the advancing army. Unfortunately, their confidence in the ability of the Polish Army to resist the Blitzkrieg was unfounded. All of Poland fell rapidly before the Germans. Roman and his family returned to Cracow, where they were segregated along with the rest of the Jewish population. The Jewish ghetto was ringed with barbed wire by the Nazis.

Over the next few years, the Jewish population of Poland was systematically murdered by the Nazis. The individual Jewish neighborhoods were raided, and people were kidnapped en masse and removed to concentration camps. As these raids progressed, the area of the Jewish ghetto, as well as the population, was reduced, and the remaining people were forced to crowd into ever tighter quarters. The young Roman Polanski lived with six or more other people in a single room.

On one of the German raids, Polanski's half sister was taken by the Germans. After that, feeling the threat grow closer and closer, Roman started sneaking out of the ghetto every time a German raid appeared to be imminent. He would hide outside the perimeter until the raid was over, then return to his parents.

After one of the raids, Roman returned to find that his mother had been taken to Auschwitz, where she subsequently died. The boy learned that his mother was pregnant when she was taken away to be killed.

Shortly before another raid, Roman cut his way through the

barbed wire surrounding the ghetto, as usual, and hid outside until the raid was over. But when he returned he discovered that this raid was to be the last, and that the Germans were marching everyone away. Roman got back in time to see his father being taken away by the German soldiers. He tried to speak to him, but his father signaled the boy to run away. The eight-year-old Polanski narrowly escaped the "final liquidation" of the Cracow ghetto.

Hiding out with friends and relatives in the rural areas of Poland, Roman managed to survive the rest of the war. The first family to which he escaped was one of several to whom his father had already given money for his son's care. When Roman moved on to the next prearranged foster family, the alcoholic wife squandered the money that had been left for him. So the boy went to live with a Catholic peasant family, where he was brought up as a Catholic. Although it was dangerous, the boy still snuck into town now and then and sold newspapers to make money. He spent the money going to movies, despite the fact that the movies were in German. Anti-intellectual Germans had written on the walls of the theater: ONLY PIGS GO TO MOVIES.

After the Soviet Army liberated Poland, Roman moved back to Cracow. An uncle found him in the street one day and took the boy to live with him. When Roman's father miraculously returned from the Mauthausen concentration camp, the boy was overcome with joy.

Conditions at first were far from comfortable. Roman and his father, uncle, and other friends and relatives lived twenty to a room. Later, when his father remarried, Roman and his stepmother did not get along. So Polanski left to live with another family.

Roman's uncle provided a tutor for the boy up to the fifth-grade level. When he returned to the equivalent of high school, he worked on the side as a child actor. At fourteen he played the lead in a play called *Son of the Regiment*. The play was a big success, and he received so much acclaim that he decided to undertake a theatrical career.

As Roman's interest in the theater increased, his interest in schoolwork decreased. After graduation from high school, at his father's urging, he went to technical school, where he studied electronics. While there he continued to work in radio and theater. Despite the fact that Roman's father impressed on his son the importance of having a "practical trade," the boy did very poorly in technical school except for one subject, drawing. With the help of his teacher he transferred to art school.

After a year of art school, Roman applied for admission to acting school, but was rejected for political reasons. Without his student deferment, he was subject to being drafted into the army. To avoid the draft, he lived like a gypsy, moving from home to home so that he never had a fixed address where the draft could catch up with him. In many ways, it was similar to his war years. There were times when he slept in train stations.

Roman's break came when he got a part in a movie, which enabled him to once again make contact with a man he had known earlier in the theater, a man who was now a professor at the National Film School. With his help, Roman was accepted into the National Film School, where he learned to direct movies. His talent soon came to the fore. Three of the short films he made in school were exhibited and won prizes at international festivals. Finally, in 1960 he made his first feature film, *Knife in the Water*. The film was an international success and, though his two-year marriage to a Polish actress was disintegrating, Polanski's career was off and running.

In 1966, while directing and acting in a spoof of vampire movies, *The Fearless Vampire Killers,* Roman met the young American starlet Sharon Tate, who played opposite him. They fell in love. In 1967 Polanski went to Hollywood to direct *Rosemary's Baby.* He also shot some seminude photographs of Sharon for *Playboy* magazine.

Commenting about being typed as a horror-movie specialist, Polanski said, "It wasn't surprising. I was already typed as a horror-movie director because of *Repulsion.* I had never intended to concentrate on that genre—it had simply seemed the most saleable when I was broke. But as so often seems to happen, accidental choices turn into the back stories that color the rest of our lives."

Polanski was, of course, unaware of the tragic irony in his statement. Not only was the horror that had given such dark hues to his early life, and which now lent his movies a chilling sense of reality, about to reinvade his life, but some "accidental choices" were going to make it possible.

Polanski and Sharon Tate were married in 1968. Sharon became pregnant early in 1969. Although the couple planned to live in California, Roman was working on a movie in Great Britain, so they lived there until that summer. Because they wanted the baby to be born in the United States, they rented a house in the secluded hills of Benedict Canyon, in the Bel Air section of Los Angeles. They had planned to return together, but Roman's work on the picture wasn't done yet, and by the time it would have been completed, Sharon would be too far along in her pregnancy to be allowed to travel. So she went ahead without him and he planned to follow her as soon as his picture was complete, sometime around mid-August.

But another cast of characters had already assembled that would prevent that lovers' reunion from ever taking place.

CHARLES "TEX" WATSON

Charles "Tex" Watson was born December 2, 1945, and raised in a small town in rural Texas. He went to church every Sunday, got all A's and B's in school, and wet the bed occasionally. Tex's brother was the high school football hero. Although he went out for football and basketball, Tex really shone in track, in which he held a state record.

In the Watson family, the mother was the boss. Tex never went against her wishes and always did what she wanted, without question. "She expected a lot of me," he said. "She expected me to be good—the best." Toward this end, his mother selected his clothes, his college major, and his girlfriends. If Mom disapproved of one of the young ladies Tex dated, he promptly dropped her. Because she seldom approved, he had few girlfriends in high school and college.

Tex's father was a quiet, somewhat passive man who owned and operated a combination grocery store and gas station. Father and son spent a lot of time together. His father taught Tex how to fish, build models, and fix automobiles. Tex also drank beer with his father, although they had to make sure Mom didn't find out.

As a teenager, Tex worked as a gas station attendant at his father's station, and part-time at the local onion-packing plant during the summers. He spent his spare time building hot rods—one of which he named after his mother. In college, at North Texas State, his grades were as consistently good as in high school, and his record during that period is clean—except for one incident in which he and a college buddy stole some typewriters from their former high school. According to Tex, they stole the typewriters, "just for something to do," and after keeping them a couple of weeks, returned them. No charges were filed.

A year or so before graduation, Tex left college and went to work as a baggage handler for Braniff International Airlines. He took advantage of employee passes and discounts to visit a friend in California. Tex liked what he saw and decided to move there. His parents didn't want him to go, but when he told them he was making the move in order to go to college in California, they went along with his plan.

Once in California, Tex got a job as a wig salesman and enrolled in a California state college. But though he made some sales, the job didn't pay very much. The pressure to earn a living required him to work too many hours to allow time to study and attend classes. After only a few months in school, Tex dropped out.

One day in March 1968, Tex was driving along Sunset Boulevard in Pacific Palisades when he saw a hitchhiker. He stopped to pick the man up. It was Dennis Wilson of the Beach Boys rock group. Tex was amazed to have such a world-famous celebrity riding in his car, and he was even more amazed when Wilson invited him to his home. There, Tex met some new friends, people who were guests at the house. There were several young women, a few young men, and one older man who seemed to be the leader. His name was Charles Manson.

Tex fell in quite easily with his new friends, and started living at the Wilson home, too. Not only were the women affectionate, but the drugs were plentiful and free. Tex experimented with LSD, mescaline, psilocybin, and others, and started smoking marijuana regularly. The free and easy drugs and sex were a heady combination for this "small-town boy," as Tex described himself. Suddenly he was in a different world, a world of celebrities, for whom Manson also supplied drugs. "I couldn't hardly believe what was happening," Tex said. "I couldn't believe that I met Dennis Wilson. My whole life changed."

All his life Tex had been shy with girls, and had felt inadequate and insecure. But his contact with the young women who lived with Manson changed all that. As he started spending more and more time with the Manson Family, his contact with his family back in Texas dropped off. The women he was now living with showered Tex with affection. As this affection made him feel ever more powerful and secure, he adopted increasingly more of the philosophy of the Family and looked up to Manson as his leader. "He pulled me toward him with his girls. I wanted them to want me," Tex said. He was in awe of Manson and believed, as most members did, that Manson knew him better than he knew himself. "He could see right through me," Tex said, "and convinced me that it was wrong to try to hang on to material things, and that the only things that mattered were love, and giving and belonging. For the first time in my life I felt like somebody."

For the first time in his life, Tex felt that he "belonged." So much so that he gave all his possessions to Manson and the Family. Finally, in August 1968, Tex moved to the Spahn Movie Ranch to live with the Family. The ranch, at the sparsely populated northwest end of the San Fernando Valley, was a run-down collection of "Old West" buildings and stables owned by the aging, near-blind George Spahn. Spahn let the Family live there, and in turn the Family, in its own fashion, took care of him and the ranch.

Once at the ranch, the drugs and sex "treatment" Tex had received earlier was intensified. Manson would encourage women to have sex with Watson, and they always obliged. All of Tex's sexual inadequacies were exposed, and Manson and the women seemed to help him overcome them. On occasion, Manson himself fondled and babied Tex—and then sent him to have sex with a woman Manson had preselected for him.

A man who had lived at the ranch for awhile and then left said that Tex was a "quiet, happy-go-lucky type of person" who spent most of his days working as a mechanic repairing Manson's dune buggies and the motorcycles of visiting bikers. Watson took orders from Manson just like everybody else in the Family. "Every morning he'd tell us what he wanted us to do that day."

After a few months, Tex grew afraid of the effects all the drugs might be having on him. In December 1968 he moved away from the ranch and went to live with a friend in Los Angeles. When the friend was drafted, Tex went to live with the man's girlfriend. But the woman not only sold drugs, but used them constantly. It seemed as though Tex couldn't escape the drug culture. Nor could he escape Manson. Out at the ranch, Manson scavenged parts from stolen cars to build dune buggies. Tex's skills were vital to the effort, so Manson was not about to let him stay away. In February 1969 Manson found him and convinced him to move back to the ranch.

Around that time, Manson started preparing the Family for what he called "Helter Skelter," which was to be a bloody war between the white race and the black race. Manson convinced the Family that the war was imminent and that they would be the only survivors of the conflagration. But first they would have to lose all their fear. To desensitize them to fear, Manson took them for wild dune-buggy rides through the hills. To prove that he could even "take the fear out of animals," he tossed kittens up in the air time after time. At first the animals were scared, but eventually, according to Tex, "it didn't bother them." None of the cats ever scratched Manson. They became docile and submissive, the way all the Family members would have to become, Manson told them.

Drugs were a major part of the program. Tex correctly suspected that Manson himself did not take anywhere near as many drugs as he handed out to the Family. In his own words, Watson described the drugs he and the others were taking: "LSD, mescaline. . . . I didn't take any heroin or any reds or yellows. We had peyote and cannabinal, STP. Everybody had it . . . and the girls too, they always had a bagful and Charlie himself would pass it out with whatever he thought the person needed. Later I took speed and whites and bennies and uppers. Then I started sniffing white powder. That made me feel like I was wired up. There were three or four different things at one time. You could see all the stuff in your body. It was electronic like with electric flashes and no feeling."

One day, as Tex was on his way to the motorcycle shop at the ranch, he walked into the kitchen, where a woman offered him a cooked potatolike root vegetable that had been pulled out of the ground near the ranch. It was belladonna root, a source of power-

202 ──────────── ALONE WITH THE DEVIL

ful natural hallucinogenic substances (and atropine). Tex "ate it like a baked potato—it didn't taste bad." But its effects stayed with him for days. The full force of the drug started to hit him later, when he was hitchhiking. He was reduced to crawling on his knees. "My mouth was foaming cotton, my body was sort of red and I fell down three or four times. . . . The last thing I remember was blaring down the road in the daytime. The next thing I remember the police were dragging me out of some car."

Tex was carried—because he couldn't walk—to the Van Nuys jail, where he hallucinated through the night and into the next morning. He saw little people from outer space come out of their flying saucers. The other inmates in the lockup didn't appreciate Tex's visions or the conversations he was having with them. Three of his cellmates beat him up and left a gash over his eye, which required stitches.

The police let Tex go the next morning. Nevertheless, for ten more days his mind would suddenly go on brief belladonna trips, away from reality.

In addition to drugs and sex, a major part of the Family program planned by Manson was eliminating their fear and resistance to killing. Manson led the Family in "visualizations" where they imagined they were killing people. Manson told them there was no such thing as bad and no such thing as wrong. Also, Tex recounted, "there was no such thing as death, so it was not wrong to kill a fellow human being." The Family would gather around Manson, who would sometimes sing his original songs, accompanying himself on the guitar. "He'd play the guitar and sing songs, then he'd place his thoughts in us," Tex said. And then they would go through exercises in which they would kill "imaginary people," who were visualized sitting on chairs in the middle of the group. "He'd tell us that they were already dead, and that the only people that were, were at the ranch."

Tex and the other residents of the ranch seldom left. "Charlie never wanted us to leave the ranch. It was drugs, drugs, drugs . . . bags of acid and speed. The girls would go out and hitchhike and meet new guys and bring them to the ranch and get the drugs. There were a lot of people coming and going from the ranch all the time."

One of these new arrivals was Leslie Van Houten.

LESLIE VAN HOUTEN

Leslie Van Houten was born in Altadena, California, on August 23, 1949. In addition to an older natural brother, she had several younger adopted siblings—Korean war orphans. She grew up in nearby Monrovia, where she lived in the same house and went to elementary school, junior high, and high school. In all three schools she played the sousaphone and drums in the school band. Although she excelled in extracurricular activities, according to her mother, "her grades were never good enough for me."

Leslie was always a good girl, although her mother did say that she was "sort of feisty." She knew everything that was going on in their neighborhood, and seemed to have a hand in most of it. According to her mother, Leslie was fun to be with when she was small. "She had a wonderful sense of humor. She was always small and kind of thin. . . . In the sixth grade she learned to play the sousaphone. She could hardly hold it up, and anytime anyone saw her they just about died laughing, it was so funny. It was hard for her to play because it was so big. . . .Yet she was always the one who went around shaping up the boys that were fighting, and making them stop, and sending them home." Leslie enjoyed hiking, needlework, and reading. In fact, she and a girlfriend started their own lending library.

Leslie's mother worked as a volunteer for the local Presbyterian church, where the choir counted Leslie among its members. Not only did Leslie and her family attend services regularly, but during the summers, when they weren't hiking, camping, or going to the beach, Leslie attended church school where her mother taught.

Leslie seemed to know how far she could go without upsetting her parents. "So I never did what I wanted to because I knew it would upset them," she said. "Until I started learning how to sneak and not have them catch me. And then I started sneaking things, to do what I wanted to do without them finding out."

Leslie was very active in school activities. She was a member of Campfire Girls, Future Teachers, Job's Daughters (an auxiliary of the Masonic Temple), and student government. Her first two years of high school she was voted homecoming princess. "I liked winning," she said, "and I always won. So every time there was something to try for, I'd try and I'd win. I saw it through, but it wasn't as interesting as trying to win."

In 1963, when Leslie was barely fourteen, her parents divorced. Her mother believed that the divorce was a severe blow to her daughter. Leslie, herself, said that "At first the thought shattered me because I always thought people were supposed to be happy if they got married. But then I caught them arguing a couple of times. And I asked my father if it would make him happier, and he said 'Yes.' And I asked her, and she said, 'Yes.' So I figured if a divorce made them both happy all the time, that they should go ahead and do it."

For a while after the divorce, Leslie's mother took her children for group therapy. However, because Leslie appeared so normal and adjusted, the therapist hardly ever questioned her. After five or six sessions, the therapy was discontinued.

But despite her well-adjusted exterior, all was not right with Leslie. During her final two years of high school, her participation in family activities, church, and school functions dropped off severely. At around this time, she started taking drugs. Bobby, a special boyfriend, introduced her to marijuana and LSD. Leslie said she didn't take drugs to get back at her parents, but because "it was just there." "Like here is a pretty guy and he comes up to you and he says, 'Do you want a tab of acid?' and you say, 'Sure, I will try it.' It wasn't escape. It was complete curiosity."

Once she began using drugs, Leslie dropped out of school activities. "I started losing interest very rapidly," she said. She was not voted homecoming princess during her junior and senior years of high school. Her interest in academic subjects dropped off, too, and her grades took a nosedive. "I was having more fun just going out and being with people who I felt close to than sticking my nose in a book. I couldn't keep my interest in anything that wasn't moving, colorful, and entertaining."

As Leslie spent less and less time on school activities, she spent more time on Bobby, who had been a student at Monrovia

High until he was expelled. "Half the time I didn't go to school for seeing him." When she was sixteen, Leslie became pregnant and had to get an abortion.

Although she had been on a college-bound track during her first two years of high school, any college plans Leslie may have had were left behind when she unofficially "dropped out" during her final two years of high school. She seemed to be in the throes of adolescent rebellion, but was actually more than willing to become selflessly devoted to a will other than her own. Around graduation time, she and Bobby became interested in a religious cult called the "Self-Realization Fellowship," or SRF, located in Pacific Palisades. "Bobby just said he wanted to be a monk for it," she said. "If you will be a monk for it, I will be a nun for it."

And become a nun she did. For eight months, Leslie not only stopped taking drugs, but she also stopped seeing Bobby, talking to men, smoking, drinking, and eating meat. Totally devoted, she asked the people at the SRF what they wanted and needed. They said they needed a secretary, so she enrolled in business school. She went to live in an apartment in Manhattan Beach, just downstairs from her father's apartment, and "I either meditated or did shorthand for eight months."

Leslie's old competitive instincts kicked in and she quickly became the best secretary in the school. She could take 160 words of shorthand and type sixty-five words a minute without error. "I was just like a complete machine at it. I was perfect," she said. But Leslie soon became bored with the SRF. By the time she graduated from business school in June 1968, the SRF and Bobby were no longer part of her life. She mechanically went through the motions of applying for a job, and even registered with an employment agency. But her heart wasn't in it. When she was offered a job at a bank, Leslie turned it down and continued to accept support from her parents. "All my life I had gone to school. All my life I had been put into a set routine," she said. "I waited for the years when I would be released from my parents to where I would be living on my own, and to get a nine-to-five was just like going right back into the same routine, or never leaving it. I wanted to get away."

Get away she did. Shortly after graduation from business school, Leslie—who had started taking LSD again—went to a cattle ranch in the desert with two other women. She and her friends lived on the cattle ranch for awhile, then Leslie left to live in the Haight-Ashbury district of San Francisco, which was the center of the "drug counterculture" of the late 1960s. Leslie found life in the Haight very frightening. "It was a change from all the things that I heard when I was younger," she confessed. "It started out, supposedly from what I heard, there was lots of love on the street, and by the time I got there it was all a bunch of—it was just all gutter, the whole thing."

While in San Francisco, another Bobby came into Leslie's life —Bobby Beausoleil, a young drifter who fancied himself an actor. Bobby was at the time living with two other women, Catherine (Share, a.k.a. Gypsy), and Gail. Leslie joined the trio because "I felt such a good feeling around them, and it was a feeling I had all my life been looking for, to be in someone else. In fact, when I was a little child, I remember I used to look in the mirror and wonder why I couldn't be happy with other people as I was within myself. And when I met these people, it was like I was seeing the people that I had always wanted to be with, to have a good time, and they lived for the moment in everything they did. It was so obvious, their complete freedom and just wish to experience. It was like a little caravan of people where we were cowboys."

Leslie fell in love with Bobby Beausoleil "almost immediately." So did Gypsy and Gail.

The caravan of four decided to leave San Francisco for lusher pastures, and so took off on what was to be an odyssey to Oregon. The first leg of their journey took them south, to Bobby's parents' home near Santa Barbara. There, they built a house tent on the back of their truck. "So wherever you wanted to stop, you just undid the ropes, and your house was right there." But despite the practical design of their homemade camper, the quartet was not very good at either making plans or carrying them through. "Nothing was planned, everything happened for the moment, at the moment. Just freedom. Where someone would ask us to come over, we would go over. There was no idea for tomorrow, because we never, you know, we didn't know tomorrow would even ever be there. Everything was pleasurable."

Not surprisingly, the group never made it to Oregon. Instead, they wandered up and down the coast of California, staying with friends or parents, or camping out on the beaches to the south or in the dense woods north of San Francisco. Along the way, Bobby would play his guitar and the girls would sing along with him. They also took LSD, marijuana, hashish, mescaline, and other drugs. Bobby would tell stories, too. Some of them were about a man named Charles Manson.

All through her sojourn, Leslie had kept in constant touch with her mother by means of frequent phone calls and letters. Before leaving the San Francisco area for the last time on their way north, Leslie called and told her mother that she was going to "drop out" and "I just told her that I was going to do whatever I did and that she might not hear from me for a while." The call was a difficult one. Leslie's mother became very angry, and the two argued over the phone. Finally, both hung up alienated and upset.

All was not joyful between Leslie and the others, either. The three-women-to-one-man arrangement fostered jealousy, tension, and conflict, which eventually erupted into outright bickering and fights. One of the women, Gypsy, finally grew tired of the constant tension and left for Los Angeles. Leslie, too, was growing bored. While the group—now a trio—was staying in the San Jose area, Leslie heard that a group of people from a Los Angeles commune were traveling nearby and their bus had broken down. Gypsy had spoken very highly of these people, so Leslie went off in search of the broken-down bus.

She found the bus, its owners, and Gypsy, too, in a prune orchard, and was immediately accepted into the group. Leslie fit right in. "It was like I had known them forever. It was like walking into a group of old friends."

The bus was finally abandoned and the group hitched a ride on a diesel truck back to their commune near Los Angeles, in the northwest corner of the San Fernando Valley—the Spahn Ranch. Once there, Leslie was introduced to the leader, Charles Manson: "He just walked up and smiled real nice, you know, and I just smiled back. And he wasn't any different than all the others. But I could feel much strength in meeting him. I felt very good feelings toward him."

Leslie also met Susan Atkins (Sadie), Patricia Krenwinkel

(Katie), Squeaky Fromme, and Ruth Morehouse (Ouish). Bobby Beausoleil was a frequent visitor, too.

In some ways, life at the Spahn Ranch became a kind of counterculture Disneyland. In keeping with the "back to the land" fantasies fashionable in the late 1960s, Leslie enjoyed the fact that "it was like my very own country house that I took care of, and it was a very down home place where you had to pump water in the morning so you would have water for the evening, and it was a good feeling." Other chores included taking care of the horses, which were rented out to visitors, cleaning out the barns, cooking, and other household duties. At times there were as many as twenty-five people at the ranch, and as few as twelve. For a while they had four little children and three babies living there.

When they weren't helping to run the ranch or take care of George Spahn, members of the Family would go on trips, or "adventures." From time to time they played different roles in what came to be known as the "Magical Mystery Tour," a fantasy derived from the music of the Beatles. "Usually on weekends I was a cowgirl," Leslie said. "Dressed up like one, talked like one, and rented horses out to people. When the kids would come up to rent a horse, you talked to them like they were on a ranch way out in the middle of, you know, the Midwest."

Leslie also played the role of a "motorcycle woman." When the bikers came to the ranch, which was frequently, Leslie would help them overhaul and repair their bikes, and sometimes the bikers would take her and the other women on motorcycle outings or trips.

Though she enjoyed the rural flavor of her life at the ranch, Leslie did not enjoy the city of Los Angeles, which she characterized as "a giant-sized monster." Nevertheless, going down "into the stomach" of the "beast" of Los Angeles was something she and the others had to do from time to time. To get food, she and the other women would go on "garbage runs," in which they would go to the back doors of supermarkets, where the box boys would give them ripe fruits, vegetables, cheese, milk, and baked goods. Some people gave them money, some gave them automobiles. Leslie also panhandled now and then, but wasn't too good at it.

For about three months, Leslie and other members of the Family went to live on the more or less deserted Barker Ranch in the desert near Death Valley. The desert was even more idyllic than the Spahn Ranch. It was much farther from any city and, as she recalled, "just a complete peace. The only thing you could hear would be the hum of the air." When Family members got tired of Los Angeles, they would go to the Barker Ranch. Some of them, particularly Manson, would even go off into the desert around the ranch for days at a time. Leslie enjoyed the role of desert ranch homemaker. "I liked to stay around and do the diapers, and I liked to bake bread." She was the "manager" of the Barker Ranch. She stayed there the longest of all the Family members and delegated chores to visitors.

Eventually, Leslie and the other returned to the Spahn Ranch, where the previous isolation of the commune seemed to be breaking down, in part by design. The Family opened up a freewheeling kind of "nightclub" in which people could come and listen to music or make their own. Leslie and the others called their new venture the "Helter Skelter Club" and painted the name on a huge mural along the back wall, on doors, and also on the jug they passed around for donations. The club had to close down, however. "We kept giving away all the soda pops and everything," Leslie said. "So George told us we would have to close it down because we weren't making any money on it."

There were other problems that sometimes disturbed the peace of the ranch. The Family constantly had to deal with men who were attracted by the stories of freewheeling sex and drugs at the ranch, but who weren't especially willing to really join the Family and share other aspects of their counterculture values. According to Leslie, the men often had to protect the women. "We took care of the men, we cooked for them, we did everything we could to make life as it is supposed to be for them, a good life. And they would protect us against the big guys that would come up on the 'stumblers' and would end up falling around and kicking things over and trying to steal this and that from under our noses." The "stumblers" Leslie refers to were "red devils," or Seconal, a barbiturate sedative which, according to her, "really messes people up."

Yet Leslie did not feel "messed up" by all the LSD and other drugs that she and others took at the ranch. "LSD doesn't make you sloppy," she defended, "it makes you alert. You just see things for what it is when you are on LSD." And what Leslie saw in her life with the Family at the Spahn Ranch was a lot of fun: "It was a good feeling of just existing, being with your brothers and your sisters is what it was. Nothing was hard labor, even when we had to dig a hole and put a big waterpipe in, it was still fun to do it. Everything was."

By April 1969, Leslie had not had any contact with her mother since the call from the Bay Area in which she fought with her about dropping out. But one day that spring Leslie was picked up by the police for hitchhiking in the San Fernando Valley, not too far from the Spahn Ranch. She phoned her mother, who picked her up at the police station, which was about an hour's drive away, and drove her home to Monrovia. She spent one night at home, and, the next day, told her mother that she was leaving to see a friend in Hollywood. Her mother asked her to leave a phone number, but she did not. Leslie returned to the Family. Her mother did not hear from her until many months later, when Leslie was once again in police custody—this time for a much more serious crime than hitchhiking.

THE TATE MURDERS

The night of August 8, 1969, Charles Manson called Tex Watson over. "He was smiling, total perfection," Tex recalled. "I would do anything he asked me to. I was the same person he was. He computed me to go with three girls and kill people. He handed me a knife and a gun and told me to make it as totally gruesome and bloody as we could. . . . As we drove along I could hear Charlie's voice inside my head, computing what he had said, every moment: 'Go up to the house where Terry Melcher used to live, kill them, cut them up, hang them on the mirrors!' He did not know who would be there."

The people there included Jay Sebring, thirty-five, an internationally known hair stylist; Abigail Folger, twenty-five, the coffee heiress; Wojicieck "Voytek" Frykowski, thirty-two, Folger's boyfriend; and Sharon Tate Polanski, twenty-six. There was never any evidence that either Watson or any of the Family women who went along that night actually knew any of their victims. At one time, Terry Melcher, Doris Day's son, used to live in the house. Manson and Tex had been there before, with Dennis Wilson. Melcher had once offered to help Manson get a start in the record business and had put him in touch with a recording executive. The contact never bore any fruit.

Selected to go along with Tex were Susan Atkins, Patricia Krenwinkel, and Linda Kasabian. Manson had given them their instructions too. He told them to write on the walls, preferably in blood, to make it look, to his way of thinking, as if black people had committed the murders—in order to bring on "Helter Skelter." Manson had grown tired of waiting for the end of the world race war he predicted, so, as far as Family members were concerned, he decided to quicken the pace of history.

Linda Kasabian drove them to the house. Linda had first come to the ranch in July, and had met Manson as he worked on a dune buggy parked in a grove of trees. Manson asked Linda why she had come. "I told him my husband had rejected me and that Gypsy told me I was welcome here as part of the Family."

Later, Linda experienced a "love orgy" at the ranch: "Well, we all shed our clothes, and we were laying on the floor . . . and it was just like . . . it didn't matter who was beside you, if it was a man or a woman, you just touched each other and made love with each other and the whole room was like this. It was sort of like just one. . . ."

Tonight, Linda was going to experience another kind of orgy, another attempt at oneness.

When they arrived at the house, Tex and the women parked the car next to a nearby telephone pole. Watson, who had been riding in the backseat, got out of the car, climbed up the pole, and cut the telephone wires leading to the house. Then they drove the car to the bottom of the hill, parked, and started walking up the hill toward the house.

The house was surrounded by a fence. Tex and the women climbed over it and started up the driveway. Suddenly they were bathed in light as a car came down the driveway. At Tex's direction, the women scurried to hide in the bushes while he walked down the middle of the road to meet the car. The car stopped. Tex approached it with his .22-caliber, long-barreled, Western-style revolver aimed at the driver's head. The driver, eighteen-year-old Steven Parent, who had been visiting the person who rented the guest house in the back, begged Watson, "Please don't hurt me, I won't say anything."

But Tex squeezed off four shots at almost point-blank range, and then reached in over Parent's lifeless body and turned off the ignition. Then he bid the women to come out and help him push the car back down the road, out of sight.

Watson told the women to go around the sides and back of the house to see if any windows or doors were open. Linda, although she did find an open window, came back and told him she could find no easy way into the house. But Tex found one, anyway. Linda waited outside as he slit a screen with his razor-sharp knife and climbed inside, and then came around and opened the front door to let the others in. Voytek Frykowski was lying on the couch, asleep. As he woke up, Tex walked up to him and stood over him as he stretched out his arms and asked, "What time is it?"

Tex stuck the barrel of his gun in the man's face and said, "Be quiet. Don't move or you're dead."

"Who are you and what are you doing here?" the man asked.

"I am the Devil, and I am here to do the Devil's work," Tex replied. "Now where is your money?"

"My money is in the wallet on the desk."

Tex told Susan to get the wallet. She couldn't find it, so he told her to search the rest of the house to see if there were any other people there. Susan left and soon came back herding Abigail Folger, Jay Sebring, and a very pregnant Sharon Tate into the room.

Jay Sebring asked, "What are you doing here?"

Tex told him to shut up and then ordered them all to lie down on their stomachs in front of the fireplace. Pointing to Sharon Tate, Sebring protested, "Can't you see she's pregnant? Let her sit down."

Sebring refused to lie down, so Tex shot him. Then he ordered Abigail Folger and Sharon Tate to lie down next to the wounded man. Tex tied a rope around Sebring's neck, then Sharon Tate's neck, then Abigail Folger's. He asked them if they

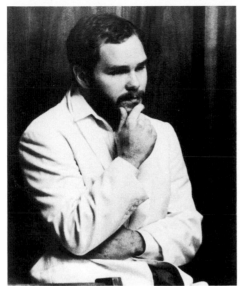

AP/WIDE WORLD

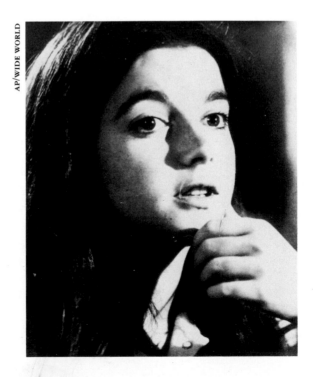

AP/WIDE WORLD

With her appearance in Poltergeist, *Dominique Dunne's (right) acting career was on the rise—until her lover John Sweeney (above) refused to let her go on living without him.*

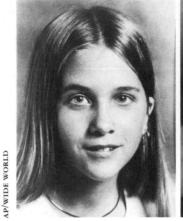 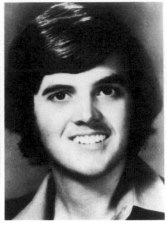

Within hours of having brutaly murdered Vriana Dean, twelve, and her brother Brian, eighteen (above), psychopath John Zimmerman (below) asked the author for help in getting out of jail. Ironically, without certain information obtained during the psychiatric interview, the killer might have been set free.

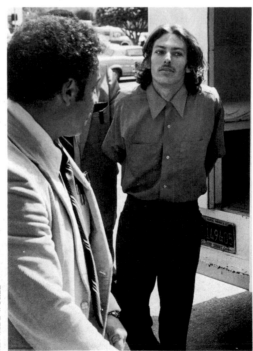

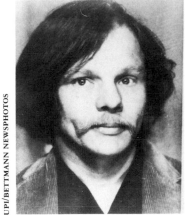

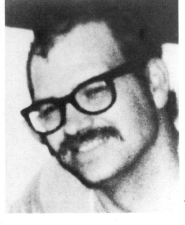

Despite the knowledge that Lawrence Bittaker
(above left) and Roy Norris (above right) were
violent, dangerous man, they were set free
to go on a crime spree, the grotesque results of
which still haunt veteran police officers and
prosecutors who dealt with the case. Bittaker
had no sense of the repulsiveness and the horror
of his crimes. He is shown here (below) after
being held in contempt of court for refusing to
answer questions about an alleged burial site.

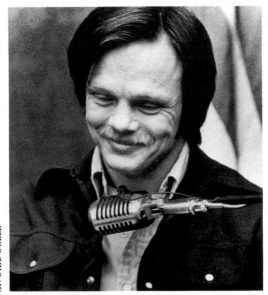

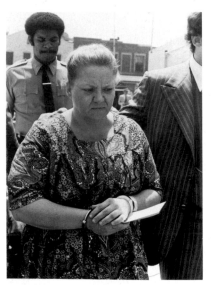
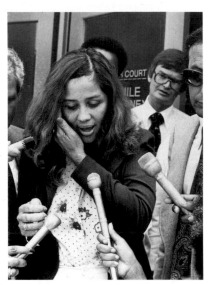

*Norma Jean Armistead (left) wanted a baby
so badly that she was willing to commit murder
in order to steal one. Mary Childs (right) was
one of the victims of Armistead's cruel and
ultimately violent baby-snatching scheme.*

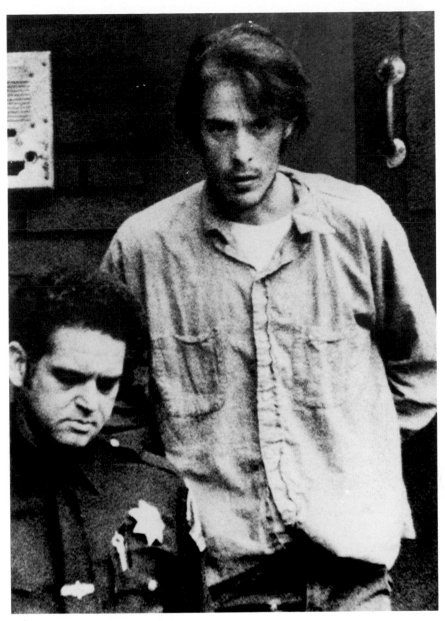

Even though his parents and the authorities knew that Richard Chase was willing and able to kill in order to satisfy his unsatiable craving for blood, he was not prevented from committing the grisly crimes that earned him the title "Vampire of Sacramento."

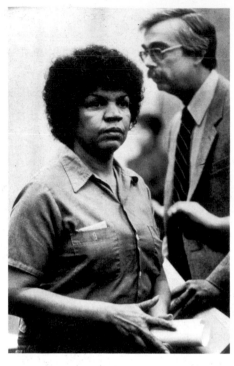

UPI/BETTMANN NEWSPHOTOS

The seething rage that drove Priscilla Ford (left) to wreak death and destruction on the sidewalks of Reno, in what came to be known as the "Thanksgiving Day Massacre," may not subside until she keeps her appointment with the Nevada gas chamber.

AP/WIDE WORLD

Though she killed her two infant children in full view of several witnesses, Fumiko Kimura (right) served very little time in jail for her crime and is today a free woman.

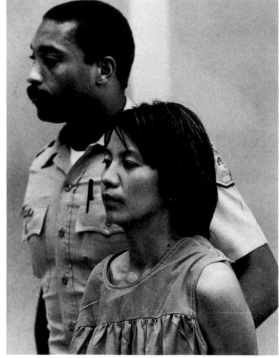

The Manson Family

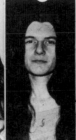

2

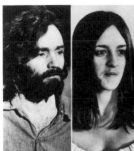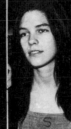

1

*Charles Manson was privy to the
psychological secrets that enabled
him to turn more or less normal
adolescents into bloodthirsty killers.
(1, left to right) Manson, Susan
Atkins, Patricia Krenwinkel,
Leslie Van Houten. (2) Charles
"Tex" Watson. (3, left to right)
Atkins, Krenwinkel, Van Houten.*

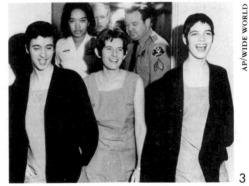

3

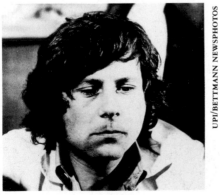

*Roman Polanski (left), haunted
by the Manson Family's murder of
his wife, was later charged for
sex crimes.*

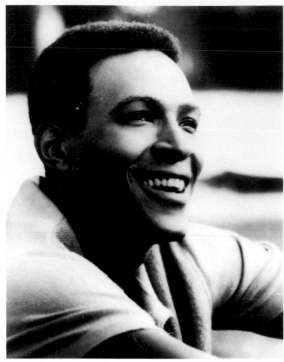

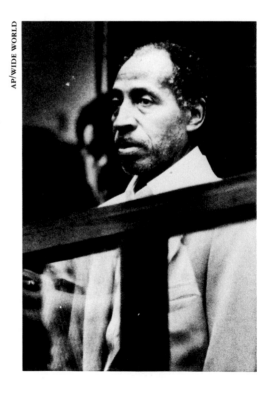

*Marvin Gay, Sr. (right) was
a man of God, a minister,
and the killer of his own son.
Was it the devil, self-defense
or insanity that brought him
to cut Marvin Gaye's (above)
life tragically short? Or was it
a previously unsuspected
factor discovered by the
author?*

had any money. Abigail said she did, but only $72. "I just went to the bank yesterday," she said.

Susan took the money from Abigail and put it in her pocket. Then Tex ordered her to tie up Frykowski with a towel from the bedroom. As Susan was doing that, Tex went over to Jay Sebring and started stabbing him viciously with his knife.

A dog came to the window, looked in—and ran away.

Done with Sebring, Tex ordered Patricia Krenwinkel to turn off all the lights in the house. Then he took the end of the rope that was tied to Sharon Tate, Abigail Folger, and Jay Sebring's body and threw it up over one of the exposed beams in the living room. He pulled hard on the rope, and the two women had to stand up to keep from being choked by the rope.

"What are you going to do with us?" one of them asked.

"You are all going to die," Tex answered.

As Sharon and Abigail began to plead for their lives, Tex ordered Susan to go over and kill Frykowski.

But Frykowski fought back. He grabbed Susan's hair and pulled as hard as he could. Susan cried for Tex to come and help her—and then Frykowski got away from her and ran to the front door, screaming for help. Tex raced after him, wildly stabbed at the big man, and hit him over the head with his gun. He hit him so hard that he broke the gun butt and damaged the gun so that it would no longer fire. Frykowski fought hard for his life and managed to get out the door and run onto the lawn, screaming. He fell into the bushes, and then got up and started to run across the lawn.

Just down the hill from the house, a group of seventy children from the Westlake School for Girls was camping out with five counselors. One of the counselors heard Frykowski's screams as Tex and his razor-sharp knife caught up with him on the lawn: "Oh God, no! Stop! Oh God, no, don't!"

Linda Kasabian, who had been waiting outside, heard men and women screaming and walked back toward the house in time to watch Frykowski's last moments. Susan Atkins ran out of the house and joined Tex in savaging the man's body on the lawn. Linda cried out to Susan to "please make it stop!"

"It's too late," Susan said.

Then Tex told her to go back and kill the women in the house. Linda ran back to the car in horror.

Back inside the house, as Tex and Susan approached the two women, Sharon Tate begged for her life: "Please let me go. . . . All I want to do is have my baby." Susan grabbed her by the hand and put her arm around her neck.

Just before Tex started stabbing Abigail Folger, she looked up at him and said, "I give up, take me." Then he stabbed her repeatedly—but she broke away and ran out on the lawn. Tex chased after her, caught her on the lawn, and viciously stabbed her again and again.

Then he went back inside. By Susan Atkins's own description, "Katie [Patricia Krenwinkel] and I were standing by Sharon and she was out of her mind."

Sharon Tate Polanski and her unborn child were the last to die. The word "pig" was smeared on the front door with Sharon's blood.

Tex, Susan, and Patricia ran down the hill to the car. As they approached, Linda started the car. Tex charged up to her and said, "What do you think you're doing? Don't do anything unless I tell you to do it!" Then he got in the car, pushing Linda out of the driver's seat, and drove away. He allowed Linda to steer while he took off his bloody clothes. The women changed their clothes, too.

As they cruised along Mulholland, Tex pulled the car over and parked near another house.

At approximately 1 A.M., August 9, Rudolph Weber and his wife were awakened by the sound of running water. Someone was using their hose. They got up and went to investigate, and saw four people standing in the street using their hose to spray each other. It was very dark. All Weber and his wife could make out was that there were three women and a man and they were maybe in their late teens. They continued to playfully wash each other's hands, arms, faces, and feet, oblivious to the approaching Webers.

But then Mrs. Weber yelled, "Who's there? My husband is a sheriff!"

Tex looked up. "Gee, I'm sorry, I didn't think you were

home," he said politely. "We were just walking around and wanted a drink of water. We didn't mean to wake you up or disturb you." Then he and the women started walking away, back toward their car. Mr. and Mrs. Weber walked after them. Mrs. Weber started yelling at them, calling them names, such as "filthy hippies," "sluts," and "tramps," while Mr. Weber followed the four down the hill, shining his flashlight on them all the way.

Tex told the women to just get in the car. As he started the car, Rudolph Weber came right up to the car and reached in and tried to turn the car off. However, Tex was able to put the car in low gear and drive away.

On their way back to the ranch, they threw the gun, the knives, and the bundle of bloody clothes out of the car, over a hill. Then they stopped at a gas station, where Tex told them to wash themselves off again. In the rest room, he looked in the mirror, "trying to find out who I was. I wasn't anyone. I wasn't Charles Watson. I was an animal. The end of the world was there. I was the living death."

About an hour and a half after the murders, they arrived back at the ranch, where Manson was sitting, naked, waiting for them. The women went to their bunk house, and, a little later, Tex came in with Manson. Tex repeated what he had said when he entered the Tate house: "I am the Devil here to do the Devil's work."

Manson asked them if they had any remorse. They all said, No.

THE LaBIANCA MURDERS

The next day, August 9, 1969, Manson came into the bunk house, called together Tex, Linda, and Patricia, and told them they were going to go out again. The previous night's murders had been discovered and the pictures of the grisly murder scene were everywhere on TV and the front pages of newspapers. The Family was part of that vast audience. Although only they knew the "plot" behind the murders—and the rest of the world could only wonder why anyone would commit such atrocities—the pieces of Manson's "Helter Skelter" plan seemed to be falling into place.

There was only one problem, however, and this is what Manson wanted to talk about. The previous night's business had been far too messy. Tonight, Manson was going along with them to show them how to do it right.

Leslie Van Houten was also summoned for this night's mayhem. Leslie had taken LSD that day, as she had done quite often since her boyfriend, Bobby Beausoleil, had been arrested and charged with murder in the death of a man who had done business with the Family.

Manson told them to get a change of clothes and prepare to leave. Tex spoke up and said that the weapons they'd used the night before had not been very good, and that they needed better ones. Manson handed Linda some leather thongs and jumped into the driver's seat of Linda's yellow 1959 Ford. The knives and swords were stashed under the driver's seat, and they drove off: Manson, Tex, Leslie, Linda, Patricia, Susan, and a man named Clem. First, they stopped at a gas station, where Manson bought gas and cigarettes. When he came back to the car, he ordered Linda to drive.

Manson directed Linda to get on the freeway and head toward Pasadena. Then he told her to get off at the Fair Oaks exit. They cruised along quiet residential streets until Manson told her to pull over and park. They were in front of a small, one-story house. Manson got out of the car and told Linda to drive around the block and then return to this exact spot. When she and the others returned, Manson was standing on the curb. He got in the car and said that he had looked through the windows of the house and seen children's pictures on the walls and decided not to do it there. Then he said that they would not be able to let the children stop them, "for the sakes of the children of the future."

They sat there for several minutes. A few houses down a man and a woman were getting out of their car. Manson and the others watched them . . . until Manson said that the man was too big and told Linda to drive away.

Then, according to Linda, the Family "drove and drove and he took over driving for a while. Then I just remember driving up a hill and it was pretty high because I could see a lot of city lights, and we stopped in front of another house which was a big house, a more expensive-looking house. And we looked at the house and then he said something about the houses were too close together."

Next, Manson and his murderous crew drove to a church parking lot. Manson got out and said he was going to find a priest or a minister. But the door of the church was locked, so he came back and they drove off. They "got back on the freeway, drove for a long time, and Charlie drove," Linda recalled. "Then, I remember near the end of Sunset Boulevard, he had me take over driving. I was driving and he told me to take a right onto this dirt road, which I did, and went up the dirt road. It was real dark. I couldn't see too much and I turned around and came back. We stopped in front of a house. I remember there was a barn or some kind of a building like that to my right. To my left there was a house but I couldn't really see anything. It was dark. And then we drove on and got back on that main road.

"Then I took another right and there was expensive-type homes, and he had me take rights and lefts and rights and lefts and then we got to a point and he told me to turn around and go back the way I came. We got back onto the main road and I remember driving up a really big hill, a winding hill, and on top there was a gate that was locked and I turned around and came back the way we were going."

Although Linda was lost, they drove on more or less aimlessly until the lights of Sunset Boulevard came in sight. Back on Sunset, heading back toward the city, a white sports car caught Manson's eye. He told Linda to follow it, "and at the next stop light to stop and he was going to get out and kill the man." At the next light, Linda pulled up next to the white sports car, and Manson started to get out of the car. But then the light turned green and the white sports car sped away. Manson got back in and gave Linda more directions, until they pulled up in front of a house in the fashionable Los Feliz section of Los Angeles, near Griffith Park. Linda looked at the house and recognized it.

About a year earlier, before she had joined the Family, Linda had visited the house with her husband and friends. Apparently, both Linda and Manson knew the man who owned the house. "I was really surprised that we stopped there and I said, 'You are not going to that house, are you?' And Charlie said, 'No, I am going to the house next door.' And he got out of the car, and I saw him walk up the driveway that looked like to Harold's house. Then he disappeared. It was dark."

Linda and the others lit up cigarettes while waiting for their leader to return. In the time it took them to finish one cigarette, Manson returned. He summoned Tex, Leslie, and Patricia out of the car and, as they stood beside the car, told them that there were two people in the house, a man and a woman, and that he had tied them up. He said that the previous night's panic had occurred because Tex had let the people know they were going to be killed. Tonight, with smiles and a very quiet manner, Manson had told the man and woman not to be afraid, and had reassured them that no one was going to hurt them. As a result, they were very calm. He told Tex, Leslie, and Patricia, "Don't let them know that you're going to kill them. Don't cause fear and panic in these people."

Then he told them to go in and do what they had done the previous night, and then to hitchhike home. Manson got in the car and, with Linda, Clem, and Susan, drove away, leaving Tex, Leslie, and Patricia in front of the LaBianca home.

Tex went into the house first, then the women followed. Although she claimed her memory was fuzzy because of the LSD she had taken that day, Leslie recalled that, "When we got in the house, the people were all tied up. We all just looked at each other for a few minutes, a few seconds. The woman looked at us and she said, 'We will give you anything.' " The family dog came out to greet them, wagging her tail. Patricia petted the dog, surprised that it wasn't afraid of her. The dog followed them into the kitchen, where they ate some food from the refrigerator.

Then, according to Leslie, leaving Tex and his victim, Leno LaBianca, forty-four, in the living room, "Patricia and myself and the lady went into the bedroom, and the closet door was open, so we were looking at the clothes. She had some very pretty clothes. And then she said, 'I won't call the police! I won't call the police!' She kept saying that." Then Patricia left the room.

Leslie was uneasy. Something seemed very wrong to her: "I wasn't even sure what was happening. I don't know if afraid is the right word. There was that feeling you get."

Rosemary LaBianca, thirty-eight, was uneasy and afraid, too, and when she heard her husband's death screams from the other room, she tried to defend herself. "She picked up a great big table lamp and it looked like she was going to throw it," Leslie recalled. "I looked through the corner of my eye and I saw the lamp coming down, so I blocked it. I got it away from her, and we fought for a few seconds and I got her on the bed and ripped the pillowcase off the pillow and I put it on her head." During the struggle, Leslie kept saying, "Please be still," to Rosemary LaBianca.

Patricia Krenwinkel came back with some kitchen utensils, including some knives. She threw down the utensils and went to Leslie's aid with the struggling Rosemary LaBianca. The three women wrestled, and Patricia and Leslie subdued their victim but they couldn't bring themselves to stab her. They called Tex in from the living room, where he had just finished off Leno LaBianca. Tex had no such qualms, and without hesitation stabbed Rosemary LaBianca in the back several times. As Mrs. LaBianca's blood ran, Leslie and Patricia joined in. "We started stabbing and cutting up the lady. I don't know if it was before or after she was dead, but I stabbed her. I wasn't thinking about anything while I was stabbing. I don't know if she was dead. She was laying there on the floor." Leslie kept stabbing long after Rosemary LaBianca had stopped yelling for the police. As Leslie later told a Family member, at first she didn't want to do it, but the more she did it, the more fun it was. "I was obsessed with the knife. Once it went in, it just kept going in and in and in."

Then Leslie got a towel and started wiping everything off. "I just got obsessed with the thought of the fingerprints, because in the movies and things, when things happen you always get a towel and wipe off fingerprints." Leslie felt compelled to wipe off not only things they had touched, but also to open drawers and wipe off things they had not touched. Patricia came and took the towel away from her and led her out of the house. As they passed through the living room, Leslie "saw a man lying there, and I saw writings on the wall." DEATH TO PIGS and RISE were written on the walls, and HELTER SKELTER on the refrigerator door, in the victim's blood. In addition to the words on the wall, written in blood, the word "war" had been carved on Leno LaBianca's stomach, and a double-tined carving fork had been left sticking into his body.

The three took showers in the house, changed into clean clothes, and then hitchhiked back to the Spahn Ranch. When Leslie arrived, she took off her clothes and burned them, along with a purse and a rope.

AFTERMATH

After the murders, Tex was sent from the ranch on a mission to scout for a new home for the Family. While away, he was picked up by the police and questioned—not about the Tate-LaBianca murders, but about some stolen cars. The police had not yet connected the Family with the murders. As a matter of fact, they were not even working under the assumption that the two murders were connected despite the grotesque similarities between them! But the police did suspect the Family had something to do with some cars that had been stolen around the San Fernando Valley. So Tex was questioned and released.

Apparently, his close brush with the authorities frightened him, so he fled California and went home to Texas. He moved in with his mother and father and "I tried to be Charles Watson again."

Nevertheless, Tex was not above trading on his past experiences. He bragged to an old girlfriend that he had been living on a ranch in California, with "a whole bunch of girls—thirty girls and only three guys." Tex took up with the woman, who said that he was essentially the same when he came back from California as he was before he left, except for one thing: he seemed a bit more "animalistic" when they had sex.

Back in California, on August 16, 1969, just eight days after the murders, the Los Angeles County Sheriff's office raided the Spahn Ranch. More than twenty people were arrested, including Leslie Van Houten. All of those arrested spent seventy-two hours in custody, then were released. The police were looking for stolen cars, not murderers, at the Spahn Ranch. None of the officers involved in the raid—though the ranch was thoroughly searched—noticed any connections between the writings on the walls and doors at the ranch, including the almost ubiquitous HELTER SKELTER, and similar messages written in blood at the murder scenes.

After the raid, members of the Family split up. Leslie and Patricia stayed in the Los Angeles area for a while. On September 18, Leslie was arrested for making department store purchases with a stolen credit card. She was soon released. She and Patricia fled to the Barker Ranch in the desert, where they were eventually arrested on October 19, 1969. At the time of her arrest, Leslie was using the alias "Louella Alexandria." The police had never really picked up the murderers' trail. The case was "cracked" when Susan Atkins bragged about the killings to a fellow inmate while in jail for another crime.

After her arrest on murder charges, Leslie contacted her mother. Mrs. Van Houten had not heard from her daughter since the previous April, when Leslie had spent the night in her girlhood home. Leslie's mother visited her daughter once a week at the Sybil Brand Facility for Women, where she was kept in custody. "One of the things that has been most surprising to us," Leslie's mother said, "is that people we knew, friends, have sent perhaps a hundred letters or more to me speaking of their concern for Leslie. They have been very supportive."

One of Leslie's attorneys asked Mrs. Van Houten, "How do you feel about your daughter now?"

"I love Leslie very much."

"As much as you always have?"

"More."

"When Leslie was living with you and while she was living with her father at the beach, was there ever any hint or the slightest hint to you that something like this would happen to your daughter?"

"For myself, I never would have believed it."

"Do you still believe it?"

"I don't believe it."

Leslie's first attorney proceeded to prepare an insanity defense for his client. At first, Leslie more or less cooperated with him. But her cooperation did not last, for she was to be tried along with Manson, Susan Atkins, and Patricia Krenwinkel. Once Manson gained access to the other defendants, a defense was planned that would, basically, shift blame away from him, the leader, and onto Leslie and the others, his followers. To this end,

Leslie and the other defendants followed Manson's lead. If any attorney didn't want to go along with the plan—and most didn't, since it meant not adequately representing their client—he was fired. During the course of the trial, Leslie was represented by four attorneys.

So Leslie fired her first attorney, claiming that he was not truly representing her. "He was going to claim that I was nuts. He said, 'I will get you out. We will make these tapes, Leslie, and we will take everything that Susan Atkins said in her story, and then we will put it on tapes and play it for some psychiatrist to see if you are crazy.' " Leslie said that she did not believe she was mentally ill. I was one of the psychiatrists for whom this tape was played, and I had to say that I agreed with her. Although the horrible nature of the crimes led many people to believe that Leslie and the others must have been insane, there was little in the tapes to suggest either actual legal insanity or a major psychiatric disorder. I had been called in to evaluate her and determine whether or not she was competent to stand trial. I made the very limited psychiatric-legal determination that she was competent.

However, this is not to say that I didn't have other pertinent psychiatric information that might greatly reduce Leslie's responsibility for the murder. As a matter of fact, I did—and I would eventually examine her again and ultimately testify to that effect.

Once Manson gained control of the defense team, Leslie became even less cooperative with her attorney's legitimate efforts. Falling into step with the Family's mind-set, when asked if she felt sorrow, shame, guilt, or regret for the murder of Rosemary LaBianca, Leslie retreated into pious platitudes: "Sorry is only a five-letter word. It can't bring back anything. What can I feel? It has happened. She is gone. What can I do? What can I feel? You can't undo something that is done. If I cry for death, it is for death itself. She is not the only person who has died."

In many respects the trial became a sideshow put on by Manson and the Family, with the criminal justice system willingly participating. On the first day of the trial, Manson came in with an X carved on his forehead. On the second day, not only did Leslie and the other defendants come in with identical X's carved on their foreheads, but Family members demonstrating on the sidewalk outside the courthouse had similarly mutilated themselves. Of course, the Family had only graphically demonstrated how far they were willing to go to follow their leader's wishes.

When Leslie testified, she never implicated Manson in any way. In fact, she even said that he did not go along on the night of the LaBianca murders. And she told other lies to help protect him. On January 25, 1971, all defendants—Leslie, Manson, Patricia Krenwinkel, and Susan Atkins—were found guilty of first-degree murder. On March 29, after the penalty-phase trial, the jury returned with the death penalty.

After her death sentence, Leslie told a probation officer: "What's to say about it. It happened. I didn't kill anybody. Only reason I feel I'm sentenced to death is because I didn't talk against Charlie. I think he's a decent man." She also said that although she had no desire to kill anyone, she would have no difficulty doing so again if she really wanted to.

Leslie's first conviction did not stick. It was eventually reversed by the appeals court. When one of her attorneys mysteriously disappeared during the trial (he was later found dead— drowned in a wilderness flash flood), the trial judge chose to continue the trial with a new attorney. This, according to the appeals court, cast a shadow over her conviction, because she had lacked continuous competent counsel. The case was remanded back to the superior court and a second trial was scheduled for her.

Meanwhile, it took police in California several months to link Tex with the Tate–LaBianca murders. Once they tracked him down, there was one major complication: The sheriff of the county in which Tex was living was his second cousin. Tex did not try to flee and agreed to give himself up. On the day of his scheduled surrender to local authorities, he went for one last fling at the lake. As his girlfriend recalled, "He was always a real open, friendly person. The day he was arrested, we made out at the lake and he was real depressed and I knew something was wrong, but I didn't ask any questions. He was going back to California. . . ."

Tex showed up as promised and was officially placed under

arrest at the Collin County sheriff's office on that December day in 1969. He was accompanied by his father's uncle. His attorney immediately set into motion legal maneuvers to fight extradition to California.

While Tex was held in custody in Texas, he had a TV, portable radio, portable record player, and a Styrofoam cooler. His mother brought him cottage cheese, fruit, prune juice, grape juice, and other food. "My parents came to see me every other day," Tex said. "They brought me a big grocery sack full of food I could keep down." His mother also did his laundry for him. Tex kept his spare pants hanging from a clothesline, to keep them neat.

Most of the time Tex lay on his bunk, with the TV on, often with the sound turned way down. He read newspapers, particularly his hometown papers. His favorite magazines were *U.S. News and World Report* and *Life.* He shaved every day and showered sometimes twice a day in hot weather. On especially hot days, he might also change his shirt twice. Tex was respectful and courteous to the prison guards. One guard reported, "The whole time he was there, you couldn't ask for a more ideal prisoner."

Tex was asked if he had to do it all over again, whether he would have left Texas. "No, I wouldn't. I'm sorry I ever came to California. I'd like to go home to be with my parents right now. I'm truly sorry I met up with Charles Manson and all those people. Because of what happened with the murders and all that. I can't believe I'd do something like that. I pray every night for forgiveness."

Tex was finally extradited to California in September 1970. His mental and physical health immediately deteriorated: "I get out of breath easily and I have pains in my chest and in my heart and it's hard for me to breathe sometimes. When I think about some of the things that have happened I get frightened. I often wake out of my sleep with bad dreams and I tremble and feel weak when somebody shouts at me. I guess my body is in pretty weak condition. I frequently get tired in the morning. My appetite isn't very good. I seem to have an upset stomach a lot. I get sick to my stomach and I have indigestion. My intestines don't work well and sometimes I get pain in my stomach."

Most of Tex's physical complaints centered around his diet. Watson appeared unable to eat meat, bread, or potatoes. When these items were placed before him he claimed he felt sick. He complained that if he were only given the "right food" he would regain his health: "If I could get a proper diet, I'm better with things that I can eat. Fruit and vegetable juices. I can eat dried foods a lot. Mother used to bring me that in jail in Texas. I can't eat sugar or oily things. Somehow I can't keep them down." Tex traced his trouble keeping certain foods down to his first experience eating belladonna root at the ranch. Tex finally provided prison authorities with a list of the foods he could and would eat.

These physical symptoms Tex experienced were, in part, a reaction to the stress he was experiencing. I suggested that he was also exaggerating in order to develop a psychiatric defense. Tex was exhibiting emotional symptoms, such as paranoia and depression, too. He started expressing what was going on in his mind as a battle between control by his parents and control by Charles Manson: "Charlie would always tell us what to do. . . . I try to keep writing every day to my parents to keep my mind with them and on them instead of on Charlie and the girls. Sometimes I was in between, and the people were pushing Charlie on me so much and I wanted to be with my parents . . . and the confusion was too much. I didn't know which was right, my parents or Charlie, because Charlie took control.

"I get real jittery in the cell. A couple of guys bother me because they think I'm going against Manson and a lot of people in 'high power' go for what Manson says and it's hard for me to keep from being nervous and jittery. I'm not going along with Manson. Down in the cell there's this loud confusion, and these people for Manson are talking about people 'being snitches and how snitches won't live long' and all this stuff. And I get sort of pulled back into Manson's world by all this talk. I'm trying to keep in my parents' world and not in between them and Manson." Most of the time in custody, Tex was quiet and kept to himself. He appeared depressed and anxious.

Finally, Tex was moved from the county jail to Atascadero State Hospital, where his emotional and physical health improved. Nevertheless, officials at Atascadero said that Tex did not appear to respond very well to psychotherapy. His answers were "evasive, noncommittal, and covertly hostile." In the examiner's opinion, he "feigned amnesia." Tex apparently forgot many of the details of the murders, particularly the fact that he was in charge both nights. He said he was "out of it" and the women were in charge. The evidence suggested he was not only in charge but, far from being out of it, he also acted with precision all the time. His amnesia was usually correctable. When reminded of details, he was able to remember and talk about them.

Tex's answers were not always covertly hostile, either. He was very sensitive to discussion of the act of killing, and became angry when pushed to talk about it. "I could kill you easily" he once retorted to an examiner.

In trying to explore the mind of this murderer, examiners asked Tex to answer questions that amounted to self-descriptions. Putting his answers to these questions together gives us a look at how Tex viewed himself, or wanted himself to be viewed.

"I'm extremely shy and sensitive. I make friends easily, though. Yes, I've taken dope regularly . . . just up there at the ranch. My enemies go to great lengths to annoy me. I wish I had somebody to tell me what to do. I have to do things very slowly in order to be sure I'm doing them just right. It's hard for me to make up my own mind sometimes. I'm usually quiet at a party. I think my emotions are usually dead.

"I love children. Sometimes I think my life has been a failure. I lack confidence and I wish I were a child again. I'm exceptionally orderly. I'm a Methodist."

Tex Watson's basic defense was a claim that he acted under orders from Charles Manson, which he was compelled to obey because of the drug-induced confusion in his mind. The murders were just a particularly violent episode in a life that was "one big trip between March and October of 1969."

After examining Tex Watson, I came to the conclusion that this was a psychiatrically valid position.

I was called in to examine Tex before his first trial, and to examine Leslie before her second. By now, Leslie's attorney was also a member of Tex's defense team. Another one of the many ironies in this case was that I was originally called in by the prosecution but I wound up testifying for the defense.

The law normally makes fine distinctions between types of killings, and the mental states required for each type have sophisticated differences. From the mid 1960s through the 1970s, the distinctions in California were even more refined than most. Normally, in order to win a first-degree murder conviction, the prosecution must establish that the defendant had the mental capacity for the crime. But at the time of the Manson trial, in California, case law stated that first-degree murder required not only a state of mind capable of premeditation, deliberation, and harboring malice, but also one which was able to *meaningfully and maturely* reflect on the gravity of the act. This created a higher, more sophisticated mental plateau that had to be reached before murder charges could be sustained.

I spent several hours with the defendants and advised the prosecution that it was going to be difficult to reach that plateau. Though as a citizen I wanted to see the Tate–LaBianca murderers punished as much as anyone did, I had to advise the prosecution that, in my opinion, there was evidence of diminished capacity, at least according to California law at the time.

When Leslie and Tex and the others committed the crimes, their brains were literally pickled in drugs. They were taking all kinds—LSD, amphetamines, pot, downers, and others—almost continuously. They were high twenty-four hours a day, even when they went to sleep. A person taking the kinds of drugs the Family did would almost automatically have lacked the mental capacity to meaningfully and maturely premeditate, deliberate, and reflect upon the gravity of an act. Therefore, if this psychiatric information were carried over into the legal decision, a first-degree murder conviction would not be possible. In Leslie's case, I further believed that she was so spaced-out that she may have also lacked the mental capacity to harbor malice. Therefore she could not be proved to have the mental capacity for either first- or second-degree murder. Manslaughter yes, but not murder. Without establishing malice, she could be found guilty of only manslaughter.*

* To attempt to make logic out of this convoluted area of the law boggles the mind. Simply stated, it is possible for an individual to intentionally consume drugs that are illegal and that impact on his

In the meantime, the defense team had learned of my opinion. The law requires that the prosecution inform the defense of any and all evidence, pro or con, that it gathers. Failure to do so is a "reversible error," which means that an appeals court could throw out the conviction and order a retrial. The defense does not have to reciprocate, since the Constitution does not require a defendant to assist in his own prosecution. So I met with the defense team, told them what I thought, and they decided to put me on the witness stand.

As a citizen, I was troubled because I knew that my testimony could increase the likelihood that the killings would go insufficiently punished. What made me uncomfortable was the way my medically correct testimony was going to be used by the system. The truth was again getting lost in the nit-picking of legal issues.

The defense attorneys and I had many intense philosophical discussions about this. I told them quite plainly that I was about as comfortable with this testimony as a surgeon would have been if put in the position of saving Adolf Hitler's life on the operating table. Ethics require a physician to do his or her best, *medically,* regardless of the social, legal, or personal consequences. It was my responsibility to tell the truth as far as my medical opinion was concerned, even though I felt that they should all be severely punished.

My testimony was disturbing personally not because of the medical information it contained, but because of the way the legal system applied the information. If you want to carry through on the logic, what person who kills another person can "meaningfully" and "maturely" reflect upon the gravity of the act? The greatest thinkers of every age in human history have labored over "meaningfully" reflecting upon the gravity of death. Were we

_____

or her thinking and behavior, and then employ a defense that the initial crime of taking the drugs produced a state of mind that voided the mental state required for a specific crime. So if you or I take a powerful, mind-altering drug such as LSD, PCP, cocaine, or countless other chemicals, and we then take the life of another human being—but because of the drug lacked the ability to deliberate, premeditate, or harbor malice, we could not be held responsible for first degree murder. The use of drugs cannot totally negate responsibility, i.e. produce a state of insanity or unconsciousness—this would shock the conscience of the law. However, a reduction to involuntary manslaughter is not only conceivable but realistically attainable. Imagine, the commission of one crime becomes the defense for another, more serious, criminal act.

then to demand the same level of philosophical and psychological maturity of every killer?

The courts at that time were. Mind you these were not legislated standards. No elected officials voted these standards. They were put into effect entirely by the courts, the California Supreme Court in particular.

Knowing my opinion, the prosecution naturally didn't want to use me in court. They were going for first-degree murder convictions and didn't want a psychiatrist on the witness stand who was going to say that the defendants were not mentally capable of committing first-degree murder. However, I told them, there was an alternative basis on which to prosecute the defendants on first-degree murder charges. I suggested that they charge them with first-degree murder committed during the course of another felony, in this case robbery.

Leslie and her companions had stolen some food and household articles from the LaBianca home. Obviously, the thefts were minor compared to the enormity of the murders, but the law said that a killing committed during the course of a robbery did not require malice or deliberation and premeditation to be first-degree murder. Proving the mental elements of robbery were a lot easier than proving the mental elements of first-degree murder. I advised the prosecution that the defendants most certainly did have the mental capacity for robbery, that is, to permanently deprive an owner of property.

But the prosecution chose not to go that route at Leslie's second trial. They wanted to hit hard and win on pure first-degree murder. I guess they felt that this was a high-visibility case with lots of political overtones and the jury would come in for first-degree murder no matter what, which is what they had done the first time around.

Perhaps they were also encouraged by the result in Tex Watson's trial. In his case, I had examined him and told his attorney that in my opinion, despite his drug-induced haze, Tex had the mental capacity to harbor malice, but lacked the ability to meaningfully and maturely reflect on the gravity of the crimes. This would have reduced his level of responsibility from first- to second-degree murder. I testified to that effect—but the jury did not let my testimony sway them. In fact, they essentially ignored it in reaching their conclusions, which is their right as the "trier of fact." Watson was found guilty of first-degree murder and sentenced to death.

But in Leslie's second trial it didn't work out that way. As a matter of fact, the jury not only failed to bring in a first-degree conviction, but it almost set her free! Half the jury wanted to convict her of manslaughter. Since she had already served enough time in prison for manslaughter, she would have walked out of the courtroom a free woman.

But the other half of the jury was just as adamant on convicting her of murder. So, lacking the unanimous verdict that is required, we got a hung jury. A third trial was scheduled.

For the third trial, the prosecutor decided to take my advice and go for murder in the course of a robbery. The defense, of course, knew the prosecutor's plans. I advised the defense attorneys not to use me. I would continue to say that Leslie did not have the mental capacity to harbor malice or meaningfully and maturely reflect. But if asked whether she had the mental capacity for robbery, I would answer yes. That would be sufficient to convict her of first-degree murder, if the jury accepted the psychiatric testimony.

Leslie's attorneys decided to take the gamble anyway. They put me on the stand as a defense witness. When the prosecutor's chance to cross-examine me came up, sure enough, I was asked the question, Did Leslie Van Houten have the mental capacity to commit robbery? I answered yes.

Now the jury had a simpler task, and Leslie was convicted of first-degree murder. When the jury was later asked about its decision, three of them admitted that without the "murder in the course of a robbery" theory, they would not have been able to convict her of first-degree murder. Leslie was once again sentenced to death.

But the U.S. Supreme Court made a white elephant of this and all other death sentences when it subsequently outlawed the death penalty on constitutional grounds. Leslie's and the other Manson Family sentences were automatically reduce to life in prison, with parole. Although the Supreme Court later made it possible for states to reinstitute the death penalty, it could not be restored retroactively, only invoked in new ones. In 1980, the "meaningful and mature" rule that allowed many murderers to go free with little or no punishment, and which almost did the same for some of the Manson Family murderers, was rescinded by legislative action. A law commonly known as the Victim's Bill of Rights removed the requirement that premeditation and deliberation be "meaningful and mature." Murderers no longer have to be philosophers. Today, the very same testimony I gave would not have diminished their capacity or legal responsibility one bit.

Whether or not the Manson Family murderers were "brought to justice" is a moot point, and winning the argument one way or the other—or even imagining an outcome in which they were actually executed—does not ultimately satisfy all our questions about this case. What we really want to satisfy is not our desire for vengeance or our thirst for justice, but our curiosity, our desire to understand why it happened in the first place. What was it about these people that drove them, or allowed them, to commit these awful crimes?

The tendency is to look for some special madness, some loose screw, some important personality defect to explain the horror. There is none to be found. They were, with the exception of Manson (who had already spent more than half his life in prison), all-American boys and girls. When I examined Leslie Van Houten and Tex Watson and Patricia Krenwinkel, I found nothing that could not be found in millions of other young men and women. I felt no discomfort at being in the same room with them. In fact, they were quite likable. If you didn't know what they had been involved in, you would be pleased if one of your children brought them home to meet them.

Then why?

One psychiatrist blamed it on something called *folie à deux,* which is a shared psychosis. In other words, the Family "caught" Manson's craziness. He was then able to transfer his own delusional ideas and abnormal behavior patterns to them.

Folie à deux is an attractive explanation, except for one fact: neither Manson nor any of the murderers were psychotic. There was no psychosis to "catch." The Family had a purpose in committing the murders—to start a race war, "Helter Skelter." That goal may have been unrealistic, it may have been grandiose, but it wasn't fundamentally psychotic. Remember the milieu in which this all took place. From the mid to the late 1960s, every city in the United States sweated through a "long, hot summer" on the brink of race riots. There was hardly a major city that was not touched in some way during that period with full-scale riots in which entire neighborhoods became war zones, complete with bombings, sniper fire, pitched battles setting police and National Guard troops against mobs of rioters. Entire city blocks burned down to charred rubble. Most of these riots were ignited by events far less provocative than the Tate–LaBianca murders. It was not psychotic at all to imagine that pinning such atrocities on a gang of black people could ignite an interracial conflagration.

The answer to the Manson Family and the Tate–LaBianca murders begins with Linda Kasabian's statement: "I believe that we all have a part of the Devil within us—it's just a matter of bringing it out." We all do have a willingness—even an appetite —to kill within us. All it takes is the right combination of factors to raise it to the surface.

Usually, the prime candidate for Devil in this case is Charles Manson. Manson has been called everything from criminally insane to sadistic to sociopathic. I can't offer a diagnosis because I've never examined him. He rebuffed any psychiatric defense. But it doesn't make any difference. Focusing on Manson is missing the important point: Manson needed Leslie and Tex and the others just as much as they needed him. Manson was, without a doubt, their leader. And they probably would not have become involved in such horror without his direction. They may have been playing out a scheme that was hatched in his mind, but Manson, and whatever went on in his mind, was still only part of the mix.

True, Manson was the necessary yeast, the catalyst, and, by nature, the unique ingredient in the recipe. There are thousands of Leslie Van Houtens and Tex Watsons for every Charles Manson, and it takes only one Manson to lead thousands—even millions—to commit crimes of this nature. But without willing followers, such "master criminals" are limited to only as much mayhem as they, alone, can commit.

Charles Manson was not the first of his kind, nor the last.

Consider the Family not as a wanton band of renegades but as a tribe, a valid—if somewhat grotesque—subculture. Again, look at the milieu of the 1960s. Hippie tribes, communes, and ashrams sprouted like weeds all over the country. It was almost a rite of passage for many young people to become involved in some kind of tribe that set them in some opposition to the "establishment." All of these tribes substituted their own special values, rules, habits, and goals for those belonging to the society at large, which the converts had rejected. All the tribes responded to a very deep-seated need on the part of their converts to "belong." Most of them, to varying degrees, involved some kind of religious, mystical, or satanic framework, through which the members tried to explain the world. Many, though not all, involved their members in drugs. The more intense among them became similar to miniature countries, so severe was their alienation from the rest of society. When their alienation became severe enough, many of them considered themselves, literally, at war with everyone who wasn't like them.

Of course, not all of them actually went to war against society. And though saying the Manson Family was constantly drugged may be enough to psychiatrically and even legally reduce their responsibility, it still doesn't explain why they finally turned their alienation into violence. Plenty of communes were just as drug-crazy and every bit as angry and hostile to the "establishment," and yet didn't go around slaughtering people.

Independently, none of these kids would have done what they did. Adding Manson did the trick. There were plenty of commune leaders who, as long as they could get plenty of sex, plenty of drugs, and plenty of people to do their bidding, had all they really cared about. But not Manson.

Equally important is the fact that Manson could not have done it alone. He wouldn't have had the soldiers, the human raw material, ready and eager to be led. But in order to lead them, he had to tailor his strategies to harmonize with their rebellion, dissatisfaction, expectations, fantasies, and, finally, their own murderous rage.

Hitler by himself could not have started World War II. Eichmann by himself would not have brought about the Holocaust. It may make us uncomfortable to put Manson in such company, but the dynamics are pretty much the same. The subculture defines what behavior it will accept, what behavior will be considered normal and productive. Manson and the Family did not see themselves as criminals, they saw themselves as "another country," as a tribe at war with another tribe. During World War II, SS men murdered thousands—millions—because their leader ordered it and the tribe's beliefs said it was good to do so. They were all—including Leslie and Tex—"just following orders."

Which is exactly the defense their attorneys wanted to use—but were prevented from using by the Family's last-ditch solidarity with Manson. But though that strategy of refusing to blame their leader may have been legally suicidal, psychologically it was a survival mechanism. Once the individual members of the Family were removed from the constant support of the group, once they were removed from the constant drug-induced haze of the group, once they were extracted from the chemical and psychological brine that had pickled their minds—they were suddenly in a position to realize what they had done. And what they had done was so monumental, their psyches weren't able to face it. In order for them to survive the knowledge of the enormity of their acts, they had to retreat into the comfort of the Family, the same misguided value-system that had allowed the atrocities to happen in the first place. The only way they could deal with the wrongness of what they had done was to psychically go back to where it wasn't wrong.

We are all not so different from Leslie, Tex, and the others. When any culture or tribe goes to war against another, it must incorporate into its values that it's not wrong to kill the enemy, and must feel superior to its enemy. During World War II we did that with the Japanese and the Germans, and the Germans did it with the Jews, gypsies, and homosexuals. As far as the Manson Family was concerned, they were at war.

But all wars end, or, at least, wind down. And so it was with this one. A 1972 psychological report described Leslie: "With a wide smile and a rather thin, gangly build, Leslie looks several years younger than her stated age (twenty-two)." Leslie spoke easily to the psychologist, and seemed to want to make a favorable impression. She said she wanted to somehow help the cause of prison reform, and hoped that if she could become an example of a "worthwhile person," she could thereby justify the abolition of the death penalty.

Leslie, herself, said that "My life was taken away from me and now it has been given back." She was obviously beginning to reconsider her convictions regarding the evils of society. If she could be moved from the Special Security Area of the prison to the Main Campus, Leslie could look forward to making new friends.

The custodial staff of the prison noted much progress in her: "She is friendly and outgoing in relationships to both staff and her peers. . . . If upset, she has been known to become snappy; however, she is usually apologetic soon afterward. Leslie enjoys weekly visits with her mother and has frequent visits with friends. All her visits are warm and those with her mother seem to indicate improved relationships. . . . She is interested in keeping physically fit, exercising and working outside in the flower garden in the Special Security Unit yard. She had also shown a great deal of interest in silk-screen printing classes. She practices her skill in typing; crochets, sews, and does needlepoint work. She is currently trying to learn to play the guitar."

On August 9, 1974, five years after the LaBianca murders, Leslie appeared for the first time before the Women's Board of Terms and Parole. The X scar on her forehead was beginning to disappear. Though she was not granted parole, the board filed a very favorable report: "Leslie has shown a talent for short stories, screen printing, and, most recently, oil painting. She has participated in the Santa Cruz workshops on weekends and has developed an active interest in the women's movement. She is enrolled in two Chaffey College courses to be given this fall." Leslie was perceived as "a bright, vivacious, cheerful woman who is sensitive to the needs of others. Concrete thinking has returned and along with it has come a realization of where she is and why. She has made a serious attempt with Pat [Krenwinkel] to reconstruct the past in order to understand herself, and a great deal of her depression is due to the resulting insights. She states that her thinking stops short of the crimes and that she fears a total breakdown when she inevitably reaches that point. She sees her former lifestyle with objectivity and realizes that, in her words, 'I blew my life in one night of senseless violence.' "

Leslie went on to take more college courses and eventually became editor of the *Clarion* newspaper at the California Institute for Women at Frontera. She and Pat Krenwinkel collaborated on a book, which was published. She became a member of the Clarion Conscience Club and performed community services, including reading for a blind girl. Her mother, brother, and sister were visiting her on a regular basis, and she was speaking by phone with her father once a month.

By mid-1976, the scar on her forehead was barely perceptible. Leslie was still struggling with guilt over the killings, and she understood that she had not felt any guilt for the first two years because she was too fragile to really own up to her responsibility. Finally able to talk about and reflect on the effect Manson had on her, she said, "The justification he gave us was that if we did it, it would serve the world. He said that if we did that, a revolution would start and everything would change and the tuned-in people would have a free and happy life. The longer I am away from him, the more I see the way he wielded things. I don't want anything to do with him. He knew the mind. We were young and impressionable. He got us loaded on acid and you know that is a mind opener. He knew how to affect your mind. No sense makes sense. On acid he would talk about the Beatles, and when you're down that was the only album we had that would keep the trip going *[The White Album]*. He was always happening. He was the one who was moving the whole thing. There couldn't be peace on earth unless he was out there conducting the orchestra. . . . The only thing, I wonder if he really believed it or just did it to get even for something."

The examining physician concluded: "At the time this young woman involved herself in circumstances leading to the offenses and the aftermath which followed, the time was the late 1960s. Abuse of psychedelic drugs was widespread and openly advocated by certain sectors of the academic community as well as by the communications and entertainment media. Value systems were under open assault, with rebellion and revolution being openly advocated. These conditions have ebbed and paled with the passage of time. Ms. Van Houten has disassociated herself from that situation. She has ability and potential and is considered motivated to develop her positive assets. The overall prognosis in terms of her becoming a productive and contributing member in the community is considered to be favorable. From a psychiatric point of view, there are no contraindications for parole consideration."

Of course, there are other considerations beyond the psychiatric. Leslie was denied parole in 1976, and in every year since then.

The question we have to ask is what purpose does parole play? Is it forgiveness? Does it function properly in society for an act of this enormity?

Parole has many purposes. First, we don't have a jail system big enough to hold all prisoners for the entire length of their sentences. There have been campaigns to parole thousands of people early when prison populations swelled to capacity. The second, and perhaps more important, reason is that we have to have some order within the prison subculture. If an inmate knows he's going to spend ten years behind bars and he won't get out a minute sooner for good behavior, why should he cooperate? Parole provides a reward for good behavior.

The third reason we have parole is to support our belief that there is such a thing as rehabilitation, that we can make an attempt to return people to society by encouraging them to behave in a more social rather than antisocial manner. Of course, our willingness to believe in—or gamble on—our ability to rehabilitate depends on the crime. It's one thing to say, Let's parole after one month in prison someone who shoplifted a pair of gloves from a store, and another to say, Let's parole after twenty years someone who took part in the murder of seven people. Is society willing to accept that?

Here is where the politics of parole comes in. The parole board always considers the political effects of releasing a prisoner, as well as the pragmatic effects. Some people are not parolable for psychological or pragmatic reasons, and some are not parolable for political reasons. Consider Leopold and Loeb, the men who kidnapped and killed young Robert Franks. Leopold was killed in prison. Loeb was not paroled for more than thirty years. He'd been a model prisoner all those years. Yet even when he was released there was an outcry. Obviously, he was not the same man who walked into prison thirty years earlier. But because his case was politically hot, his release attracted enough attention to stir up an angry reaction. I'm certain that during the years Loeb was in prison, dozens of killers and kidnappers were paroled after serving far less time, and with far less fanfare and public anger.

For the same reason, Sirhan Sirhan will probably never be released, despite the fact that hundreds of inmates who killed one or more people will be paroled after serving far less time. Charles Manson will most likely never be released. But it's politics that keeps him behind bars, even though there are valid psychological reasons, too. Were it not for the notoriety of the case, Manson probably would have been released long ago. Remember, he was convicted as a conspirator to the murders. He did not participate in the actual killing of any of the victims. But parole boards tend to be more responsive to politics than to either psychology or the finer legal distinctions. And it's politics that's working against Leslie Van Houten and Tex Watson.

Working for Leslie and Tex is our tendency to temper justice with mercy. The system traditionally does not like to think of itself as vindictive or cruel—even to the point where concern for the victims of crimes is placed lower than concern for the criminals. It's only been within the last few years that victims and their relatives have been allowed to testify at parole board hearings.

I believe that, though it is a politically difficult case, Leslie may eventually be granted parole, and that Tex Watson might follow her back into society before too long.

AFTERMATH—ROMAN POLANSKI

Such mercy has not been the destiny of Roman Polanski's life.

After the murders, California became unbearable for him. Roman threw himself into his work, but his next two films were not successful. In 1973, the same producer who hired him to direct *Rosemary's Baby,* Robert Evans, called him to Hollywood to direct *Chinatown.* Polanski had enormous apprehension about returning to California, but his career and his bank account needed a successful picture. He returned to Hollywood and *Chinatown* was a financial and a critical success.

Nevertheless, the next few years were not easy for Roman. He began work on what he hoped would be his best film yet, a comedy-adventure called *Pirates.* After spending the better part of a year writing the script, Polanski set about assembling a cast and obtaining financing for the picture. That task, however, did not go smoothly. Two things haunted Polanski: the fact that his prior successful movies were horror films and *Pirates* was a comedy-adventure and, perhaps more important to his psychological life, the memory of his wife's death.

Polanski was haunted by guilt over Sharon's death, and the psychological poison ate away at him inwardly, in painful contrast to the fast-lane life he lived publicly. "I was welcomed everywhere as a 'jet-setter' and given unending parties," Polanski remembers. But the celebrations were empty to him. And as the parties failed to chase away the nagging sense of gloom and fill the void in his life, Polanski found little to give or receive from others. "I found it harder and harder to establish meaningful relationships with women," he said.

Not only did Roman's love life suffer, but the "packaging" of *Pirates* hit snags. Other projects, such as the movie *The Tenant,* served as diversions. But the film did so poorly that it added to Polanski's difficulties getting *Pirates* into production. What he needed was another successful movie to give him the necessary psychological boost. It would also take the "failure" stigma from his image. So when Columbia Pictures offered him the chance to write and direct a movie made from a best-selling novel, Polanski jumped at the chance. He finished a draft of the screenplay in early 1977, while living in Europe, then returned to Los Angeles to begin post-production work. The name of the picture was to prove cruelly prophetic: *The First Deadly Sin.*

Polanski, as another diversion, had undertaken a project to photograph young women for *Vogue Homme,* a French men's magazine. He told a friend about the project, and the friend told Roman he should consider photographing his girlfriend's sister. Roman's friend reminded him that he had met the young woman's mother a year earlier, in a Hollywood bar. She was an actress who, at the time, was trying to get another agent.

Roman agreed there might be possibilities here, and called the mother to discuss them. She was excited about it, and invited Polanski to her house to meet her daughter. When he went to the house, he showed the prospective model, her mother, and her boyfriend an edition of *Vogue Homme* that featured some of his photographs.

On February 20, 1977, he returned to their home and, with the mother's help, selected some clothes for the photographic session. Then he took the young woman into the hills behind her home to photograph her. The mother did not go along. "I took some pictures of her," Roman recounted. "I asked her to change. She took off her blouse. There was no embarrassment. So next time, I asked her if she would pose without her top." Polanski shot several topless photographs, but then asked his model to put her top back on, because there were some motorcyclists watching them.

Polanski developed the film and decided that the pictures weren't very good. He set up an appointment for another session.

On March 10 Roman returned to pick up the model for another session. This time, he took her to a house in Benedict Canyon, not very far from the home in which his wife had been murdered. There were other people present at this session, although the young woman's mother had remained at home. Roman shot several photographs of the young woman, both with and without her top, until the end of daylight. Polanski remembered that Jack Nicholson's house was nearby and that the light might be better there. He remembered that Nicholson was out of town, but that his friend Anjelica Huston might be there. Roman called the house. No one was home. He was able to reach the caretaker and asked her if he could take some pictures at the house. She told him to come right over.

In the car on the way over to Nicholson's house, the young woman became very talkative. Polanski said, "She was always very talkative when her mother was not there. She mentioned that she liked champagne. She said she once got drunk at her father's house. We talked again about her modeling. We talked about the use of drugs, and she said she had once used Quaaludes, which she stole from her mother. She talked about sex and said she first had sex at eight with a kid down the street, and later her boyfriend."

At Nicholson's house they were met by the caretaker, a neighbor woman who not only took care of Nicholson's house when he was away, but also the third house, which was owned by Marlon Brando. Roman was thirsty and asked the caretaker if there was anything to drink. She told him to look in the refrigerator. He found a bottle of champagne and asked if he could open it. The caretaker said he could, and took out three long-stemmed wine glasses. While they were drinking the champagne, the caretaker noticed that Roman and the young woman were acting like lovers. To her, the woman looked about eighteen years old. Her impression was that this was just another starlet trying to get into the movies.

Roman and the starlet went to work taking pictures. "While I was photographing her on the deck," Polanski said, "she saw the steam from the Jacuzzi. We went inside. She took her blouse off, and I took pictures." In the middle of the session, the young woman called home to tell her mother where she was. Her mother asked her if she wanted her to come pick her up. The young woman said she was all right and she did not need a ride home just yet. According to Polanski, "She told her mother about the Jacuzzi and that she was going in."

Roman jumped into the pool and invited the young woman to come in, too. She declined: "She said she had asthma." Even now, after eight years, the terror of his wife's death haunted him. All it took was the sound of a car and, perhaps, the fact that they were in the vicinity of the murders, to get him started: "I heard a car coming. I was apprehensive. Some maniacs used to come around the compound."

The car went away, the feeling passed, and Roman and his model went into the bathroom together. Polanski broke a Quaalude into three parts, then wondered out loud if he would be able to drive if he took the pill. He went ahead and took part of it and offered some to the young woman. Having already experimented with the drug when she was younger, she accepted it.

The photography session continued, moving on to the hot tub. His model undressed and Roman took several nude photographs of her. She then got out of the tub and told him that she wanted to go home because she had asthma and needed to take her medicine. Roman told her to go into the bedroom and lie down.

Roman followed her into the bedroom. "The whole thing was very spontaneous," he said, "it was not planned." He lay down next to her and started kissing her. After performing cunnilingus on her, he began to have sexual intercourse with her. "She never objected," he said. Polanski withdrew before ejaculation, and then, according to the young woman, performed an act of anal intercourse.

Suddenly there was a knock on the bedroom door. A woman's voice asked, "Roman, are you in there?"

It was Anjelica Huston. Polanski got up from the bed, went to the door, and spoke briefly with her, then returned to the young woman on the bed and attempted intercourse.

A short time later, Polanski and the young woman left the bedroom and talked with Anjelica Huston for a while. Then Roman drove his starlet home. When she entered the house, he heard her tell her mother, "If he says anything about asthma, I told him I had asthma."

Roman showed the mother the photographs from the first session. When she discovered that some of the photographs of her daughter were topless, she refused to sign a release. Roman left.

Later that night, the young woman's boyfriend came over. She told him what had happened at Jack Nicholson's house, and her mother overheard the story. Enraged, the mother called her accountant to ask him to recommend a lawyer. He gave her an attorney's name, but also told her she should call the police right away.

The next day, March 11, 1977, Roman Polanski was arrested in the lobby of the Beverly Wilshire Hotel. His film was confiscated and his room searched. Police found Quaalude tablets. A grand jury later returned a long list of charges against him, including furnishing Quaalude to a minor, child molesting, unlawful sexual intercourse, rape by use of drugs, oral copulation, and sodomy. Roman Polanski's starlet was only thirteen years old.

Anjelica Huston testified that the young woman did not appear to be only thirteen, that she could have been twenty-five.

"She did not look like a thirteen-year-old little scared thing. She seemed quite tall to me, a pretty well-developed girl. I would not have thought she was thirteen." About Polanski, she said, "I don't feel that he would sodomize, forcibly sodomize and rape an unwilling girl. I don't feel that about him. I have seen him as a man with compassion, not a man who would forcibly hurt another person. I really don't. He is very opinionated, and he has a strong character, but I don't think he's a bad man. I think he's a very unhappy man."

The testimony went quickly downhill from there. The young woman was asked how long Roman's penis had been in her vagina. She answered: "I can't remember how long, but not a very long time."

When the story broke, Columbia Pictures fired Polanski from *The First Deadly Sin*. Dino DeLaurentiis hired him to direct *The Hurricane*, but Polanski worried that even that project might be in jeopardy. And when the story became an international headline—a German newsweekly published a photograph of Polanski with prison bars superimposed over his face—both Polanski and the girl and her family began to receive vicious hate mail, particularly from Germany.

One day in August 1977, Roman went to visit Sharon's grave. While at her grave, he heard a familiar sound—a motion picture camera. There was a German photographer in the bushes. Roman got angry, charged the man, and took the camera away. Unable to remove the film, Roman took the camera to the cemetery office. It was returned to the photographer that night. The man tried to press charges against Roman for grand theft and assault and battery, but the D.A.'s office rejected the charges.

On August 8, 1977, eight years almost to the hour from his wife's murder, Roman appeared in court and pleaded guilty to charges of unlawful sexual intercourse. The plea was the result of an agreement worked out between the parties. The attorney for the young woman and her mother accepted the plea bargain, ostensibly to avoid the possible harm a trial and the publicity might inflict on the young woman. Her identity was kept secret by both sides and by the press. The girl and her family stated that by pressing charges they did not want Polanski to be "thrown into prison," but rather hoped that he would admit to the wrong-doing and submit to a court-supervised rehabilitation program.

But Roman *was* in danger of being thrown into prison. Once the plea bargain was accepted, the criminal proceedings were halted. However, it was only a temporary interruption so that psychiatric tests could be performed to determine whether or not Roman Polanski was a mentally disordered sex offender. I was called in on the case. The judge wanted to send Polanski to the prison at Chino to be evaluated by the psychiatric staff there. He could be held in custody for ninety days. I argued that this was not a good idea and was not necessary. Nevertheless, Roman, who had been free on bail, was taken into custody and sent to Chino.

If I had found Polanski to be a mentally disordered sex offender, it could have meant that he would wind up in a mental hospital for an indefinite period of time. But I did not find him to be one. In my report I said that Roman Polanski was not a mentally disordered sex offender and that on psychiatric grounds he was not a danger to the health and safety of others. I also said I did not believe he required any psychiatric hospitalization. Informally, I advised not sending him back to Chino. Polanski had served forty days there and was out on bail pending a decision in his case. There was a good chance the judge would send him back there for the remainder of the ninety-day sentence. I don't think Polanski would have been required to serve more than another fifty days, but in a highly publicized case of this nature anything was possible.

The ironies in this case started to sink in. Least of all was the fact that I had examined two of the people who had taken part in the murder of this man's wife—and now I had examined him. But the really monstrous ironies were in Polanski's life. Roman Polanski had been pursued by horror all his life. He had managed to escape the Nazi horror as Europe came under its death grip only to see his mother taken away to be killed as she carried an unborn child. The horror had finally caught up with him not in a country overrun by a savage army, but in the United States of America, where he had sent his wife and their unborn child. He had seen his culture and family decimated by the Nazi mentality, where people were committing violence because their leaders "told them to"—and then he ran into the very same thing, but in a country where freedom is the rule.

Now, that country, which was known as the "land of the free," the sanctuary for so many refugees fleeing from unjust incarceration, was about to make another one of Roman Polanski's nightmares come true: it was sending him to prison.

Chino has been called a "country club" among prisons. It is a minimum security facility. However, to Roman Polanski, the qualitative differences between a "country club" prison and any other were negligible. To him, a prison was a prison and the idea of spending time in a prison invoked deep-seated, extremely powerful anxieties. The fear he felt was the same he experienced as a child narrowly escaping time after time the Nazi death squads come to round up people for the concentration camps. His forty-day stay did little to calm his fears. And as he faced the prospect of going back—for a possibly much longer stay—the anxiety was intolerable. Roman Polanski felt threatened as deeply and as devastatingly as if the SS troops were banging on his door, having come to take him away.

So he fled. He jumped bail and escaped to Europe, to live in self-imposed exile, a fugitive from the United States. If he ever returns and is caught, he will face prison not only for his original charges, but for the more serious crime of jumping bail.

I wonder if the criminal justice system will ever show him any mercy. Is society willing to accept the return of Roman Polanski? From time to time there are flurries of publicity about ongoing efforts by the director's friends and representatives to reach an agreement with the D.A.'s office that would allow him to return and face probation rather than prison. Public response to these efforts is usually negative. Letters to the editor following a recent story about Polanski were almost unanimously against forgiving him, and made generous use of such words as "reprehensible, criminal, pervert, raping, and molesting," none of which really apply to the man or to the psychiatric facts of his case.

So just as politics is working against Leslie Van Houten and Tex Watson, it also works against Roman Polanski. Judging from my experience with this crazy system of ours, my guess is that the people who murdered his wife will freely walk the streets of Hollywood long before he does.

EPILOGUE

In early 1986 I was approached to take part in the production of a TV documentary about the psychological background of killers and any possible changes these people had undergone while in custody. In May of that year I wrote a letter to Tex Watson at the California Men's Colony in San Luis Obispo, and asked him if he would like to participate.

Tex wrote back and said that if I wanted a case that "testifies of the changes that have been undergone during custody, I am a classic case."

The letter came typed neatly on letterhead from the "Abounding Love Ministries." In the upper left-hand corner of the page was a picture of two hands reaching up and plucking a bunch of grapes from the vine. Below the logo was "1 Thes. 3:12," a reference to a verse in the New Testament, and below that, the names of the officers of the organization. The president of the Abounding Love Ministries was Charles D. Watson. The vice president was Kristin Watson, his wife. At the bottom of the page, printed in the same blue ink as the logo and the letterhead, was the message: SERVING OUR LORD JESUS CHRIST, MINISTERING TO CHILDREN, ADULTS, PRISONERS.

In his letter, Tex went on to say, "Lately, as you can see from the ministry my wife and I now have, we are Christians. I am now married with two boys. I am not over-zealous in my Christian talk, so please do not worry that I would come off fanatical. I am very well-grounded theologically, and have it well-balanced psychologically. I have studied both quite extensively. Over the past years I have had many psychological groups which I would be able to comment on as well as my Christian experience, and the dependence that I now have in God. I believe we could do a great interview."

I looked up the verse Tex's stationery referred to in the New Testament, 1 Thessalonians, 3:12. As I read it, I couldn't help but remember how the Manson Family had excused their brutal crimes by saying they had acted out of love—love for the world, love for the children, love for the future, love for Sharon Tate, Jay Sebring, Abigail Folger, Voytek Frykowski, Steven Parent, love for Leno and Rosemary LaBianca—and that if you act out of love, you're beyond blame:

And may the Lord make you increase and abound in love to one another and to all men, as we do to you, so that He may establish your hearts unblamable. . . .

CHAPTER

8

"NO FURTHER DANGER TO OTHERS"

One of the hottest battlegrounds in psychiatry and law is whether we are any good at predicting just how dangerous a particular person really is. Will a thief steal again? Will a rapist attack again? Will a killer take another life? Will a criminal graduate to more serious and violent crimes? Our record is not at all good. The public perception that dangerous people are often set free sooner than they should be is unfortunately correct.

But psychiatrists don't set criminals free: judges, juries, and parole boards do. While there are some courtroom psychiatrists who use the legal system as an arena for their particular political or psychiatric agendas, the criteria for early, and sometimes premature, release are legal, not medical. In some instances it *is* possible to predict with a significant degree of accuracy just how dangerous a criminal is. But in my experience, when psychiatric testimony conflicts, courts pay attention only to testimony that tends to support what they've already decided to do, based on earlier, independent judgment. When a court puts a dangerous criminal back on the street based on psychiatric testimony, you can bet there was plenty of opposing expert testimony that warned of the danger. The court was simply exploiting the psychiatric report consistent with its own desires.

The plain fact is that our criminal justice system itself promotes the premature release of known dangerous people, whether they are mentally ill or not. All manner of criminals, from petty thieves to rapists and murderers, are routinely released after serving only a fraction of their sentences even if the authorities strongly suspect that another crime will be committed soon after they are set free.

In one such case I examined a man who had been convicted of second-degree murder for killing a six-month-old baby during a burglary. The defendant's parents testified that they believed he was mentally ill and required treatment rather than punishment. They fully believed they were testifying on his behalf—but he did not. The young man not only denied that he was mentally ill, but in open court denounced his parents and swore to kill them. He was convicted and sentenced to twelve years.

Over the next seven years, the young man was closely observed not only by prison authorities but by state hospital psychiatric personnel. Although his general behavior was good, he continued to express his hatred for his parents. When I evaluated him, I stated without hesitation that he represented a distinct future danger. But my opinion was ignored and the young man's sentence was reduced as a reward for his "good behavior."

Within a month of his release he killed both his parents, as promised.

In my opinion, the system was not willing to prevent those killings. Even if the young man had not been set free early, he would have been released at the end of his twelve-year term, no matter what anyone said about how dangerous he might be. Our criminal justice system is simply not able to take responsibility for protecting society against "future danger." Neither are many forensic psychiatrists, who believe that such testimony is beyond their scope of knowledge.

I don't think it's a shortage of knowledge that puts dangerous criminals back on the streets. Based on my experience, I believe that psychiatrists can and should render opinions on this issue, provided they are careful not to exceed the limits of the information at hand. And if the criminal justice system can then itself stay sane long enough to use the information, a lot of dangerous criminals might be kept behind bars and a lot of awful crimes might be prevented.

Unfortunately, the system is not up to it, and the horror of the resulting crimes is doubled by the fact that they could have been prevented.

The case of Bittaker and Norris is a good example. I examined Lawrence Bittaker four years before he teamed up with Roy Norris, and I indicated that this was a very dangerous man with a clear recidivistic risk. Unfortunately, my opinion was disregarded. If it had been considered and acted upon, a grisly murder spree that was in many ways more horrible and cruel than the Tate–LaBianca killings could have been prevented.

Lawrence Sigmund Bittaker, who would one day tell a prison cell mate that he wanted to be "bigger than Manson," certainly started off on the right foot with regard to outdistancing his idol. Like Manson, Bittaker spent more than half of his first forty years in prison.

Lawrence was born September 27, 1940, in Pittsburgh. Abandoned by his natural parents, he was adopted by George Bittaker and his wife. George was an aircraft worker, and the family moved around a lot. Lawrence grew up in Pennsylvania, Florida, Ohio and, finally, California, where, at the age of seventeen, he quit school after being involved with the police and juvenile authorities. The Long Beach police arrested him for hit-and-run, auto theft, and evading arrest. After serving time at the California Youth Authority facility, the nineteen-year-old was released. From that moment on, Bittaker's record is littered with felonies, burglaries, robberies, assaults, and misdemeanors. The highlights include the following:

Within days of his first parole, Bittaker got arrested again. This time, he was arrested in Louisiana by federal authorities for transporting a stolen vehicle across state lines. In August 1959 he was sentenced to eighteen months in the Federal Reformatory in Oklahoma but was soon transferred to the medical center for federal prisoners in Springfield, Missouri.

Bittaker was released before he served his entire term, and soon was back in trouble. In December 1960 he was convicted of robbery in Los Angeles. In May 1961 he was sent to prison for an indeterminate sentence of up to fifteen years. He was paroled at the end of 1963, after serving barely more than two years. Not surprisingly, two months later he was arrested on suspicion of robbery and parole violation. In October 1964 he went to prison for parole violation—but was paroled again in June 1967. Within a month Bittaker was back before a judge for misdemeanor hit-and-run and petty theft. He was sent back to prison for a five-year sentence.

Bittaker served fewer than three of those five years. He was released in April 1970. Within a year, he was arrested for burglary, and in October 1971 was sentenced to six months to fifteen years for the related parole violation. Released early again, Bittaker was arrested in 1974 for assault with intent to commit murder. I was called in to examine him and determine his "mental state"—his sanity at the time of the offense—and whether, if insane at that time, he had regained his sanity.

Bittaker had walked into a supermarket and tried to walk out with a piece of meat, which he had stuffed into his pants. One of the supermarket clerks observed the apparent shoplifting and pursued him. When confronted by the clerk in the parking lot, true to his character, Bittaker pulled a knife and stabbed him.

Before I examined Lawrence Bittaker I reviewed his records. Not only were they littered with crimes, but also with a potpourri of psychiatric diagnoses. In 1961 he was described as being very manipulative and "having considerable concealed hostility." Although the examining doctor said Bittaker had "superior intelligence," he also labeled him "borderline psychotic" and "basically paranoid." Such diagnoses, whether accurate or not, tend to stick to an individual like glue that never dries. Then, as the individual shuffles through the system, he gathers more of the same vague labels, which no one ever really takes too seriously.

So in 1962 it was added that Bittaker had "poor control of his impulsive behavior." In 1966 a psychiatrist said Bittaker, still manipulative, admitted that stealing cars made him feel important and bragged that he had stolen "too many cars." Nevertheless, Bittaker insisted that his ever-lengthening list of crimes was created "under circumstances that were not totally my fault." He explained that he had been mistreated, misunderstood, and falsely accused through his entire life. Another examining doctor said he was borderline psychotic, that he had no insight into his emotional problems, and showed no willingness to change. Bittaker was given antipsychotic medication.

I didn't need these records to figure out Lawrence Bittaker: Interviewing him was enough to tell me he was a sociopath. He tried to evade responsibility by saying that he was intoxicated by tranquilizers and beer and that he had no recall of the incident at the supermarket. "I supposedly went into the supermarket—I put meat in my pants and went out the door," he said, with the accent on "supposedly." All he claimed to remember was going to the supermarket for some milk and waking up at the Hollywood police station. "I can't seem to keep my nose out of trouble," he told me, and blamed all his problems on alcohol. Although Bittaker claimed he had been under the influence of drugs and alcohol during most of his past crimes, he denied that he abused them.

Lawrence Bittaker was not "borderline psychotic" when I examined him, and probably had never been in the past, either. In fact, he admitted that he had faked psychotic behavior while in custody. No, Bittaker was not insane. He was a classic psychopath or, in more modern terms, a sociopath, or antisocial personality. Sociopathy is a character disorder not usually categorized as a mental illness. Lawrence Bittaker was incapable of learning to play by the rules, he would never learn by experience, and would just keep butting his head against the barriers of acceptable behavior. With luck, these attacks against society would remain relatively petty in comparison to what sociopaths have been known to do (for example, Zimmerman), and Bittaker would just bounce in and out of jail for the rest of his life.

But, I warned, the risks were much higher that Bittaker would move on to worse crimes. This was a highly dangerous man, with no internal controls over his impulses, a man who could kill without hesitation or remorse.

Bittaker went back to prison and, once again, wound up in a prison mental hospital, where he was given tranquilizers. In 1977 an examining physician said that Bittaker would "more than likely" commit more crimes—but, remarkably, also said that there was no psychiatric reason why he should not be granted parole! In July 1978 a staff psychologist noted, correctly, that Bittaker was a "sophisticated psychopath" and that the prognosis for parole was "guarded at best." Nevertheless, in November 1978 Bittaker was released from prison.

Prisons have often been called "colleges for criminals," where inmates, rather than being rehabilitated, only learn more sophisticated methods of crime. That much is true. But an even more sinister thing happens in prison: Inmates form partnerships that raise their combined potential danger far beyond what each would be capable of alone. We have laws against conspiracy for the very reason that two or more people sitting around talking about a crime are much more likely to commit the crime—and even worse crimes—than any individual acting alone. When two or more criminal thoughts connect, the eventual criminal act can be magnified to horrific dimensions. Lawrence Bittaker made such a connection with Roy Norris.

Norris, like Bittaker, was a many-time loser. He was born February 2, 1948, in Greeley, Colorado, and never moved away until he was seventeen, when he quit school to join the navy. Norris was stationed in San Diego, but served four months in Vietnam in 1969. He experimented with heroin for a few weeks but never became addicted. Whenever marijuana was available, he used it.

In November 1969, Norris was arrested for forcible rape and assault with attempt to commit rape. He had attempted to force his way into a woman's car in downtown San Diego and rape her. Not inhibited in the least by his arrest, a few months later, in February 1970, while on bail and awaiting disposition of the rape charge, he walked up to a woman's home and asked to use the telephone. When the woman sent him away, Norris went around to the living room window and tried to break into the house. Failing there, he succeeded in opening the kitchen window, but the woman summoned the police before he could harm her.

In 1970 the navy gave Norris an administrative discharge for "psychological problems." Medical officers diagnosed him as a severe "schizoid personality." Once out of the navy, he continued where he left off. In May 1970 he stalked a young woman walking near the San Diego State College campus. Norris went up to her, started talking to her, then suddenly, from behind, repeatedly struck her with a rock until she fell to her knees. He then pounced upon her and bounced her head up and down on the concrete sidewalk.

Norris was charged with assault with a deadly weapon and was eventually committed to Atascadero State Hospital as a mentally disordered sex offender. He spent almost five years there, and was released in 1970 on five-year formal probation. The doctors at the hospital said Norris was "no further danger to others." It took him only three months to prove them wrong. Norris forcibly raped a woman in Redondo Beach. The twenty-seven-year-old victim was walking home from a restaurant after having an argument with her husband. Norris drove up beside her on his motorcycle and asked her if she would like a ride. She declined. Not to be deterred, Norris parked his motorcycle and fell in step beside her. First he tried to give her a hug. When she tried to pull away from him he grabbed her scarf and twisted it tighter around her neck. Then Norris said to her, "I'm going to rape you." Because the woman was afraid he would harm her if she resisted, she did not attempt to flee. Norris dragged her into some trees and tall bushes and then raped her.

The woman called the police but they were unable to find her attacker. One month later, however, the woman spotted Norris riding his motorcycle around town and immediately called the police and gave them his license number. He was arrested, charged with rape, convicted by a jury, and sent to state prison.

During his last year at the California Men's Colony at San Luis Obispo, 1978, Roy Norris met Lawrence Bittaker. According to Norris, Bittaker saved his life on two separate occasions; therefore, he was bound by the "prison code" to maintain his friendship with Bittaker and cooperate with him. Of course, in true sociopathic fashion, this bond was only adhered to when it was convenient, for Norris was at least as dangerous a psychopath as Bittaker. Together, the two men became an extremely deadly combination. They spent a lot of time talking about what they were going to do once they got out of prison. Norris and Bittaker found they had a lot in common, including a mutual interest in dominating, hurting, and raping women. While in prison together they often talked about rape. Bittaker said if he ever raped a woman he would kill her and leave no witnesses.

Bittaker was released from prison in November 1978. Two

months later Norris was released, and while living at his mother's house he received a letter from Bittaker. At the end of February they renewed their friendship at a Los Angeles hotel. Bittaker was working as a machinist and Norris, who had been trained in electronics while in prison, got a job as an electronics technician. The two ex-cons began spending weekends together in the South Bay area of Los Angeles. It was spring in Southern California, and although rainy, dreary days were always possible, most days were sunny and balmy, perfect for the beach.

And that's where Norris and Bittaker spent most of their leisure time. They would drive up and down the Pacific Coast Highway, then park and walk up and down the strand watching the young bikini-clad women on the beach. Sometimes they would go up to them and talk to them, sometimes they would snap photographs. Eventually, they decided that if the opportunity arose, they would kidnap a young girl and rape her.

Bittaker decided they would need the right kind of vehicle to carry out this plan. After looking around, he finally settled on a 1977 silver GMC cargo van. The truck had a sliding door and no windows on the side. Both men figured the sliding door would make it easier to steal things. They could "pull up real close and not have to open the doors all the way." It would also make it easier to kidnap young women, they agreed.

The two men soon found, however, that it would hardly be necessary for them to force young women into their van. There were plenty of young women who would get in voluntarily. From February to June, Norris and Bittaker picked up more than twenty female hitchhikers. They did not assault any of them, but they were only biding their time, preparing. Part of the preparation was finding a place to take their victims once they kidnapped them. Toward the end of April, Bittaker drove Norris to a remote area in the San Gabriel Mountains above the city of Glendora. As they drove up into the mountains away from the city, they reached a remote fire road and Bittaker stopped the van. He got out of the van, taking a crowbar with him, approached the locked gate, and furiously struck at the lock until it shattered. Then he replaced it with his own lock. Now they had a place to go where no one would bother them.

June 24, 1979, "started innocently enough," according to

Bittaker, who wrote a detailed account of their activities over the next few months. Bittaker had slept in his van, parked at the trailer park where Norris still lived with his mother. The two men spent the morning improving the bed in the back of the van. With wooden braces and a plywood base, they supported a twin-size mattress three feet off the floor across the back. They kept tools, clothes, and a cooler in the storage area underneath.

At around 11 A.M. they drove to the beach. It was, according to Bittaker, "a nice Sunday to cruise around the beach area, drinking beer, smoking grass, and flirting with the girls. We had no set routine," he continued, "and ranged from Pacific Palisades up through Redondo Beach, Hermosa Beach, Manhattan Beach, to Venice and Santa Monica. Neither did we always ride, but would scout the beach sidewalk on foot in Venice, camera in hand and grass in pocket, shooting pictures of the scantily clad and lovely wheeled young ladies zigging and zagging through pedestrians on those sunny summer days, and stopping to chat with any presentable girls that were unescorted and seemingly friendly and approachable. We'd also cruise Pacific Coast Highway, offering a ride, a toke, or a Coke from the cooler to the girls and couples we picked up."

Bittaker and Norris passed the day that way until around 5 P.M. when, cruising down the streets of Redondo Beach, Norris "noticed a blond girl walking down a side street." (According to Norris, Bittaker saw her first and said, "There's a cute little blond.") They had spotted sixteen-year-old Cindy Schaeffer. Cindy was not one of the "scantily clad" beach girls. She was walking home to her grandmother's house from a senior high fellowship meeting at Saint Andrews's Presbyterian Church in Redondo Beach. She had left early and decided to walk home rather than call her grandmother for a ride. She was wearing blue jeans and a white blouse. Unaware that she was being stalked by the two men in the silver van, Cindy stooped to play with a cat that had crossed her path. Then she continued walking and crossed the street.

The van pulled up alongside her and Norris asked her if she wanted to get in, go for a ride, and smoke some grass. Cindy said she didn't, and kept on walking. Bittaker and Norris didn't give up, however. They followed Cindy from a distance. She passed a group of men gathered on a street corner drinking beer, and Bittaker noticed that the men offered Cindy a beer, but she walked right by. Then she reached a residential street where there was little traffic.

Because the street was packed with cars parked in front of the houses, Bittaker pulled up ahead of her and stopped the van in front of a driveway. Norris opened the sliding side door, got out, and waited on the sidewalk as Cindy approached. When she reached him, they exchanged a few words and then Norris grabbed her and started to drag her into the van. Cindy screamed three times before Norris covered her mouth, got her into the truck, and slammed the door shut. Bittaker stepped on the gas and the van roared away, leaving behind one of Cindy's shoes, which had come off during the brief struggle. Then he turned up the radio full-blast to drown out Cindy's muffled screams. On their way up the street, they passed the group of men drinking beer on the corner. While Norris put tape over Cindy's mouth and bound her hands and feet, Bittaker found the freeway and headed for the mountains.

In his account of the night, Bittaker wrote that "throughout the whole experience, Cindy displayed a magnificent state of self-control and composed acceptance of the conditions and facts over which she had no control. She shed no tears, offered no resistance, and expressed no great concern for her safety. I guess she knew what was coming."

When they reached the fire road, Bittaker opened the gate and they drove to a remote spot. "Now we have a little party," Norris said, as the two men started smoking marijuana. Bittaker asked her several questions and learned that she lived with her grandmother in Torrance, that her mother was in Mexico, and that she had a boyfriend back in Wisconsin.

The two men grew tired of talking, ordered Cindy to remove her clothes, and then started fondling her. "I'll go first," Norris said, and then told Bittaker to take a walk and come back in an hour. While Bittaker was away, Norris raped Cindy and forced her to perform oral intercourse. Then it was Bittaker's turn. Later, Norris came back for more.

In stories the two men later told police, the next thing they did was argue over whether or not to kill Cindy. Each man said it was the other who wanted to kill her while he wanted to let her go. Whether or not there really was an argument, Cindy was the loser.

First, Norris tried to strangle her, but after a minute, when he saw the anguished, terrified look in her eyes, he felt sick and stopped. Norris went to the front of the van and threw up. When he came back, Bittaker was strangling Cindy. She fell to the ground when Bittaker released his grasp on her neck. But Norris could see that "her body was still jerking . . . alive to some degree . . . breathing or trying to breathe." Bittaker remarked that it takes more than what they do on TV to strangle someone, and Norris agreed. Bittaker handed him a piece of coat hanger and told Norris to wrap it around Cindy's throat.

The two men tried to twist the coat hanger around Cindy's throat, but they couldn't get it tight enough by hand, so they used a pair of vise-grip pliers. Then, according to Norris, her body "convulsed for fifteen seconds or so and that was it. She just died."

The coat hanger was twisted so tightly that it had cut Cindy's skin and she had bled before she died. To keep her blood from getting on the carpet in the van, they wrapped her body in a blue shower curtain. Then Norris drove the van along the fire road with Bittaker walking in front with a flashlight, looking for a steep enough canyon by the side of the road. When they found one, they threw Cindy Schaeffer's body over the side. Bittaker said the animals would eat her up so there wouldn't be any evidence left.

On July 8, 1979, Bittaker and Norris were once again cruising along the Pacific Coast Highway looking for a victim. They spotted eighteen-year-old Andrea Joy Hall hitchhiking and were about to pick her up when she got into a white convertible. Bittaker and Norris decided to follow the car, figuring she would get out sooner or later. She did—and immediately started hitchhiking again.

This time, Norris hid under the bed in the back so that the young woman wouldn't see that there were two men in the van. Bittaker pulled up alongside her, opened the door, and she got in. Then he offered her a cold drink and told her she could get it herself out of the cooler in the back of the van. Andrea went back and got a drink out of the cooler. As she was returning to the front of the van, Norris came out of hiding and sprang at her back. While the radio blared at full blast to drown out the screams, Andrea fought furiously but couldn't overcome the bigger, stronger Norris. He finally subdued her by grabbing one of her arms and forcing it up behind her, causing great pain. Then he taped her mouth, wrists, and ankles. Bittaker steered the van toward the mountains.

At their remote spot on the fire road, the men raped Andrea repeatedly. Then, while Norris went to a store down the road, Bittaker took her into the hills. When Norris returned, Bittaker had some photographs of Andrea Hall to show him. Norris described the look on her face as one of sheer terror. He said that Bittaker "told me that he told her he was going to kill her. He wanted to see what her argument would be for her staying alive. He said that she didn't put up much of an argument."

When Bittaker was done torturing Andrea verbally, he did it physically. He took an ice pick and jammed it into her brain through her ear. Then he pulled it out and did the same in the other ear. But that failed to kill her fast enough, so he had to strangle her, too. Then he threw her body over a cliff.

Almost two months later, on Labor Day, September 3, 1979, Bittaker and Norris spotted their third and fourth victims casually walking/hitchhiking along the Pacific Coast Highway. Jackie Gilliam, fifteen, and Leah Lamp, thirteen, were taking a rest at a bus stop bench at the corner of Pacific Coast Highway and Pier Avenue in Hermosa Beach when the silver GMC van pulled up next to them. The girls got in the van voluntarily when the two men offered them a ride.

The girls also accepted the joints Bittaker and Norris offered them. As they were casually smoking the marijuana, the girls noticed that Bittaker had steered the van off Pacific Coast Highway to the right, toward the mountains instead of the beach, where the girls thought they were going. When they asked what was going on, Bittaker said he was only taking a slight detour to give them all time to get high on the marijuana.

But the girls didn't buy the story and started protesting that they wanted to go back toward the beach. When Leah Lamp started trying to open the door to get out, Norris came up behind her and whacked her on the head with a bat. Realizing that the entire struggle was taking place in front of several people watching from a tennis court, Bittaker stopped the van and came around and helped Norris subdue the girls. With the girls immobilized and bound and gagged with tape, the silver GMC van pulled away and sped off toward the San Gabriel Mountains.

Bittaker and Norris kept Jackie and Leah prisoner for almost two days. As they repeatedly raped and tortured them, they tape-recorded the sessions, which progressed from the girls' forced cooperation in the men's fantasies, to their whimpers of fear, to their screams of pain. When Norris raped Jackie Gilliam, he told her to act as if she was his cousin, because he had always had a fantasy of raping his cousin.

Finally, they stabbed Jackie through the ears with an ice pick. Again, it failed to kill, so they had to strangle her. They killed Leah Lamp by strangling her as well. While Bittaker tightened his grip around her neck, Norris savagely battered her head with a sledgehammer. She fell to the ground, but her eyes came open, so as Bittaker attacked her neck again with his powerful hands, Norris set upon her head with the sledgehammer . . . five, six, seven times.

They threw the bodies over a steep cliff into the bushes, with the ice pick still stuck in Jackie Gilliam's ear.

Bittaker and Norris waited almost two months before selecting another victim. This time, they found a victim elsewhere from the beach. On Halloween 1979 they were driving in the Sunland–Tujunga section of the San Fernando Valley when they spotted sixteen-year-old Shirley Ledford hitchhiking. She voluntarily got in the van when the men offered her a ride, unaware that from that moment she had barely two hours to live.

Within five minutes after they pulled away from the sidewalk, Shirley was bound and gagged with the construction tape

Norris always used. This time they decided to torture and rape
her in the van as they drove along through the streets of the San
Fernando Valley. They took the tape off her mouth and legs.
Bittaker started the tape recorder and, while Norris piloted the
van, went to work on Shirley with a hammer and a pair of pliers.
He sodomized Shirley, raped her, and forced her to perform fellatio on him—all the while beating her on the right elbow with
the hammer to make her scream.

"Start the van," Bittaker said. Then he slapped Shirley. "Say
something, girl, huh?" He slapped her again. "Huh." He struck
her harder.

"What do you want me to say?" Shirley asked.

"Huh, huh," Bittaker mocked her. "Say something, girl."
Then he slapped her three times and mocked her again, "Don't
you hit me! Huh, huh!"

Shirley moaned.

"Say something, girl," he insisted.

"Ouch."

Bittaker slapped her again, and she screamed.

"Say something." He slapped her again. "C'mon, you can
scream louder than that, can't you?" He struck her twice more,
grunting "Huh!" as his blows descended on the helpless young
woman. "What's the matter, don't you like to scream?" He struck
her repeatedly.

Shirley screamed louder and Bittaker struck her repeatedly.
"Oh no!" she cried.

"What's the matter, huh, you want to try again?"

"Oh no!" she screamed. "Don't touch me, no!"

"Huh? You want to try again?"

"Oh no, don't touch me, no, don't touch me!" she cried.

"Want to try again?"

"No, no, no, no, no, no, no!"

"Roll over, girl," Bittaker ordered.

"No, don't touch me."

"Roll over."

"Don't touch me."

"Start getting to work, girl."

"Don't touch me, don't touch me!"

Bittaker slapped her hard. "Get to work, girl."

"Don't touch me."

"I'm not asking you, I'm telling you!"

As Shirley started to cry, Bittaker ordered her to roll over. "C'mon, c'mon, c'mon." Then he forced her to fellate him and describe to him what she was doing. As she obeyed his orders, he struck her and ordered her to "Scream, baby . . . if it hurts any-time you want to scream go ahead and scream . . . scream, baby, scream some more, baby."

When Shirley had trouble screaming loud enough to suit him, Bittaker fumbled through his toolbox and came up with a pair of pliers. First he threatened Shirley with them and got her to scream more convincingly. Then he started squeezing Shirley's nipples with the pliers.

"Is the recorder going?" he asked Norris.

"Yeah," Norris replied.

Shirley screamed. "No, no, no! Oh no!" Then she wailed in pain.

"Make noise there, girl," Norris urged, as he traded places with Bittaker. "Go ahead and scream or I'll make you scream."

Shirley moaned unintelligibly.

"Oh yeah," Norris cheered.

"Oh . . ." Shirley moaned in pain.

"Scream!" Norris ordered. Then he struck her on the elbow with the hammer.

Shirley screamed. "I'll scream if you stop hitting me." Then she screamed.

"Keep it up, girl."

Shirley screamed.

"Keep it up."

Shirley screamed.

"More!"

Shirley screamed again.

"Till I say stop."

Shirley screamed, and then cried out "Oh no!" as she saw Norris going for the hammer again. As he struck her again and again on the elbow, the young woman screamed once for all of the twenty-five times he struck her. At one point, she may have tried to say something, but her voice had become an unintel-ligible mass of pain.

Bittaker asked what was going on.

"I was just beating on her elbows with this hammer," Norris replied.

Shirley screamed again.

"What are you sniveling about?" Norris asked her. Then he started hitting her with the hammer again, and the sounds of the beating mixed with the sounds of the screaming and went on and on and on. . . .

Later, when the men were done, Bittaker volunteered to kill her. "I got a section of coat hanger," he said, "and wrapped it around her throat and tied it up with pliers." He twisted the wire tighter with the vise grips until Shirley died.

Then Bittaker decided it would be interesting to see the reaction of the press if they dumped the young woman's body on someone's front lawn. So they pulled up to a house in Sunland and threw Shirley Ledford's body into the ivy, where it was found the next morning.

Until Shirley Ledford's body was found, police really didn't take much notice of the disappearance of the young women in the South Bay area. So many young girls take off with their boyfriends, run away from home, or simply disappear. . . . Cindy, Andrea, Jackie, and Leah were a few among many. As far as the police were concerned, there was nothing to do until there was some evidence. And even then . . .

Although there was a firestorm in the press, after the horribly battered corpse was discovered, all the police could do was routinely investigate the neighborhood and hope for a little luck.

Almost three weeks went by, and then that luck arrived in a series of events that gave police the break they needed.

While visiting her father in Southern California, another young woman, Robin Robeck, had been kidnapped and raped. The assault had occurred between the disappearances of Jackie and Leah in early September and Shirley in late October. Robin, however, had been released by her assailants. Although she reported the incident, she was unable to identify any suspects. Before long she returned to Oregon, the victim of an apparently unsolved crime.

Meanwhile, Roy Norris couldn't keep his pride in his recent

exploits to himself. He bragged to a former prison buddy, a man named Joe Jackson, about what he had been doing to some of the girls at the beach these past few months. Jackson immediately went to his attorney, and the two men went to the Los Angeles Police Department with their story.

Without taking any action themselves, the LAPD referred Jackson and his attorney to the Hermosa Beach police.

The Hermosa Beach police were interested, and Detective Paul Bynum was assigned chief investigator of the case. Bynum felt that Jackson's story might be true, but it was not sufficient evidence for a conviction or even an arrest.

But there was the Robin Robeck case which, with the exception of the lack of a torture-murder climax, seemed to have a similar modus operandi as the events described by Jackson. Perhaps there was a link. An investigator was dispatched to Oregon to show Robin a series of mug shots. She positively identified Bittaker and Norris as her assailants. Now Bynum had some real evidence, and the authorities went into coordinated action. For starters, Bynum called in Deputy District Attorney Steve Kay, who had prosecuted Norris on a rape charge in 1976.

Kay and Bynum realized that they were involved in a chess game, that the next move was theirs, and that it had to be fast. But it also had to be delicate and carefully planned. They had to move in before Norris and Bittaker struck again, but they also had to watch out that they didn't blow their whole case by making too aggressive a move too quickly. All they really had linking the two ex-cons to the murders was Joe Jackson's statement that Norris had bragged about the crimes. The link with Robin Robeck made the case stronger, but they still needed more solid evidence—or a confession. If Norris and Bittaker flatly denied it, and were able to maintain their denial through a trial, there was a good chance they would be acquitted.

Bynum and Kay needed more evidence. They decided to get it from the source—Norris and Bittaker. The parole department, acting in cooperation with Bynum and the Hermosa Beach Police Department, began following Roy Norris, waiting for him to slip up and violate his parole. They observed his dealing in marijuana and figured they had enough for an arrest.

With the cooperation of the Burbank Police Department, the

authorities moved in. On November 20, 1979, while the Burbank police arrested Bittaker at his residence on suspicion of rape
and kidnapping in the Robeck case, the Hermosa Beach police
arrested Norris for parole violation. Neither man was arrested for
the rape-torture murders. Yet. The idea was to get them in custody, and then press the attack.

Initial interrogations in which both men were asked about
the Robeck case proved fruitless. But Bynum had a hunch that
Norris was the weak link and would eventually provide him with
the necessary incriminating information. On November 30,
1979, Roy Norris must have suspected something was up when
he was brought to the Torrance courthouse by detectives Paul
Bynum and Tom Cray and was met by Deputy District Attorney
Steve Kay and a judge. The judge had been called in to advise
Norris of his Miranda rights, which he waived. Then Kay and the
detectives started questioning him about the Robeck rape.

But after a few minutes, Kay and Bynum changed the topic
of conversation. They confronted Norris with the fact that they
had information that he had kidnapped, raped, tortured, and murdered several young women.

Norris at first flatly denied any knowledge or involvement—
but then tried to save himself by shifting the blame for the crimes
to Bittaker. Bynum and Kay knew they had him. On the basis of
the confession and other evidence, Norris and Bittaker were subsequently charged with robbery, kidnapping, forcible rape, sex
perversion, criminal conspiracy, and five counts of murder.

True to sociopathic form, any loyalty that may have existed
between the two men immediately broke down. Each accused the
other of inspiring and leading their rape-torture murder spree.
Each accused the other of wanting to tape-record the rape-torture
sessions. Norris had the excuse that he was high on phencyclidine
during the crimes. Besides, he went on, Bittaker was the sadistic
one and Norris had to go along with his partner because Bittaker
had saved his life twice in prison, and that bound him to follow
the other man's lead and cooperate with him. It did not, however,
prevent Norris from trying his best to let his buddy take the fall
for him.

Norris ultimately succeeded in directing the heavier weight
of justice to fall upon his partner. He accomplished this by fully

admitting his role in the crimes and working out a plea bargain in exchange for information that would convict Bittaker.

In February 1980 Norris led Deputy District Attorney Stephen Kay, Detective Bynum, and a party of officers and members of the Sierra Madre Search and Rescue Team into the San Gabriel Mountains to look for the remains of his victims. He brought them to each spot and the party scoured the area along the hillsides, cliffs, and canyons. Apparently Bittaker's idea that the animals would devour every trace was almost 100 percent correct:

Not a single trace was found of Cindy Schaeffer's body.

Not a single trace of Andrea Hall's body was found.

However, at the bottom of a canyon along a dry creek bed, the bleached, broken skeletons of Jackie Gilliam and Leah Lamp were found. The girls' bones were scattered over an area ranging hundreds of feet along the canyon floor. Jackie Gilliam's skull was found with the ice pick still in it.

In return for Norris's cooperation and testimony against Bittaker, the prosecutor agreed not to seek the death penalty or life imprisonment without parole. He pleaded guilty prior to Bittaker's trial.

Before formal sentencing is carried out, all convicted killers are routinely interviewed by a probation officer in order to review the sentence and to make a recommendation to the court regarding possible probation. When Norris was interviewed, he once again accused Bittaker of being the one who tortured their victims. Otherwise, as the probation officer noted, "in a casual, unconcerned manner, the defendant fully admitted his participation in the barbarous, inhumane acts of atrocity upon the five young female victims." In the probation officer's opinion, Norris "never exhibited any remorse or compassion about his brutal, hideous behavior towards the victims. . . . The defendant appears compulsive in his need and desire to inflict pain and torture upon women. The defendant himself acknowledged to the probation officer that in the commission of rape upon a woman it was not the sex that was important but the domination of the woman. In considering the defendant's total lack of remorse about the plight of his victims, he can realistically be regarded as an extreme sociopath, whose depraved, grotesque pattern of behavior is beyond rehabilitation. The magnitude and the enormity of the defendant's heinous, nightmarish criminal behavior is beyond the comprehension of this probation officer."

Roy Norris was sentenced to forty-five years to life. He will be eligible for parole in the year 2010.

Then it was Lawrence Bittaker's turn. He was to be given a jury trial. The prosecutor was seeking the death penalty.

Bittaker was prosecuted by Stephen Kay, who was a member of the team that helped convict the Manson Family. Kay said that the brutality of the Tate–LaBianca murders "didn't come close" to these. He admitted that this was one of the few cases he was unable to deal with objectively. The veteran deputy district attorney had seen, investigated, and prosecuted just about every kind of crime imaginable, and yet he broke down in tears twice during the three-week trial.

The defendant, of course, was incapable of breaking down. In fact, while waiting for his trial, Bittaker wrote *The Last Ride,* a book telling the story of his partnership with Norris and the details of their rape-torture murder spree. The chapter titles included: "Destiny with Death," "The Beginning of the End," "Lonely Hearts Club on Wheels," and "Two for the Price of One." Bittaker's attorney said he thought his client had a death wish, not only because he wrote such a document, but then gave it to the police.

But Bittaker had a reason. Throughout the manuscript, he portrayed himself as being continually surprised as Norris led him deeper and deeper into the crime spree. If the manuscript is to be believed, Bittaker actually tried to save the lives of their victims but was, himself, overpowered or outmaneuvered by Norris.

Of course, Bittaker was, predictably, only trying to shift the blame to Norris. Throughout his trial he maintained that he was being blamed for things his partner did.

Nobody believed him for even a minute. The jury of seven women and five men deliberated for two and a half days, not because they had a tough time making up their minds, but because there were so many separate charges to consider and vote upon. Finally, on February 17, 1981, they returned with twenty-six guilty verdicts for rape, torture, kidnapping, and murder. The court clerk needed forty minutes just to read the verdicts out loud in the courtroom.

Then began the penalty phase of the trial, to determine whether there were special circumstances to warrant the death penalty. The prosecutor wanted me to examine the defendant and testify during this phase of the trial, but Bittaker and his attorney refused to grant access for an examination. So I reviewed his record and listened to the tape recording he and Norris had made of the last hours of Shirley Ledford's life. It was the most hideous thing I'd ever heard. As far as I was concerned, Bittaker and Norris had helped each other fulfill their most savage, primitive potential as sociopaths. To call Bittaker an animal, which many people would do, only lessens his responsibility and our own—by suggesting that humans are incapable of such behavior. Unfortunately, though most of us don't ever commit such atrocities, the impulses exist within all of us.

Bittaker and Norris are different from the rest of us not so much in the character and strength of their drives, but in the ineffectiveness of their inner controls over those drives. Sociopathy is not usually classified as a mental illness, but rather as a character disorder. A sociopath knows right from wrong—he simply doesn't care. He lacks the internal prohibitions, or conscience, that keep most of us from giving full expression to our most primitive, and sometimes violent, impulses. He will be self-indulgent, narcissistic, and not concerned about the rights and feelings of other people, who will be treated as objects to be manipulated, exploited, avoided, or destroyed. A sociopath is neither subhuman, mentally ill, nor out of control. He will act intentionally and purposefully, though often without long-term motives. The acts, and whatever feelings accompany them, are the goals.

Most mental disorders result from a defect in the ego or personality portion of the mind. In sociopathy, the defect is in another part of the mind, the superego (in Freudian terms), or the conscience (in everyday terms). While psychiatry can be effective treating other forms of mental disorders, there has been little, if any, success treating sociopaths. Therefore, because they know right from wrong and can control their behavior when they have to because of external restraints, the legal system does not treat them as mentally ill.

Although sociopaths tend to keep getting into trouble, as a matter of fact many of them can get along quite well in society. In several ways, society is geared to allow certain sociopaths great success, especially in careers that require one to manipulate or lie. Successful sociopaths can make it big in the business and political arenas.

And they can make big headlines when they fulfill their savage potential and commit horrendous crimes, as Bittaker and Norris did.

Of course, the law tries not to use the words like "horror," but prefers to say "special circumstances" when referring to details of a crime that might warrant the death penalty. Normally, it takes only one or two "special circumstances" to convince a jury that a murderer should get the death penalty rather than a life sentence. When the Bittaker jury came in, they said they had found thirty-eight such special circumstances in this case. Bittaker was sentenced to death.

After the trial, the probation officer had to interview not only Bittaker but also members of the victims' families in order to write a report for the judge. The mother of one of the victims broke down during the interview and could not continue. She said that she had nightmares about her daughter's death and just could not stop reliving it in her mind. Another mother said she had been tormented, too, and had not been able to sleep. She was glad that Bittaker had received the death penalty.

The probation officer said that "during the years this officer has been submitting evaluations to the court, he has had occasion to interview many individuals convicted of brutal crimes, but none to the extent of the one for which this defendant has been convicted. During the interviews with him, although verbalizing some feeling for the teenage deaths that he has caused, there is no outward expression or emotion displayed. His total attitude was almost as if he had been able to divorce himself from the emotions felt by the major portion of society." Whenever the officer tried to evoke some feelings from Bittaker, he avoided the issue by blaming Norris for the crimes. At times, the condemned man defiantly answered one question with another question.

The probation officer concluded: "This officer feels quite strongly that with the attitude displayed by this defendant, if he were allowed to return to our society there is little doubt that he would return to a life of crime, and possibly a life of violence. As a result of this feeling, one would have to assume that the best gauge of protection to our society in this case would be the amount of time he is prevented from reoffending society. The recommendation of the jury would be the most permanent protection available."

Tragically, it took the horrible deaths of five teenage girls before the system decided that society had to be protected from Lawrence Bittaker and Roy Norris.

Does it have to be that way? Can psychiatric knowledge be used to further justice and help us protect ourselves? There are two problems here: The first is medical and the second is political. The medical question is: Can we predict just how dangerous a criminal might be in the future? The political question is: Do we have the will to use the psychiatric knowledge once we have it?

The answer to the first question is that we do have limited ability to predict danger—it can be done. The answer to the second is no, we normally do not have the political will to use the knowledge once we have it.

Cindy, Andrea, Jackie, Leah, and Shirley did not need to have their lives cruelly taken from them to make us realize that. All the information we needed was at hand long before those girls were abducted. It was no secret that Norris had a compulsive, uncontrollable need to dominate and hurt women. Nor was it a secret that Bittaker was also a highly dangerous man. Just about every professional who examined these men figured out that they were sociopaths, that the fundamental machinery of conscience, responsibility, and feeling for other human beings was totally lacking in them. These men might as well have worn signs that said they were walking horror shows waiting to begin—for all the good that knowledge did within the criminal justice system.

In the case of Bittaker and Norris, it was fairly easy to predict with a high degree of reliability that they were extremely dangerous. It's not so easy all the time. Predicting danger is a raging battleground in psychiatry. The American Psychiatric Association has gone on record to question the accuracy of testimony that attempts to predict future danger, and research studies do exist that demonstrate potential inaccuracies in the decision-making process. In one famous study, a group of psychology students presented themselves to emergency rooms and mimicked the symptoms of mental illness. They said they were hallucinating . . . they threatened to kill other people . . . or themselves. Their goal was to see if their performances could get them admitted involuntarily into mental hospitals. A substantial number of them were successful. They were diagnosed as either psychotic or suffering from some other serious psychiatric disorder and written up as being dangerous to themselves and others.

The study was supposed to demonstrate that doctors could be fooled. Well, they succeeded in that. But doctors don't like to be fooled. So when the students said, "OK, we were only joking, we're not mentally ill, let us go," the physicians at the hospitals didn't laugh. And they didn't let them go, either, at least not for several days.

Another famous study found that in cases where doctors examined people and said they were dangerous, but the court released them anyway, 85 percent of them did not act dangerously within a one-year period after release.

Both these studies are flawed in many ways. The students set out to prove that doctors could be fooled and that the system could be manipulated easily. They did succeed in proving that people who are schooled in the symptoms of mental illness can convince a doctor they are mentally ill. The implication is that many mentally healthy criminals are fooling the doctors into saying they're mentally ill so they can do their time in a hospital rather than a prison, and possibly get out sooner. But this doesn't happen as often as people imagine it does. There are not too many criminals who are as well schooled as psychology students in the symptoms of mental illness.

As far as the second study is concerned, let's assume its figures are correct, and that fully 85 percent of the people psychiatrists say are dangerous will actually not commit a crime within one year after release. Are we willing to accept the damage done by the 15 percent who become recidivists? And how do we feel about the ones who take longer than a year? If Bittaker and Norris had waited a year before going on their killing spree, would it have made a difference?

Another flaw with that figure of 85 percent is that a psychiatrist will often practice defensive medicine. In many states the psychiatrist can be held civilly liable if the person is released and subsequently injures other people or damages property. So if the doctor is liable for the patient's behavior, on what side is he going to err? Is he going to tend to say someone is dangerous or not dangerous? I believe that because of this very fact a lot of doctors are saying people are dangerous when they're really not, or when the case is borderline.

And still some dangerous people go free.

Psychiatrists aren't blameless in this. Recently we had a case where a psychiatrist testified that a man who had previously threatened his mother was no longer dangerous. The judge released the patient based on this testimony. That night, the man went home and killed his mother.

The judge, on hearing of the killing, felt very upset—but, after all, the information upon which he based his decision was incomplete. The professional who made that recommendation to the judge apparently discarded pertinent information that clearly demonstrated that the subject was dangerous. Similar stories can be told about a lot of the psychiatrists and psychologists rendering expert opinions for the courts. We have very few well-schooled and trained professionals in forensic psychiatry, very few people who can be counted upon to give a medically accurate evaluation time after time. Because, generally speaking, competent psychiatrists avoid the courtroom, this is a system of marginal players.

That's bad enough, but the problem is made worse by the fact that, most of the time, the court assumes that the opinion of a marginal hitter is just as authoritative as that of a slugger. And attorneys make full use of that fact. If they can't get one psychiatrist to say what they want, they can always find another who will. And the court will, in most cases, accept both opinions equally. There are a lot of strikeouts that the court sees as home runs.

For example, there was a case where a man was convinced that his neighbor was sending radio waves at him that were constipating him. One day he went next door and killed his neighbor. He was diagnosed psychotic and found NGI, so he went to a mental hospital instead of a prison. When his case came up for periodic review, a few psychiatrists and psychologists said the man was no longer a danger to himself or others, so it was all right to release him.

I was called in at the last minute to evaluate him. I asked him about the killing, and if he thought such a thing could ever happen again.

He said it couldn't.

I asked him why.

He said it couldn't happen because he would never get constipated anymore.

I asked him why not.

He said because he had already killed the bastard who was sending the radio waves that were constipating him.

Needless to say, my recommendation was to keep this man in the hospital. With such data, how could any professional recommend release on the basis that this man was no longer a danger? Yet some had apparently done just that.

Furthermore, a lot of psychiatrists and psychologists allow their personal, social, or political opinions to color their evaluations. There are several, for example, who make no secret that they are so opposed to the death penalty that they will say almost anything to prevent a murderer from being sentenced to death, even if it means that the killer will go free. Obviously, I'm not one of the psychiatrists who say that it's impossible to predict danger. I don't think it's either possible or a good idea for a psychiatrist to be an encyclopedia of danger, but a skilled physician can certainly give information that will help the court make its decision. I can say, "There is a risk that this person will become an offender again." I can't put an exact time and place on it, but I can qualify my opinion by saying, "There is a 99 percent probability," or "a 75 percent probability," or "a 50 percent probability." Then the court can make its decision and know what kinds of odds it's gambling against.

Sometimes an accurate prediction is impossible. Jason Nelson was, in my opinion, one of those cases that would have been impossible to predict. Had I seen the tape of him teaching the class a few days before he killed his infant son, I would never have concluded that he was a dangerous man.

But while some predictions are impossible to make, even with hours of information, some can be made in a matter of minutes. When I was testifying in the Manson Family trials, I often walked in and out of the courthouse with the defense attorneys. Occasionally, Lynette "Squeaky" Fromme, one of the Family who was camped out on the corner in front of the courthouse to protest the trial, would come over and talk to us about the case. One day, after one of these meetings that went on for about ten minutes, I turned to the defense attorney, Maxwell Keith, as we were walking away, and said, "You know, Max, that girl would just as soon kill you as talk to you."

Max looked at me and asked, "What makes you think that?"

"The quality of the way she relates," I said. "She looks right through you with that icy stare."

A few years after that, Squeaky tried to kill President Gerald Ford. She's been in prison for more than a decade, and will probably remain there indefinitely. Yet hundreds of equally dangerous people who shoot at other people and miss are released after a year or less—if, indeed, they ever see the inside of a prison at all! Yet Squeaky Fromme is not kept behind bars because the system is in tune with the psychiatric reality of her danger. On the contrary, her ongoing incarceration is a measure of political, not medical, realities.

Consider the case of another "political prisoner," Sirhan Sirhan. The day after he shot Robert F. Kennedy, Sirhan was not as dangerous to society as either Bittaker or Norris after the crimes they committed prior to their rape-torture murder spree. Yet Sirhan will most likely never be released, while Bittaker and Norris were released. Likewise, there are thousands of criminals far more dangerous than Sirhan who have been and will be released back into society.

I'm not arguing that Sirhan should be released or that his crime was not a terrible one, only pointing out that in highly political cases, the system finds the will to keep dangerous people behind bars. In less-highly charged cases it usually doesn't. That's why Norris and Bittaker were released several times, despite the fact that examining physicians said they were dangerous. If the system had found the will to keep these men behind bars once it was known that they were dangerous sociopaths, Cindy, Andrea, Jackie, Leah, and Shirley would still be alive today.

It so happens that Squeaky Fromme is potentially more dangerous than Sirhan Sirhan. The fact that she is being kept in a minimum security prison—from which she temporarily escaped while this chapter was being written—demonstrates that the authorities don't really acknowledge the fact of her danger.

Why not? Why doesn't the system respond to the reality of future danger?

It's more than politics. The political answer is that a certain loss of our safety is the price our democracy has to pay for our individual freedoms. But, in my opinion, this is only an excuse for the system's own ineptness. Sure, politics interferes with the functioning of the criminal justice system. But the interference can be a positive influence as often as a negative one. The real reason why dangerous criminals go free is that the system is simply too chaotic, inefficient, and self-absorbed to do its job. While the judges and attorneys ponder endlessly the technical nuances of issues such as equal protection, inadmissible evidence, competent counsel, and an almost infinite variety of mental states, the predators take advantage of the rules to prey on us.

And even when they are finally locked up—or even condemned—the danger does not cease.

Notwithstanding the fact that Bittaker will most likely reach a ripe old age before he's executed, if he is ever executed at all, one must ask this question: Do we impose the death sentence as a response to our anguish and horror at the crime, or because we have so little faith in the criminal justice system's ability to protect society against a dangerous person?

Most people would choose the latter as the more "civilized" answer and justify it by saying that the anguish and the horror diminish or disappear for all except the victims' families once the press coverage has died down, while our need to protect ourselves does not. This is an incorrect assumption, because the desire for safety is not separate from the emotions provoked by the knowledge of the crime. The physical danger may end when the criminals are behind bars, but the psychic danger continues. Both our desire to protect ourselves from the criminals and our desire to deal effectively with the anguish and the horror their acts call forth in us are very real psychic needs, and neither goes away when the victims' bodies are buried (if they're even found) and the headlines fade. Our justice system does not adequately satisfy these needs. They linger for a long time and have a devastating effect not only on the people who are close to the cases—the victims and the law enforcement people—but on all of us.

We are not brutalized by punishing criminals such as Bittaker and Norris, but by *failing* to punish them. The horror never really subsides, and when we, as a society, *pretend* that our anguish and rage at the criminal has been adequately dealt with—when in fact it has not—the result is that we are all forced to become more complacent about the brutality. In the same way that a battered woman or child, by being complacent, invites greater violence from an attacker, society invites all comers to test its tolerance for horror.

When we learn of the crime, the rage we experience must be processed effectively. If it is not, then anxiety, anger, and more brutality will result. We not only feel less safe, but more angry that our safety is compromised. We are thus pushed closer to that inner region where our very psychic existence feels threatened— the place where our own killing rage lies ready to go into action to protect us. In some people that rage is turned outward, and more innocent victims suffer.

In some people, the rage is turned inward. Paul Bynum, the chief investigator on the Bittaker–Norris case, a veteran police officer, was so haunted by his involvement in the case that he received a disability retirement from the police force. He went to work as a private investigator—but the vivid images of torture and death pursued him relentlessly. As this chapter was being written, the media carried the story that Paul had put his loaded service revolver in his mouth and pulled the trigger. Paul was only thirty-nine years old. He left behind a wife and kids and a ten-page letter. In the letter he focused on the Bittaker–Norris case as a nightmare he just couldn't shake.

The Bible is usually quoted as saying "an eye for an eye." Even under a modern interpretation of "not more than an eye for an eye," the equation remains fair and realistic. It recognizes that we all have a basic sense of fairness and a very real need for retribution when we are harmed. Ignoring either of these fundamental concepts can be seriously damaging to society. Our criminal justice system often ignores both of them. By bending over backward to be fair to defendants, the system is often grossly unfair to the victims—and to the rest of us. Like Paul Bynum, when our sense of fairness and our need for retribution are both ignored, we become victims, too.

The final chapters of the Bittaker–Norris story have not been completed. So far, the cold box score is as follows: There are five innocent, young women tortured and murdered, five families haunted by life-long memories of horror, a dedicated police officer driven to self-destruction by the anguish provoked by his involvement with the case, his family left without a father, a society that has become more complacent to brutality—and a criminal justice system that remains insanely preoccupied with and sensitive to only its own rules and regulations.

Norris has been given a life sentence, but is eligible for parole, and may one day be free. While Bittaker is awaiting decision on his appeal of the pending death sentence, his future is uncertain. Anything could happen. And although the agony and the horror linger, society has for the moment been made at least physically safe from these two men.

But what if Joe Jackson had remained silent? What if the young woman from Oregon who was raped had met the same fate as the others and not lived to identify her attackers? What if Norris had successfully resisted the interrogations? The case might still be unsolved, and the bodies of more young women might have been added to the five already discarded from the silver van.

And what about all the others out there who, like Bittaker and Norris, have been declared "no further danger to others"?

C H A P T E R

9

KIDS CAN GET

AWAY WITH MURDER

THESE DAYS

In the criminal justice system, children are no different from adults in that they usually fare better as criminals than as victims. The scales of justice are so perversely weighted in favor of the assailant that even when a child kills a parent the horror of the crime still takes a back seat to the concern over the youngster's future. Quite often the more violent the crime, the more intensely the defendant is protected. Of the three cases that follow, the killer who came closest to not getting punished was the most brutal and cold-blooded.

In fact, it turned out to be an accident that Barry Braeseke was punished at all.

In the early morning hours of August 24, 1976, twenty-year-old Barry Braeseke drove up to his home near Oakland, California, and found the front door closed but unlocked. He walked in and, as he told police, saw the bodies of his father, mother, and grandfather lying in a bloody heap on the floor of the family room. Barry went over to the phone and asked the operator for an ambulance. He was connected to the sheriff's office, told them he wanted an ambulance, and then hung up. He went over to his father's body and touched the hand. Then he ran out of the house to the next door neighbor's, where the police were called again.

At 4 A.M. that morning, Barry was questioned by detectives at the Alameda County Sheriff's Department. He told the detectives that he had left his home the previous night around 9 P.M., while his family had been watching a movie on television. He told them he had teamed up with his best friend, David Barker, visited friends, and finally wound up at a drive-in movie until 1 A.M. Then he had dropped David off and gone home.

When the police asked Barry whether he was having any problems with his parents, he said he was not. "Everything was cool."

But everything had not been all that cool. Barry Braeseke and his father, Floyd, were not getting along. Quite often their arguments would escalate into physical confrontations. After one such fight, Barry decided to find a solution to his problem. He shared his frustration with his friends and explained that his life would be a lot simpler without his father around. Braeseke went on a quest to find someone to help him get rid of his father. In the spring of 1976 the quest ended when Barry, using his CB nickname "Yours Truly," met David Barker, a sixteen-year-old boy whose CB name was "Phantom 309."

Barry and David quickly became friends. To help enlist David in his efforts to liberate himself, Barry fashioned a story about a great sum of money his father had in the bank. He told David that with his father and the rest of his family gone, the estate would pass on to him and the two boys could live together and have a nice, easy life.

David liked the idea, and the boys started making plans. David told Barry that he had slaughtered animals, and that the way to execute Barry's family was to hit them over the head with something hard and then choke them. The boys talked about the plan through the summer of 1976. They stopped planning on August 23.

After interviewing Barry for almost an hour, the detectives decided to end the session. One of the detectives, however, had spotted a splattering of blood on the bottom of Barry's pants leg. He reasoned that the victims's blood had to be long dry by the time Barry was supposed to have arrived on the scene, and that the only way blood could have splattered on his pants leg was if he had been present at the time of the murders.

The detectives decided to continue the interview. This time, to relax Barry, they turned off the tape recorder with which they had recorded the previous interview. Then, they accused him of the murders and stated their intention to place him under arrest. Barry denied it, and then asked for an attorney.

At that point, because he had requested an attorney, the interrogation was supposed to stop unless Barry himself offered to talk. The detectives advised him of this rule, and began to type out booking forms to make his arrest formal. While they were typing, Barry leaned over to one of the detectives and said, "Hey, I would like to talk to you off the record, if that's OK."

The detective agreed to listen, and Barry started asking him hypothetical questions: "What if I could tell you where the gun is? What if some kids might find it and hurt somebody with it? Would I still go to jail?"

The detective replied that Barry was going to go to jail no matter what he said. The young man agreed to talk, and the detective turned on the tape recorder. Barry's story, in his own words, went like this.

"I don't know how I can start. It was all gonna happen before dinner. . . . I don't think I remember how it started but, somehow, I got this idea in my head that if my parents were gone, life would be simpler for me. I would live off the insurance or something like that. This was all brought up by Dave, you see. It wasn't really brought up by me. It just—I had no idea and I'd never ever even thought of the idea myself. I couldn't think up an idea like that.

"Well, I first met Dave on the CB radio. We got to be friends, and then he told me he was winning a court case of over $100,000 because some guy shot him in the eye with a pellet gun, and how he was gonna be living rich and everything else . . . and how he wanted a best friend to live with as far as sharing a room, and just having someone close—a good friend—and as he wanted me to be his roommate or something in an apartment living off his money from that.

"And in the meantime, I've been smoking crystal for—I don't know—maybe six months now. You know, when you're on crystal, you think differently. Your mind just doesn't work right. It makes you think crazy. Most of the time I associated with Dave I was either high on crystal or going to buy some crystal, or whatever.

"I was bragging, I guess, about how rich my dad was. I told Dave that maybe my dad had $100,000 in the bank, and I was an only child, and all their insurance would come to me. Then David said, well, you know how rich and happy we'd be if they weren't around and we had all that insurance money in the bank to ourselves.

"I thought about it. I said Dave, you're crazy.

"We talked about it for weeks, in a way, with Dave saying that, well, we could go up there and knock 'em out and strangle 'em. I mean, Dave would say, I've killed cows before. He's raised steers, and he's slaughtered 'em before. He likes doing it. He likes killing chickens, watching 'em run around with their head cut off. He said I could do that, I wouldn't mind doing that at all.

"Well, anyway, these conversations have gone on and on and on. But then, when I haven't had crystal, when—when I've had to work for weeks at a time . . . say I've had to work for four days straight . . . I can't work under the influence of crystal for the phone company. Of course, I didn't smoke it then, because I didn't want to lose my job. And then when I saw Dave after work or something, he would bring up these ideas, and I'd say, Oh sure, Dave. You know, I'd agree with him and go along with it and everything. But then I would never go through with it. We'd go up to my house, and Dave would say, Are you ready? And I'd say, No, Dave, something's not right, we can't do it now. And I'm just putting him off because I don't wanna do it.

"Two nights ago, I guess, I bought a quarter of a gram of crystal rolled up in parsley and a $12 joint of crystal, which is, I guess, an eighth of a gram of crystal. We split the $20 K-J and smoked all that. And then I seen Dave the day after that. Then he started talking about it again and, of course, the idea sounded neat to me because I was under the influence of a drug. I don't really know how to continue. I think I'm screwin' myself up. I'm not saying it right.

"Tonight. Tonight we came up to my house and we were talking all day long about how we were gonna maybe kill my parents, and, uh, I would go along with it with him, but I never really thought I was gonna do it. I never wanted to do it. And, uh, anyway, we—this was early in the afternoon yesterday—we were talking about it, how we were gonna do it, and then we really didn't set any plan. We just went up to my house at maybe eight o'clock in the evening. And Dave went to the tool box looking for some tools that he could knock my parents out with, and then he'd choke 'em—me, too. But then he went ahead and did that, got a tool, put it in his pocket, and gave me a tool. These were chisels."

Barry left out a few important details. For example, that night he had another argument with his father. Floyd started criticizing him for socializing with younger people. "You're not supposed to be hanging around with young kids. You're an adult."

Barry did say to his father, "Yeah, Dad, you're right." But when he returned to the garage, where David Barker was waiting, the two young men agreed: "All right, let's do it tonight." They began selecting weapons. Barry chose a heavy metal mug, David selected a chisel, and they went back up to Barry's room:

"We went up to my room to talk, saying how we were gonna do it. Then I started getting scared. I just said, Dave, hold on a minute, I think we're gonna eat dinner now, it wouldn't look right. I mean, the bodies would have food in it, you know. I mean that wouldn't look right, Dave, and he said, Oh, c'mon.

"And I said, Well, hold on, I gotta go eat dinner. And he waited up in my room while I went downstairs and ate dinner. We had prime rib and mashed potatoes. And then, uh, after dinner, I cleared my place and cleaned my plate off in the sink and uh, told my parents OK, I'll see you later, I'll be, uh—I gotta . . . I was gonna go out with Dave to, uh, the Walk-In. I was gonna take him down to the Walk-In so he could have a job interview. My parents said, OK, be home at ten. I said, All right, I'll be home at ten. Um . . . er . . . my mom said, You be home at ten 'cause you have to go to work tomorrow, and I said, OK.

"So I went upstairs and said, Dave are you ready to go. We went downstairs and he said, Let's watch TV for a while until we're ready. And we were sitting down and watching TV, and, uh, then I went upstairs. I just said I was gonna be changing my clothes, but I just went upstairs just to go sit on my bed. I was sitting on my bed and thinking. And then I came back down. I said, Dave, come here. I said, I can't do it this way, I just can't hit my parents over the head with a hard object and choke 'em. I can't do that.

"And then I just walked over to the closet where my .22 sits, and I walked upstairs with it. And Dave said, Good, I'd rather have it this way, anyway. And I went into my bedroom and looked around until I found some .22s, and I loaded it with eight shells. Well, I said, Dave, why don't you go down there and I'll come down when I'm ready.

"He went down the stairs and sat down and started watching TV, with the chisel in his pocket. I was supposed to come down there and take care of my dad and my mom, and he was gonna hit my grandfather.

"Anyway, I walked down there and I looked at Dave sitting at the breakfast nook. Of course, my parents' backs were turned to where Dave was sitting and he's waving me, C'mon, with a smile on his face. Then I started walking in toward the living room, and I pointed at my dad, and then I look over at Dave and I kinda just whisper, Well, and, uh, he just, I guess he just nods, and then I—I don't think I meant to do it. I just—I guess my finger jerked or something, and I just didn't mean to do it. I saw my dad, my dad's head just fall back and then my mom—my grandfather looked over at me standing there and my mom leaned forward. It was the look on her face. And I pointed at her, and I s-shot my mom. And then, Dave wasn't doing anything, and I was saying, Dave, get my grandfather. I was just—I don't know what happened to me. I—why I did that. He didn't do anything. And then, uh, my grandfather and, uh, I picked up my grandfather and threw him down on top of my mom, and I said, Go ahead and hit him and then he did and I gave Dave the gun and he shot my grandfather and then we just started shaking, just started shaking.

"From then on—all of a sudden I stopped shaking. I just

froze. I just didn't do anything. I was calm. And, uh, Dave said, Stay down here, I'll go upstairs and ransack. He went in my parents' room and took drawers out and put 'em all over the place. I went upstairs and then I went in my room. I knocked my clock radio on the ground and threw some of my things on the bed. I didn't really care, I just threw 'em out there, and said, uh, Are you ready to go?

"Dave said, Yeah, and I got a jacket and, uh, another shirt, and wrapped the gun in that so the neighbors wouldn't see me carrying my gun out of the house. We just walked out to my car and started up and drove away."

Barry told his story once more that day, as the district attorney was summoned to hear his confession. The young man admitted shooting his father and mother and assisting in the murder of his eighty-one-year-old grandfather, and then went on to tell how he and David Barker had driven around to visit friends to try to establish an alibi. They threw the rifle off a bridge in a deserted spot, and finally wound up at a local drive-in. Barry tried to shift the blame for the murders to David Barker and to the effects of the PCP. However, expert testimony, as well as the testimony of his friends, presented strong evidence that he was not intoxicated when he committed the murders.

At Barry Braeseke's trial, his defense attorney, James Drew, took a double tack. His first strategy was to try to invalidate both of Barry's confessions and throw out all evidence obtained from them, since they were supposedly obtained "illegally," after Barry had asked for an attorney. His second strategy was to reduce Barry's responsibility from first-degree to second-degree murder by virtue of his supposed "diminished capacity" as a result of smoking PCP the night before the murders. Neither of these strategies worked, at first. The trial court did invalidate the first confession, ruling that the police should have told him that there was no such thing as speaking "off the record." But the second confession was upheld, and Barry was found guilty of first-degree murder.

Then the case went to the California Supreme Court, on appeal. Barry's new attorney argued that the police had violated

Braeseke's Miranda rights, which require the police to advise him of his rights to silence and an attorney before interrogating him. This time, amazingly, the California Supreme Court bought the entire argument and reversed Braeseke's conviction. The court held that the second confession and the use of the rifle as evidence were inadmissible because both were derived from the first confession.

The case then went to the United States Supreme Court. (On a point of law both sides can appeal an unfavorable decision all the way to the Supreme Court.) The Alameda County District Attorney and the California Attorney General argued that the California court's ruling was an improper application of the Miranda rule, and that Barry Braeseke had been fully informed of his rights. The U.S. Supreme Court disagreed and let stand the state court's reversal of the conviction. Barry Braeseke would have to be tried all over again, this time without either of the two confessions and without any of the evidence gathered from them.

When the Supreme Court decision was handed down, one of the more highly publicized reactions came from Barry's original attorney, James Drew, who was the first to attack the validity of Barry's confessions. Ironically, as reported in the Los Angeles *Times,* Drew was aghast at the Supreme Court decision, and wrote to protest it: "Your recent decision in the case of People *v.* Barry Braeseke was predictable. On the other hand, it is difficult to understand how a system of laws conceived to protect innocent people can become twisted to give freedom to a person who deliberately kills three innocent human beings, thereafter confesses four times to these killings, the last confession being on national television, and with all this somehow finds that freedom awaits him. . . . I am a responsible citizen in my community and shudder to think that my family has now been given less protection by our courts. No wonder the citizens in this country refer to attorneys in a disrespectful fashion and to many of our courts with comparable lack of respect. . . ." Drew also wrote, "As a lawyer and a citizen I think the decision was dead wrong. We're losing sight of what the framers of the Constitution intended. The Braeseke decision is a super example of applying the logic of the rule to the point of absurdity."

Deputy District Attorney Michael Cordoza, who was the

prosecutor in the Braeseke case, commented on Drew's statements: "In effect, he's saying to the court, 'As an attorney, I did what I was supposed to do. But you bought it. Are you crazy?' "

The Braeseke case illustrates what a game the criminal justice system is. The issues don't center around facts, information, or reality, but on the interpretation of rules. It's not a question of whether or not the ball went through the uprights of the goal posts on a field-goal kick, but whether the referee who called it was in the right place when he made the call. Despite the fact that 100,000 people and a TV audience of 25 million people saw it go through, if the referee wasn't standing in the right place, it doesn't matter. The court is not interested in the reality of what took place, but in its own complicated and often completely artificial rules.

One of the controversies in sports is the use of instant replay. The argument against using instant replay is that human beings make mistakes and that's part of the game. The argument for using it is that we want to find out what actually happened. In a game like football or baseball, you can argue that it's part of the game to make mistakes. It's a very human enterprise—we've been doing it this way for a hundred years: Do we really want to become more accurate.

The courts are saying the same thing: We don't want to be more accurate. We want to play the game at the same level of ineptitude—or at an even greater level—by paying obsessive attention to the rules while we ignore the truth of the situation.

Because of the Supreme Court ruling, Barry would have to be retried—but using what evidence? All evidence that the police obtained after he asked for an attorney was judged inadmissible. Suddenly, none of the evidence the police had obtained was valid. In one fell swoop the Supreme Court wiped out the case against Barry Braeseke—despite the fact that he had confessed to the crime on several occasions.

But there was one confession that was not covered by the Supreme Court's ruling. Two years after the slayings, after the original conviction but while the case was on appeal, Barry was interviewed by Mike Wallace on the CBS television program

"Sixty Minutes." The segment in which Barry appeared dealt with the drug PCP, "angel dust," or "crystal," as Barry had called it. During his interview, Barry once again confessed to the murders.

Naturally, the prosecution wanted the tape from CBS, but CBS didn't want to give up the tape, claiming journalistic privilege.

Now it became a First Amendment issue as well as a Fifth Amendment issue. Should CBS give the tape? And if they did, should they give the entire two-hour interview or only the two minutes that were broadcast?

The court ruled that they had to give over everything that was shown on TV. The prosecutor was satisfied with that because there was enough of a confession to get a conviction. Braeseke was sentenced to life with parole. His juvenile accomplice was held in custody to be tried as an adult.

Braeseke's crime was clearly calculated and cold-blooded. When I examined him, I found that he had no remorse for the murders and, in fact, exhibited no emotion whatsoever for the loss of his family. It appears to have been a business deal, plain and simple.

As it was to the criminal justice system. The system is so befuddled, so caught up in its own rhetoric, that what actually happened—or may happen—loses all importance. In the Braeseke case, the system was interested only in whether the evidence was tainted or not, or whether First Amendment rights were violated—which is a totally irrelevant issue. Three lives were snuffed out, but, ultimately, the system cared about as much as Barry Braeseke did. Once again, because of the perversity of the criminal justice system, the guilty party was protected while the innocent were punished, and Barry Braeseke almost got away with murder.

In Torran Meier's case, as long as the boy remained a victim of his mother's brutality, the system ignored him. But once he reversed the situation and became the assailant and more brutal than his mother, he received all the help he needed.

One of Torran's first memories was playing hide-and-seek with his mother, Shirley. He climbed into a large toy box and lowered the lid. Then his mother came and sat on the toy box. But even after Torry gave up and let her know he was in there, she didn't get up. The toddler started to scream to be let out of the dark, stuffy box—but his mother refused. Only after the child cried for half an hour did she let him out of his prison.

From the point of view of Gus and Joyce, Shirley's parents, the trouble started even before their grandson was born. Shirley was always lively and outgoing. As a child she took singing, dancing, and acting lessons, and landed a job in a cigarette commercial at the age of eleven. It was her first and last job in the entertainment business.

When Shirley was in junior high school, her mother noticed that she had a tendency to tell lies when it suited her purposes. She had long been able to get her way by flirting with her father. But as she got older she started lying to get her older sister in trouble. She also lied to her drama teacher that she was having trouble with her mother and had moved out of the house. In fact, not only was she still living at home, but her mother was driving her to and from school every day.

At the age of sixteen, Shirley got pregnant. When Torran was born, his grandmother remembers that Shirley did not even want to hold her son. She observed that her daughter treated her baby more like a piece of property than a child who needed to be cared for and loved. For the first four years of his life, Torry was cared for largely by his grandparents.

Shirley was constantly belittling Torry's father, Dennis. She would insult him and provoke him into shouting matches he never could win. The boy never knew his father because Shirley banished him from the family when the child was one and a half years old. After she kicked him out of the house and warned him to stay away, she told Torran that his father was dead. Dennis did try to maintain contact, but finally gave up.

One evening, years later, when Shirley and ten-year-old Torry were eating at a restaurant, Dennis walked in and recognized his former wife. He walked over and said hello, and then went away. Shirley told her son that the man was "just someone I used to know."

When Torran was eight years old, Shirley gave birth to her second son, whom she named Rory, after his father. Shirley did not allow Rory Sr. to see his son until he married her. The marriage lasted only a few months. Shirley bickered, argued, shouted, and threw things at her new husband, who answered in kind. The police came to know the address rather well. Shirley and Rory were divorced in 1980.

People who knew Torran said he loved his little brother Rory and took good care of the boy, even though Shirley gave all her affection to Rory and never showed any tenderness toward her older son. Often, Rory would imitate his mother's apparent contempt for Torran. Friends noticed that although Rory could be obnoxious, the older brother was always patient and caring. Rory had diabetes and it was usually his brother who had to give him his insulin shots. Rory often had bad dreams and woke up crying in the middle of the night. It was Torran who went to the boy's bedside and comforted him and stayed with him until he was no longer frightened. Torry also disciplined his brother and tried to teach him not to ride his bike in the street.

Torry's aunt Shannon noticed that the boy often cried silently. Every time his grandparents came to take Torry home, the boy would cry bitterly. Aware that his mother absolutely prohibited any crying at all, his grandparents started making up silly games to take his mind off what was happening and prevent his crying.

Meanwhile, Shirley's life was on the skids. She was injured at work and started taking Valium. Her parents noticed her screaming and yelling a lot more than usual. And not only did she start associating with a "rougher bunch of people," but she started dressing in skimpy, provocative clothes. She seemed to be losing her sense of propriety. On one occasion she started screaming and cursing at her father in the middle of the street in front of their house.

Shirley tried to kill herself twice. Not too long after the second attempt, Gus and Joyce went to visit her and Torry one day, and found mother and son walking around the house completely naked. After that incident, Torry's grandparents attempted to get custody of him. But when Torry started to grow closer to his grandmother, Shirley began to show signs of jealousy. She was once again able to call upon her acting powers to convince the judge that she was more abused than abusing—and the attempt to liberate Torry failed.

After that, Shirley refused to let her parents see her son except when it was absolutely necessary. Between Torry's fourth and seventh years, Gus and Joyce were allowed to see him only on his birthday. But even these occasions were unreliable. On Torry's sixth birthday, when Gus and Joyce showed up with presents, they were greeted by Shirley, who yelled at them that they were not welcome. She screamed that they were trespassing and that she would call the police if they didn't leave. Gus and Joyce left the presents on the steps and left. A few days later the gifts were returned, unopened. Torry later told them his mother said he was not allowed to have a birthday party that year.

The grandparents did call Torry now and then, but the boy seemed constrained to tell them that everything was OK. Sometimes he would admit that his mother yelled a lot. One thing he never told his grandparents was that his mother was beating him regularly. When Shirley hit Torran, she would hit him in the face, on the arms and back, and sometimes in the genitals. Sometimes she threw things at him, brushes or shoes. She would shout abusive names at him, call him "faggot," and tell him he'd never be a real man.

Shirley constantly kept after her older son to do chores around the house. Many of these were normal responsibilities, but some were not. It was Torry's duty to make breakfast, and sometimes dinner too. He kept the whole house clean: bathrooms, kitchen, bedrooms, and living room. He maintained the yard and the pool. Every day, when he came home from school, there would be a letter waiting for him with a list of chores. Torry had been responsible for cleaning the bathroom since he was four years old.

Shirley once insisted that he build a six-foot-high chain-link fence around their yard to keep the dog in, after the dog had run away. But even with the normal chores, there was always an edge of madness to the intensity with which Shirley insisted that the chores be done her way. If Torry's performance was not to her liking she would scream at him to do it again.

Once, when Torran was a teenager, but not old enough for a

driver's license, Shirley called him at 2 A.M. to pick her up at a bar in Studio City, about twenty miles from their home. The boy obeyed his mother's demand, but when he got there, she yelled at him for taking so long.

Shirley's life took a turn for the better when she received between $30,000 and $40,000 in settlement of a lawsuit against a market where she had been injured. She used the money to buy a nice house in Canoga Park. But her behavior toward Torran was still erratic and violent. She still humiliated him in public and, though he performed the many chores she set for him around the house, she constantly reminded him that he couldn't do anything right. Shirley acted like a Marine drill sargeant around Torry. She rarely missed an opportunity to cut him down or make fun of him in front of his friends. Often, she would tell him he could do something or go somewhere—and then abruptly change her mind. Whenever she yelled at him, she would charge right up and stand uncomfortably close as she shouted in his face.

Though Torry always tried to please his mother, she continued to put him down. He was not allowed to complain of feeling ill, uncomfortable, tired, or in pain. When he did, his mother told him he was just looking for sympathy. On one occasion, when Shirley, Torry, and the grandparents went out to dinner, Shirley forced her son to wear a pair of shoes that were painfully too small for him. When he told her how much his feet hurt, she scolded him and refused to let him take off the shoes, for fear he would not be able to get them back on again when they left the restaurant.

By the time Torran was ten, Gus and Joyce had been allowed back into his life. When he got a paper route, they helped him by driving him around to deliver his papers. A few years later, Torry was aided by his grandparents in an attempt to escape. They bought him a plane ticket to San Francisco, which he used successfully to flee. However, his grandparents told him to call his mother just to let her know he was OK. When he did, Shirley pleaded with him to return and promised to change her ways if he did. She managed to talk the boy into coming home. And she did treat him better . . . for about two months.

In 1983 Shirley met her third husband, Steve. The couple was married by the same Presbyterian minister who married Shirley and Rory five years earlier. The marriage lasted two and a half weeks. During their courtship, Shirley was on her best behavior with Steve. But as soon as the ink was dry on the marriage license, she confronted Steve with a totally different personality. She constantly yelled, screamed, and attacked her new husband. At first, Steve simply tried to ignore her bouts of violence. On one occasion, he walked out on her when she started shouting at him in a restaurant. But Shirley got worse and worse. Her screaming fits were growing more and more violent and unpredictable. She might yell at the top of her voice for hours, anywhere, for any reason. Steve could never be sure what would set her off, and was really frightened when he noticed that she actually foamed at the mouth during these fits. And there was no escape from her once she began screaming. She would follow him all around, in the house or outside. If she happened to get angry while in the car, she would floor the accelerator.

Shirley tried to control every aspect of Steve's life. She not only criticized all his friends and former girlfriends, but also wrote nasty letters to all of the women in his personal telephone book.

Steve really felt sorry for Torran, for the boy's torment was even more severe than his own. Many times Steve would cover up for Torry and take the brunt of Shirley's wrath upon himself, just to give the boy some relief. Steve believed that Shirley really cared for her son and was proud of him. The only reason she ever gave for all the yelling was that Torry needed it in order to keep up his grades. Steve figured the pills may have had something to do with her behavior. Her medicine cabinet was always full of them, but even those weren't enough. Shirley used up an entire bottle of pain pills Steve had bought for an old motorcycle injury.

Finally, to protect himself, Steve left. He regretted having to leave Torry because he had begun to develop a real friendship with the boy. Steve told Torry he could come with him or visit any time he wanted, but he knew that Shirley would come after the boy if he ever accepted the offer. Steve felt sorry for Torran because he knew there was no way for him to get away from his mother—unless she died. Many times Shirley told Steve that she was going to kill herself someday by driving her car off a cliff.

For a few brief months, Torry had a girlfriend, Kery. According to his male friends, the girls thought Torry was a "hunk." But he was never able to bring girls home, because his mother would always criticize or insult them. Torry would sit in his car with Kery and they would each talk about their unhappy homes. Kery at first found it difficult to get Torry to talk about his mother. But once he opened up, the entire story came out. When Kery talked to Torry on the telephone, she often could hear Shirley yelling and screaming in the background. Whenever the subject of his mother came up, or when Kery pressed Torry to talk about her, Torry would instantly change from a happy mood to a cold, quiet mood. Torry told her that his mother did not like to see him smile.

Torry usually had to break up with his girlfriends because his mother "grounded" him so often that it was impossible for him to have a normal dating relationship. The "groundings" were unpredictable and sometimes enforced for the slightest reason. He could be grounded for not performing a chore in the precise manner laid out in Shirley's instructions, or for making a simple mistake. Once, he was invited to double-date with a friend to the school prom. Shirley at first gave her permission and all the arrangements were made, including the rental of a limousine. At the last minute, however, Shirley rescinded her permission because Torran had, in her opinion, received a bad grade on a test. He had to cancel his date.

When Torry was grounded he sometimes had to stay in his room after school for anywhere from a day to a month. Once, he was grounded for a month because Shirley didn't like the way he played football. When he was grounded, not only was he not allowed to use the telephone, but he was also forbidden one of his favorite activities, his computer. One of his girlfriends advised him to just "hang in there" until he was out of high school, or, if he couldn't do that, to file an "emancipation of a minor action" to free himself. Torry said he'd look into it, but never followed through.

To help cover the household expenses, Shirley took in boarders, all of whom were required to help in keeping the house clean. In addition, they had to follow Shirley's long list of rules and regulations, which applied not only to their behavior in the house but also to the specific manner in which they helped with the chores. Everything had to be done Shirley's way. Often she would enact one of her violent attacks against Torran right in front of one of the boarders. She would beat him and grab his arms and shake him violently while she attacked him verbally for some mistake, real or imagined. Torran was forced to look her straight in the face. If he turned away she would scream more loudly until he looked at her. Sometimes the boy would quietly apologize, even though it hardly ever did any good. Most of the time he merely stood silently and did not offer the least resistance, until Shirley seemed to be done. Then he would quietly walk away. Often she would pursue him and carry the attack into other rooms. Sometimes she would simply continue yelling from whatever room she happened to be in, regardless of where Torran had fled. There were times when Shirley would continue to scream abuse at her son for four or five hours.

One Saturday morning Shirley marched into Torry's room and slapped the sleeping boy square across the face, as hard as she could. Then she grabbed his ankles and yanked him off the bed so that the dazed boy was sitting on the floor, his back up against the bed. Finally, she started yelling at Torry and berating him. His crime? Out of his long list of chores that were to be performed the day before, he had forgotten one—to take out the trash.

Sometimes Torry would cry during the attacks. Most of the time he would do his crying in his room, silently.

One of the boarders finally moved out because she could no longer stand being awakened every morning by the sound of Shirley screeching insults at Torry.

Shirley saved all her affection for Rory. She hugged him, treated him gently and kindly, and played games with him. Though Torran cared for his little brother, Rory seemed to take after his mother. He usually could be counted on to say something biting or critical about Torran, in the manner of their mother. Rory liked to get Torry in trouble because he knew he could get his way when Shirley was angry at the older boy. So whenever Torran said no to Rory, the younger boy would run to Shirley, who could be counted on to attack Torran and then grant Rory whatever he wanted.

Though Torry felt some anguish over the way Shirley showered Rory with attention and love, he still took good care of his little brother. When Rory had trouble going to sleep, which was often, Torry would sit with him and read him a bedtime story.

In 1985 Shirley began to abuse Rory, too. Torry would hear her yelling and screeching in another part of the house. Then he would hear her pushing his younger brother against the walls.

When Torran was in high school, his mother was usually out on Thursday nights. On these nights, his grandparents would come over and spend time with the boys. Sometimes they would all go out to eat together. Torry really looked forward to these evenings. His grandmother would often cry when she heard stories of the way her daughter was treating the boy.

Torry joined the high school football squad, and sometimes Shirley would go to football practice and watch him play. Then she would criticize him all night about his performance, telling him that if he only hadn't made so many mistakes, the coach would like him better. But Torry was actually quite good at football, and his natural talents enabled him to move up quickly to the number-one spot on the team. When Shirley found out about her son's success, she forced him to quit the team. Torry bitterly told Kery that there could be only one number one at his house, and that had to be his mother. The boy was so embarrassed that he henceforth avoided his former teammates. He felt as though he had let them down and his quitting had branded him forever as a loser.

In March 1985 Shirley called her mother and told her that Torry no longer wanted to live at home and that she and Gus could have him if they wanted him. But she also told Torry that if he left he could never return. Torry moved in with his grandparents. Two weeks later the police showed up at Joyce and Gus's house. Shirley had sent them there to return her "runaway son."

Torry was crushed. His grandmother noticed that the boy now had a blank look in his eyes. Shortly thereafter, she noticed Torry using a foam cup holder inscribed with the message: PARDON ME, BUT YOU'VE OBVIOUSLY MISTAKEN ME FOR SOMEBODY WHO GIVES A DAMN.

Joyce and Gus shared Torry's despair, but they tried to encourage their grandson to "hang in there" until he finished high school.

It was around that time that Torry began to miss school. It

was also then that sixteen-year-old Torran started confiding in his friends his desire to somehow liberate himself from his mother. Torry didn't keep his desperation secret from his friends. Quite often he would talk to them about what was going on at home and how he wanted to get away. He even brought up the idea of killing his mother as the only way to get free of her, and asked some of his friends what they thought would be the best way to go about doing the job. At one time a rumor made the circuit at his high school that he was planning to kill Shirley. But no one ever took it seriously. His friends always discouraged him from that idea and told him to just "hang in there" until he graduated from high school and could move away.

But not all of Torry's friends discouraged him. Not all of them failed to take him seriously when he said he wanted to kill his mother: Matt Jay took him very seriously, especially in light of the fact that Matt had similar troubles at home, too.

Torran confessed that he didn't know what else to do. He had no money, since his mother took all his paychecks, gave him only a small allowance, and spent the rest on the house and on herself. The boy was too young to join the military, and when a friend suggested a child abuse hot line, Torran said he didn't think it could help him much. He was desperate, and he admitted to one of his closest friends, Skip, that if he couldn't get rid of his mother he would kill himself.

Then, suddenly, Torran didn't talk about it anymore. About two weeks later Skip stopped by to see him at the service station where he worked. In the booth where Torry worked the pump computers, Skip noticed a hangman's noose. One of Torry's other friends, Richard Parker, was also there. Torry told his friend that they were going to kill his mother that night, and that they were waiting for Matt Jay to pick them up. Skip didn't think Torry was serious.

But on that balmy October day, Torran had indeed called his friend Matt and told him that he was "going to get rid of her." He and Richard, a twenty-three-year-old transient Torry had met through Matt, had made up a plan, and Torry would need Matt to help him execute it.

Torry had fashioned the noose during the slow hours on Sundays. He was "just playing around" with some rope and found that he had made it into a noose. Then he realized he could use the noose to strangle his mother.

After work, at about nine forty-five that evening, Torran and Richard drove to Matt's house on Torry's motorcycle. Then Matt and Richard, riding in Matt's father's car, followed Torran to Ameci's pizza restaurant in Canoga Park. At the restaurant, the three young men finalized their plan.

Torran rode home on his motorcycle, and Matt and Richard followed him but parked their car down the street. Torran went into the house alone.

Shirley was sitting in the dining room. Torran said, "Hello, I'm home," and his mother immediately started complaining about his coming home so late. Torran said he'd had trouble with his motorcycle, and she told him there was some food for him in the oven. He got his dinner out of the oven, went back to his bedroom, and let Matt and Rick into the house through the window. He left them hiding in his room, with the noose, and then went back to eat his dinner. As he finished, Shirley started complaining to him about money. He told her to come into his room with him and he'd show her something.

Shirley answered by complaining about how he was always interrupting her TV shows, so Torran told her to come in when there was a commercial. When the commercial came on, Shirley got up to follow him to his room. He asked her to close her eyes as she entered the room, or to let him blindfold her. Shirley refused to close her eyes or be blindfolded, but she did say she'd walk backward into the room. Torran agreed.

Shirley turned around and backed into the room as her son opened the door. Suddenly, she saw Matt coming at her from behind the door, but it was too late. Richard swooped down on her from the other direction, dropped the noose around her neck, and tightened it. Then Torry and Matt knocked her down on the floor as Richard pulled on the noose. Shirley kicked and screamed and fought and clawed at the boys, but she couldn't win against their combined strength.

Her muffled screams woke eight-year-old Rory, who started crying for his mother. Then he got up and walked down the hall toward Torran's room. When Torran realized his brother was awake, he looked up to see the boy standing in the doorway, watching the death struggle of his mother.

Torran let go of the noose and went out to intercept Rory, and get him back to bed. But he was unable to calm him. Finally, he managed to lead Rory into the family room to watch TV. Then he went back to the bedroom to help Matt and Rick, who were still struggling with Shirley.

But then Rory started crying for his mother again. Torran went out to calm him, but the youngster refused to remain settled for more than a few minutes at a time. So Torran had to go back out to him, return to help Matt and Rick, and then return to calm Rory over and over again during the next twenty minutes.

It took that long for Shirley to stop struggling. When all was still and the boys eased back off her body, they saw that she was bleeding from her mouth and her nose. Matt dutifully held a rag under her face to catch the blood before it could stain the carpet.

Torran went out to close the garage door, then went back to help Rick drag his mother out and stuff her in the trunk of her car, a five-year-old Thunderbird. With that grisly task accomplished, he went back into the house to calm down his little brother. He realized that Rory had seen them struggling with Shirley on the floor of the bedroom, and that he probably had a good idea what was taking place.

The trio decided they would have to kill Rory too.

Torran tried to think of a method that would knock the boy unconscious quickly. The boys decided rat poison would do the trick, so they sent Matt to the store to get some. When he returned with rat poison and snail poison, Torran made a peanut butter-and-jelly sandwich laced with the poison and tried to get Rory to eat it. After one bite, the boy refused to eat anymore. When he said he didn't like the taste, Torry mixed some poison with some milk and flavoring and tried to get Rory to drink that. Again, the boy didn't like the taste.

So Torran crunched up some of Shirley's muscle relaxing pills and mixed the powder with some milk. Rory drank a little, but would not finish it.

Torry told the others that he didn't know what to try next. The three thought about it for a minute, then decided to

dispose of Rory the same way they were going to dispose of
Shirley's body.

Torran told Rory to lie down in the back seat of his mother's
car because they had to drive Rick home. Matt drove on ahead
while Rick got in the car opposite Torry, bringing a gas can with
him. They stopped to fill the can at a Shell station on their way
out to Malibu Canyon.

Malibu Canyon Highway winds through some of the steepest
canyon ledges in Southern California. Newcomers who drive
through for the first time are astonished at the rugged, treacher-
ous beauty of the landscape. Most of the road twists and turns
along the rocky face of a cliff—without the security of a guardrail
—and it's not unusual to see a tow truck cranking up its cable, the
other end attached to a car that went over the side.

Rory and Rick drove up into the canyon and found a spot
they liked, then drove back to the San Fernando Valley to retrieve
some forgotten items. First they stopped back at Torran's house
and picked up Shirley's purse, then they stopped at the same Shell
station and got $6 worth of gas for the car. Then they drove to
Matt's house. Matt came out and followed them in his father's car
to the chosen spot in Malibu Canyon.

All this time, Rory had been sleeping peacefully in the back
seat. But when they arrived at the designated spot in the canyon,
he woke up. Torran tried to get him to go back to sleep, but the
boy refused. So Torran told him he would have to blindfold him,
because they were going to Rick's house and he didn't want Rory
to know where Rick lived. Rory did not resist, even when Torran
said he'd also have to tie up his hands.

With Rory sitting in the backseat, blindfolded and hands
tied, the boys took Shirley out of the trunk, untied her, and
propped her up in the driver's seat of the car, whose engine was
still running. They soaked a rag in gasoline and stuffed it in the
open gas tank nozzle. Rick lit the rag, and Matt and Torry aimed
the car across the road, into the canyon, and put it in gear. The
car crossed the road and went up over the embankment, rolled
down the hill, and came to rest on a plateau part-way down the
gorge. Flames spread from the rag. Matt, Richard, and Torry
drove away.

Torry and his friends drove through the canyon to the Pacific

Coast Highway, then headed north, where they finally came to Kanan Road, another road that winds away from the Pacific Ocean through the Santa Monica mountains to the San Fernando Valley. Back in the valley, Matt dropped Torry and Rick off at Torry's house, then drove home. Rick and Torry cleaned up the mess in the house. They gathered up the poisons and the towels which they had used to clean up the blood on the carpet, and dumped everything in a trash bin at the Carl's Jr. in Canoga Park. Torry drained the gas can on the ground and put it back in his car. Then they drove back to the Union 76 station where Torry worked, so Rick could pick up his bicycle.

When they got there, Torry suddenly felt like returning to Malibu Canyon.

As they were driving into the canyon from the freeway, they saw an ambulance and a sheriff's car coming in the opposite direction. The boys made a U-turn to follow them, when another sheriff's car pulled up behind them. Two more sheriff's cars pulled up around them on the freeway and told them to pull over.

Little Rory had felt the presence of someone else in the car with him, then he felt the car moving. Then it shook violently and pitched downward. The boy could smell gasoline and fire and, suddenly, he could see flames out of the bottom of his blindfold. He freed his hands and tore off the blindfold. Rory saw his mother leaning against the steering wheel, with blood all over her face. He climbed into the front seat and tried to open the door, but the door wouldn't open. The flames were burning hotter and brighter around the back of the car, but there was no fire inside the car yet. Rory reached for a button to lower the electric windows. Miraculously, the window went down and Rory climbed out of the car, which was soon enveloped in flames. The boy started climbing down the hill, deeper into the canyon. But then he realized he was going in the wrong direction, so he started climbing up the hill and crying out for help.

A young man driving by saw the flames and stopped his car. He looked out over the embankment and saw the burning car, about fifty feet below. Then he heard the little boy's voice: "Help me! Help me!"

The man climbed down the embankment and helped Rory climb up to the road. Then he flagged down another car. The driver of the second car went down the hill with the young man to see if anyone was still in the car, while his wife sat with Rory. But the two men couldn't get very close to the burning car because of the intense heat of the fire. Then the police and fire department arrived at the scene.

While Rory told the story of everything he had seen and experienced that long night, beginning when he was awakened by his mother's screams, the firemen put out the fire.

Shirley's body was burned beyond recognition.

As the police and ambulance were driving away from the scene, the sheriff's deputies recognized Torry's car from a description Rory had given them. They gave chase and arrested Torry and Richard Parker.

After Torran made a complete confession, the police played a tape-recording of it for Richard Parker.

Later, Torry called his aunt Shannon and asked her to guess what had happened. His aunt asked if Shirley had been hurt. Torran said that no, his mother wouldn't be feeling anything anymore.

Torry was reunited with his father in a San Fernando Valley courtroom. His father and his grandparents vowed to support and defend Torry every step of the way.

I examined Torran Meier and rendered an opinion that although he was extensively brutalized by his mother, there was no basis for negating malice aforethought, particularly in view of what had been done to his little brother. I did suggest, however, that an ongoing heat of passion defense was viable, and could sustain a manslaughter conviction.

The defense sought additional testimony from a psychiatrist who rendered an opinion that areas of the brain that control malice, premeditation, and deliberation were impaired in Torran as a result of brain damage. If this alternative theory was accepted by the jury, Torran could, likewise, be convicted of manslaughter.

The jury, it appears, did embrace that testimony in reaching their verdict. Maybe they just felt compassion for Torran and felt that the mother brought tragedy onto herself—I don't know. They found him guilty of manslaughter against his mother and attempted manslaughter against his half brother Rory. Torran was sentenced to a maximum term of twelve years, which he is currently serving at the California Youth Authority in a psychiatric facility. With time and treatment he may be able to resolve his troubled past.

Under our system it is possible for different defendants to be convicted of different crimes for participation in the identical act. This happened when the other young men were brought to trial separately. Both pleaded guilty to second-degree murder and were given sentences of fifteen years to life.

There is no identifiable part of the brain that controls deliberation, premeditation, or malice. The doctor who gave that testimony was pushing the credibility of scientific knowledge. The only influence Torran Meier was acting under was the powerful human drive to kill in self-preservation.

The criminal justice system utterly failed to help Torran Meier—until he was driven to cross the line from victim to killer. Then the system marshalled its forces to sympathize with him and protect his rights, which had been so casually ignored earlier when a little protective intervention might have salvaged his boyhood and saved his mother's life.

In the case of Eric Chapman, the system went beyond protecting a defendant's rights when it seemed to actually become a willing accomplice in the young man's psychotic drive to terrorize and destroy his own family.

Eric Chapman's problems began to surface when he was ten years old. From ten to fourteen the tall, thin boy would usually vomit after watching a movie. From twelve to sixteen he would often experience violent shaking fits when he came home from school.

Eric described his parents as "hollow people, hypocritical, prejudiced, and narrow. They discussed divorces and breakdowns behind closed doors. They criticized almost everyone they saw. They went through an extreme anticommunist phase when I was in junior high school, and this affected my mind." Eric further described his mother as "hypertensive and nervous," and his father as "a passive man, never close to me."

During his junior and senior years of high school, Eric endured violent headaches and upset stomachs every two weeks or so. Only two things would relieve these agonies: vomiting or sexual release. Eric spent most of his free time with his girlfriend. Otherwise, he was a very isolated young man. In the presence of most other people, he felt nervous and anxious. He tended to talk too fast and too much.

When people would speak to Eric, he would become, in his own words, "hysterical and anxious." He could feel his heart racing as his face became flushed. He found it more and more difficult to concentrate on his schoolwork, or even on what the people around him were saying. Eric was constantly distracted by his own inner thoughts. At times he felt as if there was a tight band around his head, which caused increasing pressure as it steadily tightened. Eric believed his headaches were caused by his adrenal glands. He often felt himself separate from his body and turn into a bird, or a tree, or a bug.

While Eric was in junior college earning an A.A. degree in architecture, his thinking became distorted, too. He felt moral conflicts over sex and started thinking that people were robots. Eric decided that the human race was headed for disaster because of "the rampant immorality." During his last semester of junior college, he began to see explosions of white light in the daytime. He would often wake up in the middle of the night to find that his hands were on backward.

Eric's parents took him to a psychiatrist, who recommended long-term treatment and suggested that Eric not get married. Eric and his parents rejected the doctor's advice, and he married his high school sweetheart in September 1968. He said that he married her because his mother and father wanted him to and because she had a "childlike" mind. He then enrolled in California Polytechnic as a third-year student of architecture. But Eric's marriage was troubled. His hallucinations returned. The couple separated.

In 1969, Eric's doctor wrote to the Selective Service that Eric was schizophrenic, and described him as "withdrawn, autistic, infantile, confused, delusional, and hallucinating." Eric was classified 4F—not fit for military service. Treatment with antidepressant, antipsychotic medication and psychotherapy followed, but did little good.

Eric grew worse. He left school, rejoined his wife, and the young couple lived with Eric's parents while he went back to school, this time at the University of Southern California's School of Art and Design. After a year and a half of marriage, however, Eric's wife left for good. She moved into her own apartment, while Eric moved into a fraternity house. But Eric's thinking distortions grew worse. Once again he moved back in with his parents and entered into therapy. In 1970 Eric's new psychiatrist decided he was not schizophrenic, but manic-depressive. She changed his medication from antipsychotic drugs to lithium carbonate, which is specifically intended for bipolar disorders such as manic depression. She also prescribed megavitamins.

Eric responded to treatment by sleeping twenty hours a day, but he did improve somewhat. He still reported feeling "spaced out" and as though he "lacked an ego." Eric's head still felt tight, and he decided his brain was not getting enough blood. He also believed that people were unintentionally controlling him with their thoughts.

During 1970 there were many nights when Eric would show up at his parents' home and plead with them to let him sleep in their bed.

Eric's psychiatrist insisted that he merely needed to become independent and "free" of his parents, and she encouraged him to do so. At the same time, she encouraged his parents to be strict and firm with him, and they, in turn, advised his grandmother—with whom Eric spent a lot of time—to be strict with him, too.

Almost a year later, Eric went back to school again, this time at Long Beach State College. He felt a little better, but feelings of being "spaced out, hollow, and invisible" plagued him. After Eric stopped taking his medication, got sick again, and dropped out of Long Beach State, he drove a taxicab for about five or six months. He was still preoccupied with the "spaced out" feeling, and he figured that the people in his taxi were sent by his psychiatrist to spy on him. Everything in Eric's life took on symbolic meaning. He fell in love with a woman he thought was married. When he discovered she was reading a book about mental retardation, he concluded that she was conspiring with his psychiatrist.

In January 1971 he suddenly decided to go to the University of Michigan in Ann Arbor. Eric was getting messages from his surroundings that he was mentally deficient. He stopped taking his drugs and his vitamins and soon became extremely agitated. A few months later, Eric returned to California with a mission. He was determined to save his family from their problems. Then he, too, would be free.

Eric felt he had learned a few things during his therapy. He had "learned" that there were three kinds of people in the world: masters, slaves, and free people. He also "learned" that someone in his family was always trying to master him, to make him into a slave. This was the cause of his mental illness, he knew.

The young man's psychiatrist played a leading role in his delusions. When he went to Ann Arbor, he knew she was there, watching him. He called her frequently, and was convinced that she had instructed him, symbolically, to come back to Pasadena and live with her. According to Eric, "she planted electrodes in my brain during an electroencephalogram and I was being controlled by her and a computer."

Eric kept receiving the message that his illness was caused by syphilis, and that his parents were mentally retarded because of this illness. He figured that his grandfather, who was something of a playboy when he was young, had caught the disease and given it to his wife, Eric's grandmother, whom the family called "Nana." She, in turn, had passed it on to Eric's parents and to Eric himself. He believed that the syphilis could be overcome by "a strong mind," but that his parents were weaklings and that Nana had made him weak, too, by controlling and spoiling him in a destructive way. He realized, "that it was either her or me, and that killing her would cure me."

The patient figured out more of the lessons of his therapy. He knew he needed a complete catharsis of his feelings before he could get well, and came to realize that his therapist had symbolically ordered him to murder someone in his family—the evil master. But he also knew that there was a family secret which, if revealed, would make the killing unnecessary. Finally, he realized that the hypoglycemia his psychiatrist had diagnosed was really congenital syphilis.

The explosions of white light were still with Eric, and when he awoke in the middle of the night, his hands were still on backward.

When he was asked if he felt life was worth living, he replied: "I felt the whole human race was not worth living." Eric once attempted suicide by swallowing an entire bottle of vitamins.

On July 4, 1971, Eric attended a dinner at his parents' house, which was also attended by his brother Greg and Nana. When his father offered to light one of the sparklers Eric had brought, the young man became hysterical and went home to his basement apartment at Nana's house.

A few weeks later, on July 27, Eric confronted his parents with a .22 rifle that had been hanging on the wall at Nana's house for thirty years. Eric insisted that he could "save" the family because he was the second Son of God. After disarming him (the gun was not loaded), his family drove him directly to his psychiatrist's office. The psychiatrist told Eric's parents that since the gun was not loaded, she felt that Eric really meant no harm but was only bidding for attention. As far as Eric was concerned he was willing to settle for a confrontation and revelation of the truth about his family. The "family secret" was not forthcoming, however, so Eric pressed on.

On August 6, Eric attacked his father during a discussion of the family medical history. He wrestled with his father and butted him with his knees. Eric asked his father, "Why don't you fight back?" Donald Chapman answered, "I don't want to hit you, but I will if you don't stop." Eric didn't stop, so his father finally smacked him across the face with his fist. Eric calmed down and said, "Now I'm OK, thank you."

On the night of Saturday, August 7, 1971, instead of sleeping in the apartment in Nana's basement, Eric slept in a large dollhouse in a neighbor's backyard.

He had figured out that his grandmother was, at least, a good source of information about his genetic history and, at most, herself the source of the bad genes causing his problems. So he pressed his grandmother for information about the cases of mental illness that had existed on both sides of her family. Nana's husband's younger brother had been hospitalized for thirty-five years for schizophrenia. And Nana's mother had been hospitalized for six years following a nervous breakdown.

Of all his family members, Eric loved Nana the most. He knew that, despite her alcoholism, she was a very strong person. If only he could overpower her and get her to confess to being the transmitter of the bad gene, then he could save his entire family as well as himself. On Sunday morning, August 8, Eric visited her to get the answers to his questions—and found she was drinking. Eric decided that she was, after all, the source of the bad gene in his family that was causing his mental illness, his syphilis, and his mental deficiency.

Eric attacked his grandmother, and tried to physically wrestle from her the answers to his questions. In the midst of the struggle, the phone rang. Eric, by now in control, ignored it.

Nana pleaded with him to allow her to get up and go to the kitchen to finish her drink. Eric let her up but attacked her again when he thought he saw her holding a small pair of scissors.

The battle began all over again. This time he wrestled her to the floor of the rear den, or family room. He tied a pink nylon slip around her face to gag her, then grabbed her tightly around the neck.

Eric knew he needed a catharsis, to express all his feelings about his family. This could be it, he felt.

The phone rang again.

Every Sunday around 11 A.M. it was the custom for Don and Christine Chapman to call Christine's mother, Nana. The first time they called her that Sunday, August 8, there was no answer. They tried again five minutes later and Eric answered. He asked his parents what they were going to do that day. They replied that they were going to the beach, and would he like to come along. In a trembling, emotional voice, Eric answered, "Yes, I really would." His parents told him to meet them at their house and, assuming that Nana was out in the yard, told Eric to have her call them. Eric hung up the phone.

The gag had apparently worked, since Eric's parents had not heard Nana struggling to free her neck from the grip of his other hand.

A few minutes later, Eric realized that his grandmother was not responding to his questions. She just lay still on the floor under him.

Eric left the house, drove away, stopped at a phone booth, and called his parents and said, "Nana is hurt—I think you better call an ambulance."

"How badly is she hurt?" Don Chapman asked his son.

"I think she is dead," Eric replied.

"Are you sure? How did it happen?" Don asked.

"I had to kill her because she had defective genes."

Then Eric drove to his psychiatrist's house. She also called Eric's father.

Eric said, "I killed my grandmother as a better alternative than physically hurting my folks. I felt my mother was lucky to be in her place rather than my grandmother's place." Eric also said he had once given some thought to the idea of taking a knife and cutting out his mother's clitoris.

At the time of the murder, Eric had a job playing piano at a pizza parlor. "My father called them and told them I wouldn't be back. And that upset me terribly because it showed he lacked confidence in my ability to achieve on my own. And this is typical of the pattern which our relationship has had. He runs my life. . . . My brother is God and I'm the Devil—according to them. I couldn't see through the situation as a youngster, therefore, I saw them as God and became the Devil.

"I went there about 10:34 A.M. The night before, I felt I was dying. I heard the angels calling me when I was at work. I thought I was dying of syphilis.

"I tried to find out why I was sick, and I asked her if I had been breast-fed too long, because of my incessant desire for food . . . and for sex. She said, 'for three months.' Then I had the feeling that she knew something she wasn't talking about. In strangling her, I tried to force her to tell me. She had been drinking, she begged me to let her finish her drink and stated that I was killing her. She fought me. Oh, yeah, it was a tussle. She finally admitted that she believed the trouble was a bad gene on her part. I tried to reason with her as to the alternatives. I told her I could let her up, but she kept fighting me. I did let her up and she went to the kitchen and got a pair of scissors—as something to

stab with—so I strangled her again, feeling there was a lack of
sympathy in wanting me to be in good health. So I talked inter-
mittently with my mother on the telephone in the other hand to
make sure the experience did not overwhelm me. That is, I was
trying to hang on to reality. My mother didn't realize what I was
doing. She didn't know I was doing that. I acted normal on the
phone because I knew what I was doing, and I was cool."

When Eric's mother asked him why he would do such a
thing as kill his own grandmother, Eric answered, "I performed a
miracle—I set myself free."

Eric told his doctors that he "felt terrible" about what he
did, but hastened to point out that Nana had called him self-
centered and told him he had these problems because he was a
coward. She also accused him of smoking marijuana in her house.

Eric said, "I didn't want to kill my grandmother. . . . I put a
slip around her head so she wouldn't scream while I phoned.
. . . I gave her some respiration mouth-to-mouth."

Eric was originally found incompetent to stand trial and sent to
Atascadero State Hospital. While awaiting trial there, Eric, who
was involved briefly in the Baptist Church while in junior high
school, served as the Protestant chaplain's assistant.

One psychiatrist wrote, after interviewing Eric before his trial,
"During the interview, the Defendant displayed great improvement until his grandmother's murder was discussed. Then, under
the stress of this part of the interview, his defenses crumbled a bit:
He assured the interviewer that he still believes his psychiatrist
ordered him to kill someone. He is now about midway between
sickness and health. He is now competent to stand trial, having
benefited greatly from his stay at Atascadero. He was placed on
phenothiazine drugs there, and there he applied his good intellect
to the task of trying to understand what had happened to him. He
has not yet completed that task. He must still work on his symbi-
otic link to his parents. . . . With a sensible treatment plan, however, there is every reason to expect the Defendant eventually to
be restored to the community as a productive citizen."

Another evaluating physician wrote about Eric: "He is capable of explaining his psychosis and answering questions thoughtfully. However, I think much of this results from his high intellect and is a thin veneer of non-psychotic thinking. I believe he needs further treatment, with a mandatory maintenance on Thorazine or other antipsychotic medication. He states that the medications are too strong and should be reduced, and I fear he will convince someone to take him off the drugs, which I believe are necessary for his continued improvement and his long term ability to avoid schizophrenic behavior."

When Eric was finally tried for the murder of his grandmother, he was found not guilty by reason of insanity (NGI) and sent back to the mental hospital.

While at Atascadero State Hospital, whenever his medications were reduced, Eric would relapse into severe psychosis. On two such occasions, he pulled out his own front teeth. His hospital record also shows episodes of incoherence, shouting and pounding on the floor, lying on the floor silently, extreme hyperactivity, confusion and shouting, talking to himself incoherently, crying "God help me! God help me!" At times he had to be kept in restraints.

The Chapmans were informed by a psychiatrist who had once treated their son that Eric was suffering from the so-called "bad seed syndrome" and that he would not rest until he had killed his mother, father, brother, and his brother's child, too—in other words, all living blood relatives.

Eric's parents frantically wrote letters to state hospital authorities and criminal justice authorities asking that Eric be permanently committed. They also asked to be able to discuss Eric's case with his doctors. They were answered by state hospital authorities that Eric would not allow information about his case to be released to them. They were told, however, the dates for his potential release and when the potential release dates would be considered for extension, usually six months prior to the release date.

Several months after the murder of Eric's grandmother, Donald Chapman sent the authorities a complete history of his son's mental problems, acknowledged that the boy was not legally or morally responsible for his actions, and asked them to "consider the possible danger" if Eric were released prematurely.

Despite his parents' wishes, state hospital authorities released Eric in August 1978 and put him in a community outpatient treatment (COT) program in Santa Barbara, about 100 miles from his parents' home. His medication was to continue and be monitored by the COT staff. Eric, however, convinced the monitoring physician to lower his dose of antipsychotic medication. Although the first three months of Eric's release were "highly successful," his condition deteriorated rapidly once his medication was reduced. Then the situation went from bad to worse: The Board and Care home he was released to was forced to close. Eric was told to find his own room and board, and was urged to get completely off his medications so he could find a job and support himself. The doctors treating Eric encouraged him to reduce his medication so that he "might better function in the community."

On January 18, 1979, Eric traveled by bus from Santa Barbara to L.A. At two-thirty the next morning he called his brother from a phone booth and asked for a ride back to Santa Barbara. Greg gave him directions to a nearby motel and told him he would pick him up in the morning and drive him back. Then Eric's brother called his parents and told them that Eric was back in town. Eric called him back several hours later and told him his doctor had advised him to take the bus back to Santa Barbara without seeing any members of his family. Eric assured his brother he would take a cab right to the bus station, and then go right back to Santa Barbara. He also promised him he would never "shame the family again," as he felt he had done by murdering his grandmother. He assured his brother he was well and there was nothing to worry about. Greg called his parents again and told them that Eric was on his way back to Santa Barbara.

Less than an hour later, at about eight-thirty in the morning, Donald Chapman was asleep when he heard the doorbell ring. He arose and went to the kitchen, where he could see who was at the door. He looked through the curtains and recognized the silhouette of his son, Eric. He immediately went back to the bedroom and told his wife that he was going to lock the bedroom door and that if she heard any commotion to call the police. Then he went back to the kitchen.

Once again he looked out the window, but Eric was no longer on the front porch. Figuring his son was out in the street,

Donald Chapman opened the front door. He was immediately overwhelmed by Eric. Before he knew what hit him, Donald was struck repeatedly on the head with a three-by-six-inch rock. To defend himself, he grappled with Eric. The two men wrestled their way into the house and fell to the floor of the living room. Donald was able to get on top of his son and hold his arms in place. He called out to a neighbor, who had come over to the front yard from next door, and she called the police.

Meanwhile, Mrs. Chapman ran to get the only real weapon in the house, an old sword. She ran back into the living room and put it against her son's side and told him that if he continued to fight, she would not hesitate to use it on him. Eric ceased struggling.

When police entered Donald Chapman's home, in response to the call, they found Eric and his father on the floor in the living room, near the front door. Eric's father was on top of Eric, holding him down. Donald's face was covered with blood, which was still flowing from his wound. Eric's face, neck, and hands were also covered with blood. Eric's mother stood over the two men, holding the point of a long, curved sword against her son's side. One police officer got hold of Eric, and another got hold of his father. The third officer asked Mrs. Chapman for the sword. She refused to give it up. He asked her again, and she refused again. "It's mine, you can't take it away," she replied. The police officer then threatened to take it away from her if she didn't give it to him. She gave him the sword.

After being subdued by police officers, Eric announced, "I was just released from Atascadero. I spent seven years there. I just tried to kill my father."

Less than an hour after he had told his brother he would never shame his family again, Eric's mother phoned her other son and told him that Eric had tried to kill his father.

Eric's participation in the Community Outpatient Treatment program was revoked after the assault on his father. He went back to the state hospital, to await trial on charges of assault with a deadly weapon.

In June 1979 I examined Eric Chapman, at court request, to determine whether or not he 1. remained a danger to the health and safety of others; 2. had fully recovered his sanity; 3. qualified as gravely disabled; and 4. was competent to stand trial.

During the exam, Eric told me that he strangled his grandmother because "she tried to drown me when I was a baby." He also believed that his psychiatrist at the time wanted him to kill her. He explained the assault on his father by saying, "I hated him—he was a joker the way he brought me up."

"Yeah, it was a crime—a crime of passion. The Bible says to take a weapon and kill your parents. I forget where it says it but I read it after I did it. I did it just to do something silly to get back in jail. I couldn't make it in the streets because I had too much brain damage from the medication and the stress of being ill. I have schizophrenia—that means childlike and don't know what you're doing all the time. Yeah, that's me. Yeah, I told police I had to kill my parents to be free. The Bible says to help them out, and they won't make you feel guilty anymore if they're dead. Yeah, they used to make me feel guilty. Only my mother. My father was an amazing guy. He was my servant, my slave. He tried to do everything for me, but he made me a superior person who ended up in a mental hospital. He was angry at himself and me for trying to do so much for me, and not looking out for himself. He didn't get back at people who hurt his feelings—me and the guys at the office where he worked. He was a fool. He let his sister tell him to do crimes. He was the Boston Strangler and the Hillside Strangler. My mother cracked up. She had a vase that proved I'm Jesus Christ, and when I was a child I broke the vase so they couldn't prove I wasn't Jesus Christ. Nah, I wouldn't touch my mother, that's the wrongest thing you can do. I thought of hurting her once, but I just drove right past the street where we live. Yes, my father and his brother did rape murders."

Eric heard Nana's voice while he was in county jail after trying to kill his father. "I resurrected her. She's been in a nursing home ever since. Everybody in jail tells me I'm Jesus Christ, the doctors, the guards, the inmates. I look a little like Him. I used to pretend I'm Him, with a beard. They cured me of syphilis by witchcraft in county jail. . . .

"Father drove me insane, he and my mother. I took out my

anger on him. The crime triggered my motivation to get well. I hit him with a rock on his head. I did it so I could fly around the sky and come back in twenty minutes. My accomplishment could save the world. I flew through a mirror in an upright position. They're trying to decide if I'm Jesus Christ. I am. Everyone is in worse shape than I. I'm not well yet. I can replace my limbs if they are cut off. I could open my third eye and make things like bullets and hatchet blades passing through me. My third eye is a spiritual concept. . . . I'm Jesus. Everyone is tuned in and all are behind me."

Eric told me he was now asking for a lobotomy, which he thought would be a "cure" for his mental problems.

My conclusion was that Eric continued to suffer from chronic paranoid schizophrenia, that he required active treatment and should be kept on antipsychotic tranquilizing medication in a hospital setting because he was clearly incapable of adjusting on his own, even with outpatient supervision. As to the specific questions asked by the court, I replied: 1) that Eric remained a danger to the health and safety of others, particularly family members, although his transfer of hostility to others was a possibility. 2) He had not "fully recovered his sanity" within the meaning of the law. 3) He was gravely disabled. 4) He was, however, competent to stand trial, within the required legal standards.

Other doctors who examined Eric after his attack on his father also found him to be severely mentally ill, paranoid schizophrenic, and a "menace to the health and safety of others," and in need of extended hospitalization.

But the criminal justice system did not focus on that medical advice. Instead, it mirrored Eric's own craziness. Although the assault charge was filed as a felony on February 14, 1979, the case was amazingly plea-bargained to a misdemeanor. As a result, this dangerous individual was to be sentenced to only a six-month term and his mental condition was not placed in issue. Eric's family wrote letters protesting this disposition, both asking for his proper treatment and pleading for protection from the criminal justice system. The district attorney's office, a party to this plea-bargain, responded with a strange tactic, requesting the court to revoke the guilty plea. This was denied.

Before the sentencing date, however, Eric was again found

incompetent, forcing a delay in further proceedings, and he was rehospitalized for eight months. When Eric returned to court on January 17, 1980, the district attorney's office again asked to have the guilty verdict set aside. This time the court astonishingly agreed, despite defense arguments of double jeopardy. Further defense appeals were futile.

Now facing a felony charge, Eric entered a new plea of NGI and was found insane by the court. This verdict was then linked with the insanity confinement for the murder, thereby relegating all of the earlier, intricate legal maneuvering to the level of an elementary academic exercise. Eric was returned to the state hospital for further treatment.

Eric's parents finally had some breathing room. They were able to relocate and change their names and hopefully would not have to face the imminent threat of a dangerous son.

Although the majority of people suffering from paranoid schizophrenia are not acutely or actively dangerous, in some people the nature of their assorted obsessions puts the lives of others —in many instances loved ones—at risk. In April 1979 doctors at Atascadero requested an extension of Eric's commitment.

Later that year, the Chapmans sold their home and moved "thousands of miles away from California," in hopes of living safe and secure from future attacks by their son. Eric, however, correctly guessed where they were living.

In 1980, after a long phone call during which Eric made several hostile remarks toward his family, his brother wrote to Eric's probation officer: "Obviously, it will be difficult ever to completely trust Eric again as he has a capacity to convince his family, his doctors, experienced hospital personnel, and some renowned legal professionals that he is not a threat and that in fact he is quite well, when in reality he is pathetically sick and extremely hostile and dangerous to others.

"Eric's and my father sadly had to terminate his career. He has been reduced to a nervous wreck, has sold his home of thirty years, changed his name and has left the state. He lives in fear of the day that Eric is released, knowing full well that he is Eric's target."

In October 1981, more than two and a half years after the assault on him, Eric's father wrote a letter to the medical director at Atascadero State Hospital, pleading that his son not be released.

In 1982 Eric was still claiming to be Jesus Christ and that he had come to "save the world." An examining physician stated that Eric "was one of the sickest individuals I have had the opportunity to examine." Eric claimed to be "crazy" because the CIA had gained computerized control of electrodes that had long ago been placed in his brain. Eric's uncle, who had been dead for many years, was a "man from heaven" who had assisted the CIA in its plot. In addition to the CIA, the sheriff's department and the county jail also had access to the computer, which was loading classified information into Eric's brain. Eric said he had been told before he was born that he was Jesus Christ.

He also said he believed that by assaulting his father he was making the world a better place to live. His intention was not to kill his father, he said, because he believed that if he did the world would end. Eric said that his real father was his deceased uncle Gene—but he also stated that he was born by immaculate conception.

In April 1984 I examined Eric again and found him still suffering from chronic paranoid schizophrenia, with a continuing potential to become violent and dangerous during actively psychotic episodes.

At Christmas in 1985 Eric told his father: "Given my freedom, I will probably kill you."

In April 1986 Eric stated to an examining psychiatrist that he believed he had once been a hermaphrodite, but that his parents had his female sex organs surgically obliterated when he was ten years old. He believed his mother was a hermaphrodite, too. Regarding his belief that he was Christ: "Yes, I thought I was Jesus Christ. I have heard the infinite spirit talking to me. Maybe it's Zeus. I think my uncle was the real Jesus, and when he comes back as my baby he'll be Jesus Christ and I'll be escalated up to God, who would be Krishna's girlfriend in heaven. I should be a girl now, so when the time comes my uncle can put me in his palace in heaven. . . . My grandmother gave my mother a bad gene because she had fellatio with an animal. Our genes are changed with every sexual experience. . . . I think my father is the devil. I think his influence on me is affecting the whole world, because the whole world hears my thoughts. Right now I'm the son of perdition, the Grim Reaper. . . .''

That month, Eric's commitment was extended for another two-year period, until June 1988. Examining psychiatrists found him actively psychotic and in need of further hospitalization.

In March 1987, mental health authorities at the hospital (Patton) reported that Eric was improving, that he no longer believed he was God or Jesus, and that he seemed to be getting along better in the hospital. He still expressed the wish "to be put to sleep."

Although doctors then felt Eric should remain in the hospital for at least another six months, they believed that if he showed further improvement he could someday transfer to a locked community facility, where movement is controlled by the staff and residents do not have the freedom to come and go as they please. Because such units clearly violate the civil rights of the residents, they are legally regulated by the court. A more recent evaluation finding Eric to be a continuing danger to others has extended his confinement through June 1990.

In Los Angeles last Christmas they built a Tent City for homeless people. I walked past there one day—it was like a scene out of a Dickens novel. Hundreds of people knocked about dressed in rags. I would venture to say that half of those people were severely mentally disturbed—psychotic. Why are they out on the streets? We've got twenty thousand people living on the streets in Los Angeles. Why? Because it's almost impossible to hospitalize them. The laws that have been created for involuntary commitment and treatment are quite demanding and difficult to sustain. In the United States, people have the constitutional right to remain mentally ill.

Prior to 1967, when the Lanterman–Petris–Short Act (the California Mental Health Treatment Statute) was implemented, the criteria for putting someone in a mental hospital were much simpler. A person could be committed if he was mentally disordered and in need of either supervision, care, treatment, or restraint.

But then political interest groups jumped into the act and

charged that many people were being railroaded into mental hospitals. In truth, this was probably a valid commentary of practices that existed during the infancy of psychiatry.

It did not reflect current practices. But the special interests managed to have the law changed. They advocated three criteria by which a person could be involuntarily committed to a mental hospital: danger to self, danger to others, and gravely disabled. What does "gravely disabled" mean? It means unable to provide food, clothing, and shelter. What does that mean? According to the way the law is interpreted, if you can go to the mailbox and pick up your Social Security check, you're not gravely disabled, even if you think you're living on Mars.

At the time the law was being considered, I was one of the four doctors regularly consulting for the mental health court, Department 95. The mental health subcommittee came down from Sacramento for hearings on the bill—yet not one of us was invited to testify. Then the sitting judge of the mental health court was refused permission to testify, as he was against the provisions of the bill. Instead, there was professional testimony to suggest that schizophrenia was fully controllable and treatable within seven days.

This does not reflect the experience of the psychiatric community. However, the subcommittee apparently endorsed this testimony. Well, they figured, if it can be done in seven days, we'll give the average doctor double that time—fourteen days. That's how the fourteen-day hold was created. After the initial seventy-two-hour evaluation period, without further legal proceedings, a person could not be held for more than fourteen days against his will. So if a person fit one or more of the criteria, he could be held for a total of seventeen days—three days for evaluation and fourteen days for "treatment." He had to be discharged after seventeen days unless a conservatorship was initiated (for gravely disabled people), or danger-to-others post-certification proceedings were started. A suicidal patient, or one dangerous to himself, could not be held beyond seventeen days.

As a result, people were being released prematurely—still disturbed—and committing crimes, attempting suicide, or acting dangerously. The legislators were forced to go back and rewrite the law.

Because of the increasing suicide rate in recently released patients, they concluded that fourteen days wasn't enough. So they doubled it again. Now, a person who is dangerous to himself can be kept for three, fourteen, and fourteen—a total of thirty-one days. No more. A person who is dangerous to others can be kept for three, fourteen, and then ninety. In order to keep him beyond ninety days, it must be demonstrated that he committed dangerous acts while in the hospital. That's a very iffy proposition. So much so that in 1985 fewer than twenty cases of danger to others were upheld in the courts. The authorities don't bother filing them because they're so difficult to sustain!

The standards and criteria are no longer psychiatric, but legal. The problem has become a civil rights issue, not a medical one. Courts are dictating to the doctors that they have to "cure" these people in unreasonable time frames—when, in many cases, life-long treatment does not result in improvement, let alone cure. Before these new laws we had a population of thirty-five thousand in the mental hospitals of California. Now we have five thousand. Someone will look at that statistic and say, How wonderful! But a large percentage of those thirty-five thousand are walking the streets, homeless.

Someday, one of them may be Eric Chapman . . . searching for his parents.

CHAPTER

10

Madness,
murder, and
motherhood

We're all capable of killing if our psychic wholeness or existence is threatened. Of course, in some people that wholeness seems to be more precarious, and the murderous instinct a little too close to the surface for the health and safety of those nearby. We all have inner storms that we must calm, but some of us are tormented by a storm that can be calmed only by the unleashing of destructive forces. Such a person is actually compelled to kill. Most of the time, these turmoils arise out of the central issues and attachments of life, and the person is driven to kill by some inner emotion or instinct gone haywire. In my experience, even the life-giving instincts of motherhood are not immune.

New Year's Day 1980 was a memorable day in the life of Arlyne Genger, a day that brought about profound and permanent change in her life and the life of her family. If you asked her today, she would probably want to erase it, undo it.

Then again, Arlyne's life has had more than its share of such days.

Arlyne Genger was born in Los Angeles on July 29, 1943. She was the oldest of three children and was raised in an intact family. Her family's behavior was superficially correct, but behind the proper facade, there was no meaningful interpersonal relationships. "As a child I was very lonely," Arlyne complained.

She tended to identify with her father, although she sometimes believed he was "a very cruel person. He provided the things, and that's all my mother seemed to want." In addition, Arlyne believed that her mother "never had an interest in us as people and never wanted us to grow up."

When she was thirteen years old, her nine-year-old brother shot and killed their eleven-year-old sister. The killing was reported as an accident: the boy had been cleaning and loading the shotgun when it went off. However, Arlyne's brother manifested aggressive behavior again through the years, and was treated psychiatrically several times.

Arlyne's health was always poor. In the tenth grade she was out with infectious mononucleosis for three months. She also was discovered to be anemic, a condition that has followed her all her life.

Though she was of above normal intelligence, Arlyne was not able to go beyond two years at the University of Southern California. She took courses at other colleges from time to time, but never obtained a degree. She fancied herself a writer, but was never able to support herself adequately.

In 1966, Arlyne married a man fourteen years her senior. The marriage was troubled right from the very beginning. In 1968 Arlyne tried to get her husband to try marriage counseling, but he refused. They had two children, a boy who died after two weeks from congenital heart disease, and a daughter, Selena.

In 1969, her own mental illness was revealed for the first time. She was admitted to Glendale Adventist Hospital for three months, during which she received medications and electroshock treatments. In 1970 she was divorced. That year she attempted to commit suicide by running in front of some cars. She was hospitalized at the Van Nuys Psychiatric Unit for several weeks after that. Other hospitalizations occurred over the next decade. Arlyne did not respond well to treatment, mainly because she refused to take her medication on a regular basis.

Once divorced, Arlyne had to learn to fend for herself and became very adept at office work. She worked for two years as an office manager. She and Selena lived together in apartments and rented houses, while Arlyne either worked or received welfare.

At times she worked as a bookkeeper and office manager for her own family.

Her father died in 1975 of a heart attack. In 1976 Arlyne's brother attempted to kill their mother by strangulation. He also threatened Arlyne and her daughter Selena.

Because of her own steadily worsening mental illness and her failure to respond to treatment, Arlyne's relationship with her family deteriorated. She was in almost constant conflict with her mother, younger brother, and ex-husband. She eventually lost her job as a bookkeeper and office manager for her family. Finally, Arlyne lost custody of her daughter—to her own mother. Though Selena's grandmother had temporary guardianship, most of the time the girl lived with her father and his new wife in Northern California.

Throughout 1979 Arlyne's condition steadily deteriorated. At one particularly low point, after being evicted from an apartment, she was arrested for shoplifting. She represented herself in court and demanded a jury trial. The charges were eventually dismissed after she spent a total of twenty-nine days in jail.

Arlyne lived on the streets most of 1979. She also isolated herself from her family, and sought no psychiatric treatment. During the summer, she resorted to stealing fruit off neighborhood trees for food, until she was picked up by the police and taken to Olive View Hospital, where she was kept for seventeen days. But her problems getting food were not the worst of that year: Arlyne was also raped three times.

Eventually, Arlyne was forced to seek refuge in her mother's home. Still, she felt that her mother wanted to dominate her life and that she was intent on separating Selena from her. As an example, she pointed to the fact that Selena was sent to live with her father in Northern California.

It was during December 1979 that Arlyne decided that something had to be done to prevent this enforced separation from her daughter. She also became convinced that she and her daughter had leukemia. Arlyne decided that not only had her mother been instrumental in keeping Selena away from her, but that she was responsible for giving them both leukemia.

Selena was spending Christmas vacation with her mother and grandmother. Arlyne was further convinced that Selena did not want to go back to her father, and that the girl would rather be dead than be separated from her mother. Then there was the leukemia—a sure death sentence. Arlyne figured that neither she nor her daughter had anything to live for. They were better off dead. A murder-suicide pact took shape in her mind.

Arlyne had been living with her mother through the entire month of December 1980. If something was going to be done, it had to be done now. The New Year was approaching, and Selena was scheduled to go back to her father in Northern California the next day. So Arlyne had to act fast. She felt she would have to punish her mother for interfering in her relationship with Selena. Furthermore, she knew her mother would never allow her to follow through on the murder-suicide plans she had made for herself and thirteen-year-old Selena.

After a New Year's Eve party, her mother went to bed in the early morning hours of the New Year. Arlyne entered the room with a paring knife and attacked her mother. She stabbed her on the shoulder—"I aimed for the middle of the chest, but got her in the shoulder." Arlyne ran out of the room but then listened at the door and heard her mother walking around the room. "She was totally insensitive to pain, acting like I had annoyed her—like poking her with a pin."

So Arlyne went back into the room and attacked again. This time she tore into her mother not only with the knife but with her own teeth, and bit and stabbed at her repeatedly, until her strength was gone. Leaving the knife still stuck in her mother's neck, Arlyne left to find her daughter, who had been awakened by the noise, come upon the struggle, and then fled the sight of her grandmother's being killed.

Arlyne felt that Selena still wanted to follow through on their plans to die together. After all, hadn't she assured her mother that she would rather die than go back to her father? Arlyne's plan was to kill Selena by slashing her neck and then commit suicide.

Arlyne found her daughter in her bedroom. She entered the room still wearing her bloody night clothes, and blocked the door with a large piece of furniture. She told her daughter that they were going to live together forever and the way they were going to do it was by dying together in that very room.

She gave Selena five or six lithium tablets, which quickly

made the child drowsy. Then she approached Selena with a box-cutting knife, which consists of a razor blade fastened to a handle. Arlyne grabbed her daughter under the chin and said, "This will only be like a paper cut," as she drew the blade of the box cutter across her daughter's throat. Then she lay down with the bleeding girl.

But though Selena was bleeding, she didn't seem to be dying fast enough for Arlyne. She asked the girl for her arm, and then applied the knife to the girl's right wrist.

Selena moaned and went into shock. Arlyne could not continue. The bleeding stopped and she watched her daughter for several hours. Finally, Selena woke up. Someone knocked on the door and called to Arlyne's mother. But Arlyne did not answer, and hushed Selena. The people went away.

That night, when Selena was strong enough, her mother dressed her and the two left the apartment. They spent the night in the place that had been Arlyne's home for much of the past year—under a bridge on Coldwater Canyon Boulevard in North Hollywood.

The next day they went to the Burbank Airport and cashed in Selena's ticket to Northern California. They used the money to buy some food and a motel room. A day later, Selena got away from her mother long enough to call for help. The police took them both into custody.

Arlyne was initially sent to jail, where she spent six months before being found incompetent to stand trial and sent to Patton State Hospital. She did not adjust well to the state hospital. Her psychotic symptoms persisted. She displayed both paranoid and grandiose delusions, and often had angry outbursts. She not only resisted treatment, but also isolated herself from the other patients. She refused to acknowledge that she was mentally ill. Nevertheless, after several months of treatment at Patton, she was again examined. This time she was found competent to stand trial.

I initially examined Arlyne Genger on December 4, 1980, almost a year after she killed her mother. My examination was to be a comprehensive one, addressing both the issues of competency to stand trial and criminal responsibility.

There was clear evidence of a psychotic process, consistent with the description rendered by other psychiatrists. Arlyne blamed outside forces for her nervous breakdown, including her husband, the doctors who treated her, and her family. When I focused on the ten-month period when she lived on the streets, "starving," she stated "I was anemic." She went on to say, "I had to eliminate my mother to prevent a gross ugliness. I decided to slash my daughter's throat for us to die together, but the noise stopped me from killing her. I couldn't take it." Arlyne claimed that her daughter had helped her kill her mother.

When she was first hospitalized as incompetent to stand trial, Arlyne had been placed on antipsychotic medication, to which she responded minimally. That medication was discontinued, however, and it was my feeling that on December 4, 1980, she was marginally competent to stand trial. As far as her mental state at the time of the event, however, it was clear that she was delusional and highly disturbed. I concluded that she was insane under the criteria existing in the State of California and that she lacked "substantial capacity to conform her conduct to the requirement of law."

In short, she had acted because of her mental disorder. It was my recommendation that she be rehospitalized, placed on medication, and followed intensively.

The court went along with my recommendation. Arlyne was found guilty of second-degree murder in the death of her mother. This was a necessary prelude to the issue of her sanity being decided. Again, a legal fiction was in the making: First a finding of guilt, then a determination of whether or not she was, in fact, capable of committing a crime. Once the court turned to that question, she was found not guilty by reason of insanity (NGI), and sent back to Patton State Hospital.

Arlyne may never be reconciled with her daughter. Her attempts to correspond with Selena have met with no response. That may be the ultimate price she will have to keep paying. No doubt her ability to keep paying that price and accept the loss will be a major factor in her future stability. The authorities, acceding to Selena's wishes, have made it a condition of Arlyne's potential release that she never contact her daughter. Her life will not be easy.

The loss of a child by your own acts—even if those acts were committed while mentally ill—would be difficult enough for anyone to endure. But imagine the torment if your child is lost through no fault of your own. Such was the fate of Mary Childs.

Mary Childs was a happy woman. The twenty-six-year-old grocery checker was going to have a baby, and all signs were good on September 20, 1974, when she presented herself for her scheduled labor and delivery at the Kaiser Permanente Hospital on Sunset Boulevard. Her baby would be big and healthy: The admitting physician examined Mary and estimated that her baby would weigh in at about eight and a half pounds. Its heartbeat was clear and strong.

Mary went to sleep that night feeling safe and warm. Her baby would be born in this ultra-modern hospital in the heart of the most modern city in the world. Mary couldn't help feeling a little like a queen. The hospital staff was there to take care of her every wish. And the stocky red-haired obstetrics nurse who appeared to be in charge seemed to be taking an extra special interest in her.

But when Mary woke up in the early morning hours of September 21, something was terribly wrong. At first she thought it was a dream. She felt awake and yet her mind was smothered in a woolly blanket. Maybe this was just an aftereffect of the drugs the nurse had given her before she went to sleep? But could the drugs account for this horrible, empty feeling that . . . that she wasn't pregnant any longer?

Mary struggled through the drug haze to lift her head. She didn't have to lift it too high, because the big, pregnant belly she had carried so proudly these past few months was no longer there. Mary was already screaming and crying as she tore at the hospital sheets obstructing her view—but what she saw between her legs just took all the scream right out of her. For there was the shriveled corpse of a baby, its neatly cut umbilical cord already dried out into a short, withered stump. Mary was so lost at that moment that she hardly noticed the matronly obstetrics nurse standing over her with the doctors, who were shaking their heads.

And the doctors just kept on shaking their heads. The obstetrics nurse told them that when she had come around the ward, she had found Mary unconscious, with the stillborn fetus between her legs. Blood tests found high concentrations of barbiturates and other narcotics in Mary's blood. None of these drugs had been prescribed. The doctors concluded that this was just another drug addict who had abused her baby to death before it was even born. When Mary protested that she had never taken any of the drugs they found in her system, they just shook their heads some more.

Of course, an autopsy was performed on the 3-pound stillborn baby. Then four doctors came to Mary's bedside to discuss the tragedy. They told her the baby had not only been stillborn but that it had been dead for a week or so. Mary told them that this could not be so. She had felt her baby move for months, in fact, had felt it move the day before, on her way to the hospital. The admitting doctor had told her there was a clear heartbeat, she protested. The four doctors shook their heads. There was nothing they could do. They had been through scenes like this before with hysterical women. And this one was, after all, a drug addict. The only comfort they could offer her was a pat on the shoulder.

The doctors told Mary she would have to leave the hospital.

Profoundly grief-stricken, Mary Childs went home. For a while she was so distressed that she was almost constantly nauseous. With time, the shock and the horror lessened, but she was left with lingering depression over her lost baby.

On January 17, 1975, Kathryn Viramontes went to visit her obstetrician's office next to Valley Presbyterian Hospital in the San Fernando Valley. The blood test, urinalysis, lab work, and doctor's exam confirmed what she had known since the end of August—she was pregnant.

When Kathryn filled out the history form before her exam, she drew lines through the areas marked "spouse's name," "occupation," and "employer." Though she was not married, Kathryn indicated that the father of her child was forty-one years old and in good health. But that was all she would tell the doctor about the man.

Elsewhere on the form, Kathryn wrote that she had three children already: Ritchie, born in 1966; Angela, born in 1969; and Debbie, born in 1970. This was to be her fourth child and Kathryn had already decided it was to be her last. She asked the doctor if she could have a tubal ligation after the birth, which, from what the doctor could tell, would be in early June.

Over the next several months, Kathryn visited the obstetrician seven times. She was always in good health. Her blood pressure was normal and her blood count actually improved over her first visit, when she was mildly anemic. The doctor remarked that her blood would be nice and red when her baby was born. Kathryn knew it was because she had been dutifully taking her vitamin and iron supplements, as the doctor had prescribed.

Of course, Kathryn also knew that she had another friend who was helping to take care of her and encouraging her to take good care of herself and her unborn baby. She remarked to friends how fortunate she had been when Norma Jean Armistead had come into her life. Red-headed, matronly Norma Jean was almost like a mother to Kathryn. At the very least, she was like a big sister. And Kathryn really needed a good friend, especially since William Hooks, the father of her unborn child, had moved away in April. But Norma also knew all about how to take care of pregnant women and their newborn babies. She was not only a registered nurse, but actually worked in the obstetrics ward at one of the big hospitals in downtown L.A. Kathryn thought it was Kaiser Permanente. Norma had three children of her own, too: a son and daughter who were grown up, and a little baby girl named Carrie, who had been born just the previous December.

Norma was such a good friend, she even offered to induce labor and deliver the baby for her at home if Kathryn got tired of waiting to go to the hospital.

On May 13, 1975, Kathryn went to the doctor's office for her routine examination. The doctor told her that he expected the birth of her baby to be normal, without complications. The baby was growing on schedule and the heartbeat was strong and clear. He had performed a vaginal exam, which showed that the baby's head was still high, up out of the pelvis, and that her cervix was still clamped shut and firm. Considering Kathryn's history of three prior deliveries, this meant that the baby would not be born for a few weeks yet. It looked as though the doctor's estimate of the first week in June would be accurate. Kathryn went home pleased. She couldn't wait to tell Norma Jean.

Four days later, on the morning of May 17, a neighbor who lived near Kathryn's home on Van Owen Street in the San Fernando Valley, went to the door to find Kathryn's nine-year-old son Ritchie standing there, crying. Ritchie said that his mother was in her bedroom and was hurt, so could the neighbor please come over.

Another neighbor was already in the house calling for an ambulance. He had heard the boy crying and had come in to find the bedroom looking like a tornado had whipped through it. The mattress and box spring were off the bed and lying at an angle, the sheets and blankets strewn all about the room. And there was blood on the edge of the box spring. He saw Kathryn lying under the mattress and right away thought perhaps something had gone wrong with her pregnancy and she had fallen off the bed and was helpless and bleeding. He lifted the box spring and when he saw what was under there he put it back down exactly the way he found it and went to call an ambulance and the police.

Meanwhile, Norma Jean Armistead was being examined at Kaiser Permanente Hospital, where her daughter had driven her. The doctor examining Norma had a problem. She had walked into the hospital carrying an obviously newborn baby. Norma told him she had given birth to the baby en route to the hospital. She seemed past childbearing age but, of course, he had seen stranger things in his career. But when he started to examine her, he noticed the scar on her abdomen. When he called her attention to it, she said she once had gall-bladder surgery, and that her appendix had been taken out, too. Norma went on to protest that "They're trying to take my baby away from me!" and insisted that she had given birth to the baby.

Following routine, the doctor examined her internally to see if there were any lacerations in her birth canal. The doctor was surprised to find that not only were there none, but no blood at all—highly unusual for someone who has just delivered a child, to say the least. But the doctor was even more surprised when he couldn't find a cervix or a uterus! The doctor was suddenly certain that this woman had long ago had a hysterectomy.

"Norma, you didn't tell me you had a hysterectomy," the doctor said.

"You're trying to take my baby away from me, too," she yelled at the doctor.

The doctor just patted Norma Jean Armistead on the shoulder.

A week later, on May 25, 1975, Mary Childs, still in anguished mourning for her lost baby, was notified by Kaiser Permanente Hospital to come in and pick up her daughter, who was now almost eight months old. She was presented with the child and told that the baby she had found in her bed was not hers. For those eight months, her child had been living with Norma Jean Armistead, her lesbian daughter and homosexual son, and Charlie Armistead, her common-law husband. Little by little the grotesque story was pieced together by Mary and her attorneys.

Norma Jean Jackson—who had once been in a mental hospital in Texas, and had gone on to become a nurse in the obstetrics ward of Kaiser Permanente Hospital—wanted a baby. She needed a baby because she knew that it would help prevent Charlie Armistead, her common-law husband, from going back to his wife and kids. Of course, having another baby was physically impossible for Norma Jean. Her uterus had been removed years before. But she had a plan: Norma once mused to her sister that she could easily get a baby from the hospital where she was working. One of her duties, in addition to newborn care, was postmortem care of deceased infants. All she would have to do would be to substitute a dead fetus in place of the newborn baby, which she would steal for herself. Her sister registered horror at this idea but didn't take Norma seriously.

A few weeks later, Norma announced to her sister and others that she wouldn't have to steal a baby after all, because she was really pregnant now. When her sister asked her how she could become pregnant after having a hysterectomy, Norma said that it had really been a "partial" hysterectomy, and she could still have babies.

As her "pregnancy" wore on, Norma added some weight to make it look real. Because she was already overweight, it was not difficult for her to look pregnant. As the time for her to have her baby drew near, she began looking out for just the right one. Norma, a white woman, felt she needed a black baby because Charlie was black. When she saw Mary Childs come into the hospital, she knew her baby was as good as delivered.

While Mary was asleep that night, Norma barely disturbed her when she gave her strong sedatives plus a labor-inducing drug. Then, while Mary was dead to the world, Norma delivered her baby. She took a dead fetus from the morgue and left it between Mary's legs. Then she walked out of the hospital with Mary Childs's infant daughter.

Norma literally walked to another, nearby hospital with the newborn child and informed the staff there that she had just delivered it herself, at home, a few hours before. The clerk said she should have a medical exam, but Norma Jean refused. Though Norma Jean appeared clearly beyond childbearing age, she walked out of the hospital with a birth certificate naming her the mother of little "Carrie Armistead."

Norma Jean would have gotten clean away with the theft of Mary Childs's baby—except that one baby was not enough for her. She decided she needed another pregnancy to keep Charlie Armistead from going back to his family. So . . . Norma Jean "got pregnant" again.

She befriended Kathryn Viramontes, stayed close by, and kept watch as the unsuspecting woman's pregnancy progressed. Then, on the night of May 16, 1975, she injected Kathryn in the left elbow and buttocks with anesthetic, muscle-relaxing, and labor-inducing drugs. Then she stretched a seven-inch length of three-inch wide tape across Kathryn's mouth from cheek to cheek as the woman lapsed into half-sleep.

But half-sleep was not enough, for, unlike Mary Childs, who had been fully asleep and had never known what was going on, Kathryn knew what was happening, and could later identify Norma Jean. So Norma made a neat, surgically precise, and extremely effective slice across Kathryn Viramontes's throat, partially cutting her carotid artery, jugular vein, windpipe, esophagus, and the fourth cervical vertebra of her neck. Kathryn died very quickly, and while she did, the pool of blood beneath her head stopped growing as her blood pressure fell precipitously.

Then Norma went to work on Kathryn's abdomen. She lifted Kathryn's blouse to just below her breasts, pulled down her light-blue-checked Capri pants to just above her knees, then lowered her multicolored bikini panties. With the same surgical precision with which she had murdered Kathryn, Norma Jean then made a classical Caesarean incision beginning just below the navel, and running five inches straight down to the pubic area. Then she delivered the baby.

The next day, connections were discovered between Kathryn Viramontes and Norma Jean Armistead, and Norma was arrested. After her arrest, Norma called her sister three times. The first time, she told her that Kathryn had been murdered by her boyfriend while Norma was hiding in the closet, and she had delivered the baby to save its life. The second time she called her sister, a few hours later, she admitted that she had murdered Kathryn, had been arrested, and was now in custody at the Van Nuys police station. When the sister started to cry, Norma told her not to be upset, because she had given Kathryn drugs and Kathryn had not felt any pain when her throat had been cut.

Norma called her sister a third time that afternoon and asked her if Kathryn Viramontes was dead. Her sister told her yes. Norma said she had not killed Kathryn, but had killed Julie, Charlie Armistead's wife. Then she started to scream and cry that she didn't kill Kathy, and that if she did, her sister should let her stay in jail because she deserved to die.

When Mary Childs's baby was returned to her, it did not mean the end of her anguish. Mary's attorneys's investigations revealed an astonishing series of blunders on the part of the hospital. When the autopsy was performed on the dead baby found in her bed, the results were not compared to Mary's admission charts and test results. The admitting physicians were not consulted either. Had such a routine check been made, they would have known that the stillborn baby could not have been Mary's for several reasons: first, Mary's baby should have weighed at least eight pounds; the stillborn baby weighed only three. Second, Mary's baby was full-term; the stillborn fetus was premature. The admitting physician had distinctly heard fetal heartbeats when

Mary was admitted; the stillborn baby had been dead at least a week. Mary was found in a drugged condition, yet her admission tests showed her to be drug-free and she was not to be given any drugs while in the hospital. The umbilical cord on the infant did not match the cord still attached to Mary.

All of these inconsistencies were a matter of medical record. Yet the hospital did not admit foul play in the disappearance of Mary Childs's baby until Kathryn Viramontes's death and Norma Jean's arrest made it impossible to deny any longer.

Was there an intentional cover-up of the fact that Mary's baby had disappeared because of the hospital's negligence? One of the doctors who had examined Mary only one hour before the birth of her baby did not believe it when he was told that her child had been stillborn. He knew his examination had been accurate, and that Mary's baby was healthy. This physician had reported Norma Jean Armistead to the hospital officials for problems in her care of Mary Childs, and on other occasions. He had felt very badly for Mary and had wanted to talk to her, but he had been told by his superiors not to call her.

Mary Childs sued Kaiser Permanente Hospital Center for over $20,000,000. She and her attorneys charged that the doctors did know that the dead baby wasn't hers, but that they conspired to keep that fact from her and prevent an investigation into what really happened. As written in the lawsuit, she charged that the doctors and hospital "also knew that this would cause the plaintiff [Mary Childs] horror, grief, fright, shame, anger, humiliation, nausea, and embarrassment, resulting in great mental suffering and emotional distress, causing profound shock to her nervous system, causing physical injuries to her person."

In a nonjury trial, the judge awarded Mary Childs $275,000 and $100,000 to her daughter, whom Mary named Christy Ann.

Norma Jean did not stand trial right away. When she was examined psychiatrically, she was diagnosed as having Ganser's syndrome, a temporary condition that manifests itself during periods of involuntary confinement. This disorder, while not the origin of Norma Jean's criminal behavior, may have derived from her underlying hysterical condition. In Ganser's syndrome, the person assumes the role of "patient" and exhibits a variety of bizarre psychiatric symptoms and conditions. If there is some genuine underlying mental disorder, the symptoms may be exaggerated. The only problem is the person looks "too crazy." This was certainly true in Norma Jean's case. Consequently, she was found to be incompetent to stand trial and was committed to Patton State Hospital. After seven months at Patton, she regained her competence to stand trial and was sent to Metropolitan State Hospital, where she resided during her trial.

I examined Norma Jean Armistead prior to her trial. I was one of the psychiatrists who determined that she was incompetent to stand trial right away, and later, once she had been in the mental hospital for several months, gave the go-ahead. I saw her again when the issue of criminal responsibility came up. The most striking thing about her appearance was that her hair was bright orange. She was kind of spacy and appeared to be standing back and observing what was going on. Norma Jean was the objective examiner even while she was being examined. Normally, this kind of separation between the emotions and the thinking process points to some kind of mental illness. People suffering from schizophrenia, for example, are unable to coordinate emotion, logic, and thinking. But it was my opinion that Norma Jean did not fit the classical definitions of any single mental illness. She suffered features of both psychosis and hysteria. She was, first of all, suffering from an insatiable obsession to have a baby. Hysteria often produces obsessional desires, and Norma Jean had this obsession for most of her adult life. It only intensified in 1961 after her hysterectomy.

To some extent, Norma Jean's obsession affected her judgment and legally diminished her mental capacity on the murder charge, and I testified to that effect. She was, however, able to act in a goal-directed manner. A full-blown psychotic would most likely not have been able to carry through on the elaborate, long-term plots Norma Jean had to devise in order to satisfy her ever-present drive to have a baby. After all, she had to wait several months before she killed Kathryn Viramontes. The drive, or obsession, was always there, but controllable. In the meantime, she was able to function. When the time came for the drive to take over, it did—with murderous consequences.

Hysteria allowed Norma Jean to divorce any guilt from her thinking processes. By totally repressing any potential feelings of compassion or guilt, Norma Jean was exquisitely able to treat other people as objects in order to fulfill her goals. She had no qualms or remorse about stealing babies from their natural mothers, even if it meant slitting the mother's throat.

In the courtroom, where I had to present my opinion within a legal framework, I testified that Norma Jean's mental capacity was legally diminished by virtue of her psychiatric disorder. If the jury relied on my testimony, it would serve to partially reduce Norma Jean's responsibility and result in a lesser charge and reduced punishment. Such testimony may be upsetting from a layperson's point of view, but it was psychiatrically and legally accurate.

The jury, however, concluded that Norma Jean should be held fully responsible for her behavior. Apparently they felt that the heinous nature of her crimes completely overshadowed any evidence of a psychiatric disorder. They had been shown photographs of Kathryn Viramontes after Norma Jean's attack on her. In February 1976 the jury found her guilty of first-degree murder. During the sanity phase of her trial, she was found to be sane. In March 1976 she was sentenced to life in prison.

Norma Jean's case is an example of just how badly two of our major institutions can work. This time, the hospital system failed just as utterly and miserably as the legal system. All along the way, whatever could possibly go wrong, did. Even more important than what happened to Norma Jean is the fate of her victims, who were never really protected. Once it was discovered that a monstrous miscarriage of justice and mercy had occurred, the people in charge still didn't show any compassion for the victim, Mary Childs. They covered it up and didn't help her at all. It was a fairly simple matter for the Kaiser staff to discover that the dead baby found in Mary Childs's bed was not hers. It would have been just as easy for the staff of the second hospital to determine that the baby Norma Jean claimed was hers could not possibly be hers. Kathryn Viramontes's death could have been prevented if Norma Jean had been apprehended when these opportunities arose. But she was not discovered until her obsession became murderous and her trail became bloody. Even then, the medical system just crept along. It took nursing authorities until 1977 to revoke Norma Jean's nursing license.

As for the legal system, I don't believe Mary Childs's judgment came anywhere near to making up for what she went through. I examined Mary, too, for her civil suit, and found her to be profoundly disturbed by the ordeal the hospital put her through. She and her daughter were literally tied to each other by an artificial umbilical cord. They were inseparable during the day and slept together at night. No one was going to take her baby away from her again. Did her financial settlement make her whole and compensate her adequately for her loss and damages? Did it even enable her to begin to rebuild the wreckage of her life? Consider that more than half her $375,000 settlement went to pay for legal expenses.

Meanwhile, Norma Jean was not taking her sentence lying down. Though she was on psychiatric medication herself, by 1979 Norma Jean became a night aid in the psychiatric treatment unit of the California Institute for Women.

In April 1981, five years after her conviction and sentencing, Norma Jean came up for parole. The judge during her murder trial wrote a letter to the parole board in which he recommended that Norma Jean not be granted parole because: "This woman, in order to satisfy whatever desire she had to live with her common-law husband using the means to make him think that she was having their baby, committed horrendous offenses. With just that motivation, she stole a baby from its mother with no feeling of remorse whatsoever. Needing an additional support of a second baby to keep her common-law husband from going back to his wife and children, she murdered a pregnant woman by slashing her throat and then doing a Caesarean operation, removing the baby in the woman's apartment when the minor children were asleep. She left, taking the baby, leaving the bloody mess and gruesome body to be discovered by the children when they awoke in the morning. This inhuman lack of feeling conduct on the part of this inmate is so reprehensible that to return her to society is a lack of adequately protecting the public. The psychological evidence in no way excused any of her conduct as it was not related nor did it interfere with her conscious acts for the purposes she desired."

Norma Jean was denied parole. However, the system went on to make a mistake that could have resulted in her eventual release. After her parole hearing, Norma Jean was mistakenly sent to the Sybil Brand Institute (the county jail for women) instead of the California Institute for Women, where she had been staying. At CIW, Norma had been under constant medication. At Sybil Brand, she received no medication. By the time the mistake was discovered, Norma's mind had "cleared" enough for her to decide that she didn't want or need anymore medication. When she returned to CIW, she asked to remain free of medication, and her request was granted.

As Norma Jean's mind "cleared" more and more, she decided that she wanted to appeal her conviction. In 1977, her attorney had written to her that he did not know of any grounds for an appeal in her case. But Norma Jean believed there were grounds. In December 1984 she wrote to the Public Defender's office and requested that the office take on her case and help her file an appeal. Norma also asked that the office foot the $3,000 bill for transcribing the record of her trial. She believed that her conviction should be appealed on two major grounds. The first was that she believed her Miranda rights had been violated during her arrest. She claimed that she asked repeatedly for an attorney, but the detectives continued to question her. The second was that she was kept on medication that prevented her from fully defending herself in court or, after her conviction, from filing an appeal. Norma claimed that she did not remember very much after she was placed on medication while in custody.

In June 1985 Norma Jean, with the aid of the Public Defender's office, filed an application for a late notice of appeal. Such application was required because the deadline for normal appeal had long since passed.

In September 1985 her request was denied. Norma Jean is still at the California Institute for Women.

Norma Jean killed to satisfy her desire to be a mother, an ability that time, nature, and a hysterectomy had conspired to take away from her. Priscilla Ford killed because the welfare authorities of the State of Nevada usurped her motherhood.

Within hours of the TV news and wire services picking up the story it became known as the "Thanksgiving Day Massacre." On Thanksgiving Day 1980, Priscilla Ford, a fifty-year-old unemployed schoolteacher had purposely steered her speeding car onto a crowded sidewalk in downtown Reno, Nevada. When she was done, she had left a two-block trail of carnage. Six people were killed, twenty-three injured.

I was called in on the case by the prosecution because the defense had a psychiatrist who said that Priscilla Ford was a paranoid schizophrenic who was not capable of understanding that what she did was wrong.

Priscilla Ford certainly fit the mold of a person who was mentally troubled. She had been brought up a Seventh-Day Adventist, but became a Baptist because her first husband was. Her second husband was a Methodist, so Priscilla became a Methodist. Husband number three was a Catholic, so Priscilla became one, too. Needless to say, her self-image was unstable. In the decade before she went on her murderous rampage, she had been involuntarily committed to three mental institutions. Reviewing her history, there was no question that her mental problems kept her from functioning normally in society. About eight years before the Thanksgiving Day Massacre, the welfare authorities in Reno had taken away Priscilla's daughter and placed her in a foster home.

But more than being "mad" in the crazy sense, Priscilla Ford was "mad" in the usual way—she was angry as hell at society for her predicament. There was no question that Priscilla was a paranoid person. Paranoids are usually extremely sensitive to their surroundings, but their minds make the mistake of misinterpreting events in such a way as to exaggerate their threat—or make up a threat when there is none. Quite often this imagined or exaggerated feeling of danger or ill will on the part of others is translated into anger. The paranoid will then act in such a way as to provoke anger—and real ill will—from others. Priscilla Ford's anger had been building up for a long time, ever since the state had taken her daughter away from her. And on Thanksgiving Day 1980 she found herself in a flea-bag hotel in Reno, alone and angry, with nothing to be thankful for.

So persistent and powerful was her anger that the act of killing six people and injuring twenty-three others did not dissipate it. When Priscilla Ford was booked, she acted as if everyone else had done something wrong. I watched the videotape of the minutes just after she was brought into the Reno police station. The police officers were models of courtesy and restraint. From their behavior, you might think the woman being booked had done little more than bounce a check or two—not mowed down thirty people on a crowded sidewalk. Priscilla Ford, however, was hostile, paranoid, and even sarcastic. When the booking officer told her she would get a receipt for the personal articles being taken away from her, she replied, "Oh, beautiful, beautiful!" Then, in the tone of an angry schoolmarm addressing one of her students, she asked if that meant she would get the articles back. During another of her sarcastic replies she mentioned that the heavy car she had driven was more efficient than a smaller foreign car would have been.

It was obvious from the videotape that Priscilla Ford was clear-headed enough to know that she had done something wrong and that she was in trouble. When the police officer read her Miranda rights, for a moment she refused to sign a statement acknowledging that she understood these rights, but eventually she did. She also corrected the officers' spelling and grammar.

After looking at her performance on the tape, I found it hard to believe that anyone could say that Priscilla Ford did not know right from wrong. Of course, there was no question that she was mentally ill, too. But her mental illness did not prevent her from knowing the difference between right and wrong. That was the legal standard for insanity in Nevada.

Priscilla Ford's trial took five months—the longest trial in the history of northern Nevada. There was no doubt that she drove the car into the crowd, and no one claimed it was an accident. The only issue that had to be decided was just how mentally ill she was and whether the impairment prevented her from knowing right from wrong. If it did, the condition could have fully exonerated her from responsibility. So, although there were several witnesses recounting more than a decade of Priscilla Ford's life, the critical testimony came from psychiatrists, of whom I was one.

There was plenty of evidence to document Priscilla's mental problems. On the witness stand, her own attorney tried to bring out her insanity by asking her about some of the bizarre ideas she had written about in her journals. At one point, he asked her what happened to Adam's soul:

"Nothing happened to Adam's soul; it's still living," she replied.

"Who has it?" her attorney asked.

"I do."

"Anybody else?"

"No, of course not. And I can only live in one body at a time."

"What other bodies have had your soul, do you know?"

"Yes, I know many."

"Can you name some of them?" he asked.

"Jesus Christ."

"Any others?"

"Ellen G. White."

"Any others?"

"Priscilla Ford."

"Well, Priscilla Ford has your soul now."

"Do you want all the way back to Adam?" she asked.

"If you can. The ones that you know."

"I can."

"Who is Michael DiMaggio?" her attorney asked, apparently not wishing to start at the very beginning.

"The soul."

"What soul?"

"My soul."

"Tell me something historical about Michael DiMaggio."

"I was in my body as Michael DiMaggio before I was born Priscilla."

"What did you do in that body?"

"I lived only a few years, fourteen or fifteen years old."

"How do you know this?"

"I just know. I am willing for somebody to prove that it's not true."

Keep in mind that Priscilla delivered her bizarre testimony in the same crisp, sharp tone of a schoolteacher answering her class's questions. Her attorney, of course, was banking on the fact that the jury would dismiss Priscilla as a raving maniac. Later in her testimony, she said that Ellen G. White, a previous incarnation of hers, had been a "messenger of God." In her current incarnation, Priscilla considered herself an "instrument of God." Furthermore, she displayed or admitted to many of the elements of mental illness, including visions and auditory hallucinations.

But as far as I was concerned, a critical element was missing. Though Priscilla was detached from reality, it was not to the extent that she didn't know the difference between right and wrong. I testified that from her writing it was clear that "she focused on right and wrong all her life." The defense had tried to make points from her identification with Christ. But I didn't think there was any evidence that she really thought she was Christ, at least not to the extent that it prevented her from knowing right from wrong. Mentally ill people who think they are Christ generally act the way they think Christ would act. Driving her car onto a crowded sidewalk was an act of ferocious rage—and was about as far from Christlike as you can get.

And Priscilla Ford was clearly aware of that fact. Despite her mental illness, despite the paranoid psychosis that prevented her from getting along in society, she knew she was killing people when she steered her car on to the sidewalk, and she knew it was wrong. The psychiatrists testifying for the defense said that she was a paranoid schizophrenic. In my opinion, she was not schizophrenic. A person who is a paranoid schizophrenic generally reacts to imagined threats. A paranoid person responds to real events but misinterprets or overreacts. Priscilla Ford's madness, her paranoia, was a flame that heated up her angry response to the genuine failures in her life, heated them up to the point where only an act of enormous violence could hope to satisfy her. But when she committed that act, she knew exactly what she was doing. In Nevada, that meant she was legally sane and responsible for her behavior.

Amazingly, if Priscilla Ford had barrelled through a crowd on a California sidewalk, and was being tried in California, I would have had to testify that she was insane. My evaluation would not have changed one bit. But my conclusions would have meant different things in California. In Nevada, the legal test for sanity was whether or not she knew she was killing people and whether she knew it was wrong. In California, at that time, the test would have been more sophisticated. It would have required that she be able to "conform her conduct to the requirement of law."

However, we were not in California, and, after five months of testimony, the Nevada jury took only thirteen hours to decide that Priscilla Ford was guilty of first-degree murder. Then they were given the task of deciding the penalty. After twenty-six hours, they came back with a decision: Priscilla Ford was sentenced to die in Nevada's gas chamber. It was the first time a woman had been sentenced to death in Nevada. I could see that the jury was responding to the enormity of the crime. In no way did they want to risk Priscilla's return to society on parole.

When the sentence was read, Priscilla Ford showed no emotion whatever.

As this is being written, the sentence has not yet been carried out.

Even wholesale murder could not calm Priscilla Ford's murderous anger at the loss of her motherhood. In Fumiko Kimura's case, however, her deadly compulsion broke through an outwardly placid sea of calm.

Fumiko Kimura was a compulsive housewife and mother. Not only did she worry about whether the house was clean and neat enough, but she worried that she wasn't providing enough breast milk for her newborn daughter Yuri, even though the baby's plump cheeks were evidence to everyone else that the child was well nourished. Fumiko also worried about whether the house was really safe enough for her children. One day she removed all the furniture from the living room so that Yuri and Kazutaka, her son, wouldn't hurt themselves.

Fumiko was an equally compulsive and dutiful wife. She

never criticized her husband and always waited for him to come home from the restaurant he owned and operated. When he arrived home, often quite late at night, she would bathe his feet. On many of those nights, unbeknown to Fumiko, he was coming home from an apartment where he had been keeping a mistress for the past three years.

One day in mid-January 1985, Fumiko had a visitor. A woman came to her door and identified herself as Fumiko's husband's mistress. The woman, who was also Japanese-American, backed up her tearful confession with a stack of love letters Fumiko's husband had written over the years. The mistress offered to commit suicide to atone for her guilt in the affair.

Though Fumiko outwardly held herself together long enough to demand that the woman make a clean break from her husband, inwardly she was devastated. Her compulsiveness short-circuited her powerful emotions over the revelation into a profound depression. Her usually spotless house became a mess. Fumiko grew more and more despondent, even to the point where she admitted that she no longer had the desire to prepare food for her little Yuri and Kazataka. Yet she still did not criticize her husband. Instead, she took the full burden of responsibility upon herself.

As far as Fumiko was concerned, this incident was confirmation of the fact that she was a complete failure at life. Her mother and father were divorced when she was very young. Her father died and she never knew him. Fumiko's mother remarried, but her stepfather never developed a close bond with the young girl. His habit of introducing Fumiko as a "relative's daughter" lingered with her as she grew up. When she was still a teenager, her boyfriend had gotten her pregnant and she'd had to have an abortion. She then went on to fail at two marriages. The first, begun in 1976, had lasted only two and a half years. Her second husband, whom she married in 1981, was forty years old. But that did not help the union last any longer.

Now her third marriage was, after a little more than four years, apparently a failure, too. And as the days wore on, Fumiko's husband's mistress kept calling and confessing more of the intimate details of the three-year liaison. The mistress, it seems, had once gotten pregnant, had an abortion, and attempted suicide. She once again offered to commit suicide to atone for her offense against Fumiko. As with previous offers, Fumiko was non-committal.

Fumiko still did not confront her husband with her knowledge, even though it was devouring her from the inside. Instead, she contacted her family in Japan. On January 25, 1985, at around eleven in the evening, Yoko Arita, Fumiko's sister, called her older brother and told him that Fumiko had just called her from the United States. Fumiko had told her about her husband's mistress, and asked her sister to please tell their mother all about it. She confessed that it had upset her, but then told her sister that now, everything was going well. But Yoko was not convinced. She was concerned because, she told her brother, their sister sounded strange. As he was at work and it was in the middle of the night in the United States, he said he would call Fumiko the next day.

But a little while later Yoko called again and reported that she had received another call from Fumiko. This time, Fumiko had asked her if she had told their mother yet. Then she went on to disavow her claim to the family land in Japan, since she was not a true daughter of her father. "I have no right to inherit it," she said, "because I'm not Father's child." Her sister protested, but Fumiko insisted that all she wanted was for her siblings to respect her despite the fact that they had different fathers. Though earlier in the conversation she had told Yoko she was going to stay in the United States and "make it all right" there, at the end of the call Fumiko pleaded that she wanted to come back to Japan.

After the second phone call, Yoko was so worried about her sister that she told her brother she wanted to come right over and talk to him. He told her to come right away. Once they got together, they decided to call Fumiko immediately rather than wait until the next day. Once on the phone, Fumiko shared her doubts about being a "genuine" child of her stepfather. Her brother asked her where she got that idea.

Fumiko replied, in Japanese, "Because unlike elder brothers and sisters I am not as competent."

"What do you mean?" her brother asked her.

"It has to do with the ability to think and my life-style up to now."

"That is not true," her brother answered, "neither Yoko nor I are as competent as Fumiko thinks."

"Really?"

"Fumiko, you have done really well, made a good living in the United States, so far."

"Are we really truly siblings," Fumiko pleaded. "Are we really from the same parents—related brothers and sisters?"

Now her brother reproached her: "Don't think silly, stupid things like that."

Fumiko seemed relieved. "I am glad. I am a little more relieved. Recently I haven't been able to sleep so well. Recently I have a little insomnia. It seems like a light case of neurosis. . . ."

Her brother knew Fumiko was worried about her children, and told her, "You don't have to worry too much about your children. They'll do all right."

Fumiko agreed, but then asked her brother, "Am I like a prostitute?"

"Why do you say that?" her brother asked, startled.

"Just somehow . . . my way of thinking about things."

"That's not true," he said.

"That's true. There's no reason for that," Fumiko seemed to agree.

Then her brother told her, "Don't think about too many things. Get hold of yourself. Be more competent."

"Yes, I'll be all right now, don't worry. I will be sure to get some good sleep from now on."

As the trans-Pacific telephone conversation ended, Fumiko's brother extracted from her a promise to write him a letter explaining why she was so depressed. Then he asked to speak to Itsuroku, Fumiko's husband.

All the two men talked about were Fumiko's symptoms. Itsuroku confirmed that his wife had started acting "strange" about a week earlier. He had taken her to the doctor, who said the woman was "having a slight case of neurosis." Fumiko was given some tranquilizers. Now, the two men agreed to observe Fumiko for two or three days before deciding what to do.

When the conversation ended, Fumiko's brother told Yoko to summon their mother home from Okinawa, where she was visiting. They decided to send her to the United States right away to help Fumiko.

Unfortunately, Fumiko's mother was not able to leave as soon as she wanted to. Her passport had expired on that very day. Fumiko's mother went to the capital of the province, explained the urgency of the situation, and asked to have a new passport issued immediately. But though the authorities were sympathetic and agreed to get one for her as soon as they could, it was still not going to be possible for her to be at her daughter's side as soon as she had hoped.

Meanwhile, Fumiko's brother kept calling, trying to get in touch with her. But after several unsuccessful attempts, he finally connected with Itsuroku, who told him not to worry, that Fumiko was just slightly neurotic.

Clinically, Fumiko was exhibiting the classic signs of a major depression. Her thoughts and actions were slow and confused. She was unable to eat or sleep, and could not concentrate. She ruminated over her failed marriage, but could not express the anger against the appropriate object—her husband. Instead, she turned the anger inward and, ultimately, the people closest to her, her children.

On January 29, Fumiko kept an appointment at her pediatrician's office. She was concerned that she was not making enough milk for Yuri, since the infant had lost weight. But Fumiko, perplexed and confused, left the office before the doctor could see her. She had left her husband and was living in a hotel, awaiting the arrival of her mother to take her back "home." She managed to call Yoko, and once again told her she wanted to return to Japan. When she hung up, Yoko immediately called her brother, for this time their sister sounded more distraught than ever before. The brother went into action and tried to reach Itsuroku by telephone.

Meanwhile, Fumiko went to a travel agency but did not conclude any business there. Instead she wandered out with her children and went for a walk. It had been days since she had slept, and she felt alone, abandoned, and "afraid of everyone and everything."

Because she had left behind the key to her apartment, Fumiko felt that there was nowhere for her to go. She lifted Yuri out of her stroller and left it by the bus stop under a bridge, then boarded a bus bound cross-town for Santa Monica. When she arrived there, she bought the children a fast-food lunch and then headed for the beach not far away.

Meanwhile, Fumiko's family in Japan had succeeded in reaching Itsuroku and had convinced him of how desperate his wife had sounded. He said he would go out to find her and bring her home.

Back at the beach, to the people watching her walk along the sand, Fumiko looked distraught. At the ocean's edge, she picked up her son, Kazutaka, and waded into the surf holding both children. The waves broke and foam swirled around them, but Fumiko kept going into deeper and deeper water. Before long, the water was swelling over Yuri's and Kazutaka's faces . . . and then over their heads. When the water was up to her shoulders, Fumiko leaned forward and held her childrens' heads below the surface and then started gulping down the cold seawater herself. Soon she could feel her babies stop kicking and squirming, and then she drank in more of the ocean. Slowly, peace was spreading inside her body as water replaced air in her lungs.

Two college students who had been casually watching her and her children suddenly realized what was happening. They dashed into the surf and pulled Fumiko and her two children out onto the beach. As the paramedics were called, CPR was performed on Fumiko and her children. An ambulance arrived and the three were taken to the hospital.

Itsuroku arrived at the hospital and found his family just in time to hear his son and daughter pronounced dead. The man was stricken with grief and guilt. He later said that he not only forgave his wife, but also envied the intense bond between Fumiko and their children.

Fumiko was arrested and sent to the Sybil Brand Institute for Women, the women's jail in Los Angeles. She was admitted to the forensic inpatient program because there was concern that she might attempt suicide again. At her preliminary hearing, she was charged with two counts of first-degree murder—with special circumstances, which meant that she could receive the death penalty.

But Fumiko's story became front-page news in the local, national, and Japanese press. In most cases, the stories were sympathetic to her. Before long, she received hundreds of letters of support from people she had never met, but who had read or heard her story. Fumiko wrote thank-you notes to all of them. But more important, her case became a *cause célèbre*—first in the Japanese community, then in the community at large. A public drive to request leniency was launched, and petitions were circulated. More than one thousand signatures were obtained from Japan, more than four thousand from the U.S.A.

One reason why Fumiko received so much sympathy was that her act, though abhorrent by Western standards, was actually a form of ritual suicide-murder commonly practiced in Japan. While *shinju,* as it is called, is now outlawed in Japan, the culture tends to regard it with mercy rather than vengefully, as a tragedy to be endured and mourned rather than a heinous crime. In Japanese culture, the child is seen as a part of the mother, as though the umbilical cord were still attached. If the mother is disgraced or abandoned by her husband, *shinju* is an honorable and culturally accepted way to save face. A parent-child suicide occurs in Japan on the average of once a day. Parents who survive are not dealt with harshly, while parents who kill themselves and leave their children behind are criticized for allowing their children to become a burden on someone else.

But could her cultural background be used as a defense? Regardless of the cultural issues, weren't there psychological issues that transcended the cultural differences? And what about the strictly legal issues? The murder–attempted-suicide was committed, after all, in the United States, not Japan.

The deputy district attorney assigned to the case, Lauren Weis, addressed that question in newspaper interviews when she said the case was "very, very difficult." She went on: "You're treading on such shaky ground when you decide something based on a cultural thing, because our society is made up of so many different cultures. It is very hard to draw the line somewhere, but they are living in our country and people have to abide by our laws or else you have anarchy. American law ought to be able to handle it, hopefully.

"It's not the same situation as when a woman kills her kids because she's tired of having them around. The jury must decide, Is she a criminal who is a danger to society, to herself, to other kids in the future. The cultural aspect comes into it, but there are so many different cultures here. You can't really start letting people off for that sort of thing. Kimura was living in America. She can't forget that. We'd be saying to everyone of Japanese culture that it's okay to go out and kill your children, when it's not."

Publicly, the D.A.'s office was laying down a hard line. They would not plea bargain the charges down from murder.

Even Fumiko's attorney admitted that though the cultural factors may have explained—or even shaped—his client's actions, they did not excuse her. He also knew that although it made interesting stories in the press and the legal journals, it did not make for good legal strategy. Furthermore, he felt that it could backfire and turn the case into a racial scandal that would tarnish the image of all Japanese-Americans.

So much for the public statements. Privately, the D.A.'s office wanted as much as anybody to be merciful to Fumiko. But they couldn't let her off for cultural reasons. Even if another culture says it's OK to kill your children, it's a pretty big stretch to fit that behavior into our Western culture. Fortunately, our culture does have a way to deal with such aberrations in behavior: Call in the psychiatrists.

Fumiko's attorney figured—correctly—that the best way to defend his client was to prove that her mental state was such that she was not responsible for the murder of her children. He proposed that Fumiko was an extremely vulnerable woman who was overwhelmed by the harsh demands of her Japanese traditions colliding with the mores of American life. Her family was her life, and if all was not well, she believed it was her fault. Fumiko still felt a lot of shame over her two earlier failed marriages. And when she learned that her present husband was unfaithful, she interpreted that as a sign that she had failed again. This was too much for her to bear, and she became mentally unstable to the point where she fell into the deadly trance of *shinju*.

As testimony to Fumiko's intense devotion to accepting full

responsibility for the failure of her marriage, she never once criticized her husband. Throughout her entire ordeal, she defended him—even from her prison cell.

The D.A.'s office was willing to go along with this defense. Attorneys on both sides—and the judge—agreed that they wanted to reach some kind of settlement before the case went to trial. But the trial date kept getting closer and there was still no settlement.

The problem was they could not come up with a psychiatric evaluation that said and did what they wanted it to. They brought in a psychiatrist from the superior court "panel" of physicians that work for the court regularly and receive an agreed-on fee for each report. I had been a member of the panel for eighteen years, but a few years ago I resigned because the court refused to set a fee that would compensate a psychiatrist for a complete and adequate workup. The fee structure in effect barely pays for one hour of time, when more often than not five or six hours are required to come up with an accurate evaluation. As a result, the quality of regular psychiatric reports is superficial and limited. Now, when a judge or an attorney does not want to rely on one of these "bargain basement" psychiatric evaluations, they seek alternative reports.

But it took the principals in this case four strikes before they decided to do that. The first four psychiatric reports did not address the proper issues and neither the D.A. nor the judge would accept them. These reports utterly failed to understand the questions involved. The art of forensic psychiatry is knowing not only how to present a case, but also how to translate the psychiatric information into legal and lay terms so that the people involved can work with it. When the deputy D.A. saw the first four reports, she rejected them as insufficient. She couldn't do anything with them, and asked again for a workable report.

I was called in.

While in prison, Fumiko's husband visited her every day. These visits brightened her spirits, and a therapist observed that "out of this tragedy, they were beginning to realize the close bond between them." In general, however, all the psychiatric personnel who saw her noted the same thing I did—she was an extremely depressed young woman who was overwhelmed by the circumstances in her life. The poetry she wrote while she was in prison gave expression to her feelings about herself, her despair, and her beloved sea. In my opinion, though she had shown some improvement, she was still severely depressed and needed treatment. My report stated:

"Although much is being made of the possible cultural aspects of her behavior, it is clinically clear that she was suffering from a major depressive episode as a result of the marital turmoil, the constant confrontation with her failing marriage, and her post-partum state. She had reached physical and mental exhaustion. The acts of January 29, 1985, to include her apparent attempted suicide and the taking of the lives of her children, can more clearly be seen in the context of her active mental disorder and not on cultural grounds, i.e., a save face event. Within her depression, she was confused, lacked identity and appears to have functioned as an automaton. Individuals in this condition act in erratic, purposeless ways, many times without motivation or plan. It would be my opinion that her major mental disorder had so consumed her that her actions were a direct result of that condition. Accordingly, she would not have planned, deliberated, or considered her contemplated behavior within any meaningful or logical context. In summation, her condition controlled her behavior and she lacked a logical thinking process."

My report provided the necessary psychiatric input and as a result was accepted by the court and the district attorney. The D.A.'s office approved a plea bargain of voluntary manslaughter and Fumiko was released on probation.

Fumiko told me that she would have to learn to trust her husband again, and that she eventually wanted to have more children.

Fumiko Kimura, Priscilla Ford, Norma Jean Armistead, Arlyne Genger. All four were intelligent, all four were achievers, all four were mothers, and all four were killers. All four had to kill to preserve their inner wholeness—were literally compelled to kill in order to resolve the inner turmoil that threatened to tear them apart. Arlyne's inner storm of confusion drove her to kill her own mother and almost kill her daughter. Norma Jean had to destroy other women's motherhood, take their babies and even their lives, in order to feel whole. Priscilla Ford had to kill to try to satisfy the inner rage she felt over the loss of her daughter. Fumiko Kimura killed her children because she had already been torn apart inside and out by the infidelity of her husband and the apparent failure of her marriage.

Whose was the more vicious crime? Was Norma Jean's bloody murder of Kathryn Viramontes "worse" than Priscilla Ford's Thanksgiving Day Massacre on the sidewalks of Reno? Was Fumiko the most vicious killer of all as she held her babies' heads below the surf until they stopped struggling?

The criminal justice system has answers to these questions, but I'm not sure they're very satisfying. In my experience, the system treats criminals better than it treats victims, and that treatment varies widely among jurisdictions. So Mary Childs, whose baby was stolen from her, received less consideration from the same system that went out of its way to show mercy to Fumiko Kimura. And while Priscilla Ford may someday walk into the Nevada gas chamber, Norma Jean Armistead may walk out of prison a free woman.

And Arlyne Genger?

As this chapter was being revised, there were new developments in Arlyne Genger's case.

Although Arlyne initially resisted confinement and treatment, she eventually not only participated more in her treatment, but also responded to it. Over the next few years she suffered a few relapses, but made steady progress. She wrote several letters to her daughter, and once sent her an entire book about her life. Selena never replied to her mother's letters.

I examined Arlyne Genger again on November 4, 1987. I learned that she had received several recommendations over the years by the hospital staff and by other examining psychiatrists that she be provisionally released on parole. The court had never seen fit to follow these evaluations. But now Arlyne was up for release again. There was a general feeling that this could be her time. After all, the entire staff seemed to agree: Arlyne was a model patient, had not gotten into trouble, and now had been symptom-free and off medication for over two years.

Despite these recommendations, the judge presiding over

the case was not swayed by the hospital reports. He called in several other psychiatrists who had examined her previously, and I was one of them.

There was no similarity between the woman I examined in 1980 and the one that sat before me in 1987. Had I not known the history I would have been hard pressed to believe that this was a woman who had killed her mother and attempted to kill her daughter. She was emotionally stable, fully cooperative, and handled the interview intelligently and without difficulty. She exhibited none of the signs or symptoms that I had noted in my earlier examination. Indeed, by this examination alone, one could not classify her as mentally disordered. True, in the interim she'd received years of medication and treatment, and for the most part lived in the protected, unstressful environment of the hospital. This absence of stress in and of itself can alleviate significant symptoms.

And this is one of the dilemmas that society, as well as psychiatrists, must face. People who are hospitalized usually improve simply as a result of the hospitalization. It is difficult to determine how they will react to being thrust back into society, usually into that same environment that helped create their illness.

In Arlyne's case, it had been almost eight years since she was on her own. The ward community at Patton State Hospital was composed of individuals suffering from a wide variety of illnesses, ranging from mild to severe. Within that community, her life was highly structured. The staff controlled most of Arlyne's waking hours: She was told when to get up, when to exercise, when to eat, and her basic needs were provided.

In 1980 Arlyne Genger was severely disturbed. Now, in 1987, she exhibited no significant mental disturbance at all. She was no longer in need of hospitalization on psychiatric grounds.

Arlyne had not required any medication for the past two years. Her behavior had been free of incidents and she had full ground privileges at the mental hospital. Furthermore, she realized and acknowledged that she killed her mother because she was mentally ill, that she had been deserted by her family, that her daughter did not want to see her or have contact with her in any way—and that she must, essentially, start life anew.

When talking about the loss of her family and her estranged

daughter, I noticed that Arlyne did try to hide her feelings somewhat. But this was normal, not psychotic, behavior. During the
interview she made good eye contact, and her emotions were
appropriate.

Having been advised that the judge handling the case did
not have extensive experience in mental health cases, I knew it
would be a good idea to fully explain my evaluation. For my
diagnosis was that she was still a paranoid schizophrenic, but in
remission. Though she still required psychiatric monitoring and
continued treatment, she did not require hospitalization. People
are not "cured" of schizophrenia. The disease can be controlled
by medication and psychiatric treatment, or it can go into remission and lie dormant, with no signs of an active process. Arlyne's
schizophrenia was now dormant.

Could it someday awaken and again render her a danger to
herself or others? That question cannot be answered with perfect
accuracy or finality. There are too many variables. If the amount
of stress and anxiety in Arlyne's life remain low, she might not
experience any significant symptoms in the future. But if her life
becomes stressful enough and she experiences enough anxiety,
her symptoms could recur.

As I said in my report, the adjustment into a modern big city
is a very lonely proposition. Arlyne will be subject to daily failures, self-doubt, and rejection. Is it reasonable to expect that her
life could remain stress-free once she returns to the fast pace of
modern life? No—but here is where close monitoring comes in.
If monitored once a week, it would be possible to observe any
potential problems and take appropriate action—psychiatric treatment, medication, or rehospitalization. In other words, Arlyne
will have to be closely supervised.

Psychiatric patients sometimes have a negative attitude about
supervision. They often take the first opportunity to "break
away" from their doctors and then they are not seen again until
they get into trouble. Arlyne's attitude toward close supervision
was positive and cooperative. She gave no indication that she
would try to break away or be uncooperative.

Arlyne Genger was not—nor will she ever be—"cured of
herself." But, as I told the judge in my report, the risks are man-
ageable at this time, and further hospitalization will not improve

her chances. No one could guarantee her future conduct anymore than a cardiologist could fully rule out a heart attack after a "clean" examination. Nevertheless, I wrote that Arlyne Genger would "never be more ready to re-enter society than she is now."

The judge agonized over his decision for many months. Hearings were held, more expert witnesses were called, pro and con opinions were heard. It was beginning to look as though the judge was not going to release her.

Then, a few days ago, I was at the Van Nuys courthouse on another matter, walking through the first floor hallway, when a man I recognized as Arlyne Genger's attorney came up to me. "Guess what," he asked.

From the smile on his face and his obvious excitement I could tell something good had just happened. "Arlyne's been released," I guessed.

I was right. She would have to continue being regularly supervised, but she was, basically, soon going to be a free woman again.

In previous conversations, Arlyne told me she planned to go back to work and start life over again. Actually, not everyone in her family deserted Arlyne. She will have enough money to get by modestly, because her father named her the beneficiary of the interest from a trust fund. When Arlyne dies, the principal of the fund will go to Selena.

The attorney thanked me. I responded that I was just providing the court with appropriate psychiatric information to allow for an informed decision.

Just then, Arlyne came up to us. She was all smiles. If you hadn't known the background of her case, you would never think she had committed matricide. She thanked me too, in a way that suggested that I really understood her plight.

I congratulated her and then informed her I was writing a book, and that her case was included.

Just then her attorney indicated that they were pressed for time. Arlyne, though essentially free, had to catch the ride back to Patton State Hospital, where her final release would be processed. As a matter of fact, the driver was now calling her.

But she seemed to be handling that tension very well, by

almost ignoring it. This was a moment frozen in time. She would finish it before moving on.

"What's the purpose of the book?" she asked.

"Well, that we're all capable of killing. We all have it in us."

Instantly Arlyne's smile disappeared and her face grew very sharp and serious. She took my hand, including me even more closely among the people who understood, and said, "Thank you very much, Dr. Markman. . . . You're right."

Then, as suddenly as it had vanished, the full, enthusiastic smile returned, and Arlyne Genger walked away, a free woman, indistinguishable from anyone in the crowded hallway, indistinguishable from you or me.

EPILOGUE
MEN OF THE CLOTH

The cases in this book are only a small fraction of the many homicide cases I have reviewed in the past twenty years. They are representative only insofar as they demonstrate that the devil that drives some of us to violently take the life of another person does not discriminate: Killers come in all sizes, shapes, and colors. They come from all ethnic groups, sexes, ages, religious denominations, sexual preferences, socio-economic backgrounds, and mental states. Of all the crimes that exist, homicide probably best represents a cross section of America. It is a unique crime. Most of the time it is committed by people who have never committed any crimes before.

When I walk into the county jail on my way to a psychiatric evaluation, I see around me the men and women of the general prison population; and I know that if we washed them and groomed them and dressed them up in the finest clothes and dropped them off at the premiere of a new movie or a Broadway opening night, they'd still look and act out of place.

But if we did the same with the killers, most could melt right into the crowd.

Individuals committing homicides don't come from the same mold as those charged with crimes such as robbery, burglary, auto theft, rape, assault, and child molestation. While the latter group is heavily weighted psychiatrically with antisocial personalities, killers commonly reflect the character of the overall society. Stripped of their acts, that moment of supreme power when one has ultimate Godlike control over another life, another being, each and every individual exhibits the strengths and weaknesses found in us all. There is a panoply of human misery, including the psychotic frenzy of an Orlando Camacho or a Richard Chase, the depressive despair of a Fumiko Kimura, the estrangement of a Priscilla Ford, the frustrated isolation of a Kevin Green, the solitude of a Torran Meier, the rage of a John Sweeney, and the alienation of the Manson Family members. Common threads in their lives are feelings of helplessness, frailty, and lack of worth, whether one examines Laura Schindler in her desperate marriage or Arlyne Genger struggling with her family. From time to time we all experience such feelings.

Anyone can commit homicide: the person who lives next door or across the street, the person who sits across from you at lunch, your partner in business . . . your partner in bed. John Sweeney was a chef at a prestigious restaurant. Laura Schindler was a secretary; her husband a successful businessman. Kevin Green was an honor student. Orlando Camacho was a college dropout. Fumiko Kimura was a housewife and mother. Norma Jean Armistead was a nurse. Jason Nelson was a teacher and a seminarian. Priscilla Ford was a schoolteacher. Leslie Van Houten and Tex Watson were the girl and boy next door.

This generalization doesn't always apply and there are some killers, sociopaths like Zimmerman and Bittaker, who do fit right in with the general prison population and who would stand out in any crowd. But for the rest, however, the only real difference between most of the killers in this book and most of its readers is that most of the readers have not killed another human being. Yet. And while the likelihood that some individuals will kill can be predicted with a high degree of accuracy, most murders are completely unpredictable.

And yet few are random events. Once you sift back through the personalities and incidents leading up to the climactic violence, it is possible to understand a great deal about why the killing took place. But for every human drama that ends in violent death, there are hundreds involving identical personalities in similar conflicts that do not end that way.

Jason Nelson could just as easily have expressed his aggression and confusion by throwing a rock through the stained-glass window of a church.

John Zimmerman might have burglarized the Dean house but left the children unharmed.

Orlando Camacho could have descended into the depths of his paranoid delusions without beheading his young wife Elizabeth.

Kevin Green might have found a way back into the loving

embrace of his family before his exile drove him to that fateful, deadly confrontation with Roger Anderson.

Bittaker and Norris could have let all their victims go, as they did the one woman who eventually was instrumental in their capture.

Laura Schindler might have simply left Lou and hired a lawyer, rather than firing a bullet into the back of her sleeping husband's head.

But they didn't. All of the dramas in this book rose up and broke through to the most violent and deadly peaks of human conflict. And despite our best efforts to deny it, we all swim in that same chaotic sea of potentially violent emotions. We are all alone with the devil.

Even those among us who study theology and assume the role of "men of the cloth."

When priests, ministers, or rabbis commit murder, our sensibilities are aroused by the bewilderment that someone who assumes the role of spiritual and moral leader can fall into the snares of violence. Such acts emphasize the potential weakness in us all. But when the victim is also the son of the minister, the outrage and the emotional disorientation are magnified by the grisly similarities between the crime and our culture's fundamental religious stories.

The fact that a seemingly righteous person not only takes the life of his child, but does so while mimicking biblical dramas and/or claiming divine guidance, leads us to face the uncomfortable prospect that what we may believe is our birthright of civilization and moral behavior is actually a veneer stretched tenuously over a violent, molten core of immense passions, drives, and desires.

On April 1, 1984, inside the heart of Marvin Gay, Sr., a fundamentalist minister, that delicate veneer crumbled. The murderous rage that burst forth was loose for only a few moments—but it resulted in the irrevocable loss of the son who belonged not only to his family and friends, but also to millions of people all over the world who loved the music of Marvin Gaye.

Marvin had been the middle child of five born to Marvin Sr. and Alberta Gay. Marvin Sr. was a stern man, who demanded obedience and high achievement from his children. As is often typical in such taskmaster fathers, he seldom displayed any emotions and certainly did not openly express love. Marvin Jr. found love and support in his mother, who encouraged him to sing and share his talents with others. Thanks to her guiding energy, Marvin became the premier performer in the church choir.

Later in life, Marvin confided that his father never gave him the love and acceptance that he desperately needed. Between father and son there was constant strife. Marvin Sr., who could not bring himself to acknowledge his son's achievements in the church choir, also complained about his son's growing involvement in secular music. But it was through Marvin's musical brilliance that the young man found the acceptance that he never received from his father, as his talent was appreciated by a growing audience.

Marvin Gaye (he added an "e" to his family name) became one of the music industry's brightest superstars. Though he thrived on the lavish attention of his fans, he also received sustenance from his mother and his sisters and brother. A multimillionaire, thanks to his recording success, Marvin bought a thirteen-room house for his mother in an upper-middle-class neighborhood in Los Angeles. The home seemed to represent a haven for the world-roaming singer. Though his travels and travails led him all over the globe, he always returned to his mother's house.

And the travails were always plentiful. For despite his success, Marvin never seemed to find peace and satisfaction. His two marriages ended bitterly. Though he earned millions, he endured periods of bankruptcy and enormous debt. Contributing to the tragedy of his life was his passion for drugs, particularly cocaine. Cocaine not only deadened his creativity but also destroyed his health and financial security.

So on April Fool's Day 1984, the eve of Marvin Gaye's forty-fifth birthday, his life could be said to have been in shambles. He had filed for bankruptcy, owed millions to the IRS, was being sued for hundreds of thousands of dollars in back alimony by his first wife, and was desperately trying to break his addiction to cocaine.

That may have been the most difficult task that lay ahead for Gaye. Money was certainly important to him, not only for security but for stature—and to enhance his image in his father's eyes.

Marvin once bragged that he wanted to personally hand his father $1,000,000 in cash so that Marvin Sr. would have a tangible, undeniable manifestation of his son's success. But as much as he needed both money and his father's approval in order to be happy, Marvin appeared to need cocaine in order to live from one day to the next. Cocaine seemed to fill the emptiness he felt inside, while it obliterated the excruciating contradiction that a man could be so lonely and depressed in the midst of such success.

Yet Marvin was making an heroic effort to divorce himself from what could be called his "third wife," cocaine. He had succeeded before, sworn off the drug and experienced a resurgence in his creativity—until the drug was once again foisted upon him by a "friend" or a business associate.

Now Marvin was home with his family, trying again to rid his life of cocaine and the depression that made the drug so attractive. Around noon that day before his birthday, as Marvin's mother, Alberta Gay, recalled, "I was in Marvin's room sitting on the foot of his bed talking with him. My husband came walking through my bathroom and asked me where he could find this insurance letter. I couldn't hear him very well so Marvin asked him to come into the room where we were. My husband said, No, he wouldn't come in the room.

"Marvin told him, 'If you don't come in now don't you ever come in my room again.'

"Then my husband came in the room. Marvin told him get out and got up from the bed, walked over to my husband, and pushed him back. Marvin pushed him a couple of times. My husband turned and walked back to his bedroom. Marvin followed him, yelling little cuss words at him. Marvin told his father, 'I'll beat you up.'

"They both went into my husband's bedroom and I followed them. I didn't see what happened in the bedroom, I heard my husband say, 'He's kicking me, I don't have to take that.'

"When I entered the room my husband was on the floor and Marvin was standing a short distance away. I took Marvin by the arm and led him back to his room. I sat him on the foot of the bed. Marvin told me, 'Mother, I'm going to get my things and get out of this house. Father hates me and I'm never coming back.'

"I figured Marvin might have been taking some stuff today, because he was so quick to fly off. Marvin used cocaine at times. When he used it, he would fly off real quick. My husband drinks every day. I think he was drinking . . . but I didn't see him.

"I was standing about eight feet away from Marvin when my husband came to the door of the bedroom with his pistol. It's a silver-colored revolver. He's had it about a year. He—my husband—was always quick to talk about shooting people. My husband didn't say anything, he just pointed the gun at Marvin. I screamed but it was very quick. He, my husband, shot—and Marvin screamed. I tried to run. Marvin slid down to the floor after the first shot. Then my husband fired two more times. I ran out of the house and ran to my son's house next door. I told him to call the cops and the paramedics. My son Frankie and his wife called the police and then went over."

While Marvin Gaye lay dying, his father went outside, threw the gun—which his son had given him for protection—on the grass, and sat on the porch to await the police.

Marvin Gay, Sr., born October 1, 1913, had never been arrested before. He could be described as a law-abiding, somewhat rigid and opinionated individual who was difficult to live with. His relationship with his wife and children was emotionless and distant. The major purpose in his life, by his own admission, was religious teaching.

He also admitted that he had taken a drink of vodka that morning. His breath test confirmed this statement. His dead son was also tested for drugs: a significant concentration of a metabolite of cocaine was found in the blood, indicating that Marvin Jr. had, indeed, as his mother reported, "taken some stuff" that day.

Marvin Sr. claimed he had acted in self-defense. His bruises certainly supported that contention. But his subsequent statements to police—made after being told, and waiving, his rights—grew more confused and contradictory. At one point he told the police that he believed the gun was loaded with blanks. Later, he said he thought it was a BB or pellet gun. Strangely, he recollected that the shooting took place in the hallway, not in his son's bedroom, as the evidence suggested.

On April 16, 1984, the Mental Health Court requested that I evaluate the Reverend Gay's competence to stand trial. Prior to my examination, he had consented to an interview with the *Herald Examiner* and described his son as a "beastlike person" because of his constant use of cocaine. "I heard him all the time—the sniffing," Gay said. Then, describing the scuffle between him and his son, he continued, "He took me from the back and grabbed me and slung me to the floor and he started beating me, kicking me. . . . He knocked me onto the bed. . . . My hand happened to feel the little gun under the pillow."

Familiar with the newspaper interview and the police arrest report, and having spoken to the family and friends, I examined Marvin Gay Sr. My first impression was that the seventy-year-old man was confused and disoriented. He believed it was November or December, not April but, in his confusion, admitted that he knew it wasn't a holiday season. He could not recall why he was in jail. In my opinion, his condition suggested the possible existence of an organic or physical disorder affecting his brain. So I postponed any further psychiatric evaluation and recommended a complete neurological exam.

Sure enough, a CT scan at the L.A. County–USC Medical Center revealed a tumor at the base of Marvin Gay, Sr.'s, brain, near the pituitary gland. Although surgical removal of the tumor was recommended, Mr. Gay initially refused further treatment.

On April 27, I continued the psychiatric examination. This time I found him more responsive and aware. He understood that he was in custody for the killing of his son, and his narration of the incident closely paralleled his published accounts. Although I noticed no acute psychotic process, his concentration was limited and his memory subject to unpredictable gaps. I explained to him the importance of his consenting to surgery to remove his tumor. He said he would think about it.

In my report, I stated that Marvin Gay, Sr., was competent to stand trial. However, I pointed out the fragility of his condition and the potential for sudden, wide fluctuations in his mental condition, possibly owing to the tumor. I cautioned that while he might be rational and alert one day, he could easily lose concentration and memory the next—and flip-flop back and forth between these two extremes.

Did the tumor contribute to the shooting of his son? In my opinion, while it may have contributed, it was not the sole cause.

Obviously the life-long strife between father and son was a major factor. Marvin Sr.'s somewhat rigid, distant, cold stance toward his son did not help matters. On the other hand, Marvin Jr.'s use of cocaine affected his perception of reality and shortened his fuse while it aggravated the father's impatience and disapproval. Likewise, Marvin Sr.'s use of alcohol, though minimal, was enough to affect his emotional stability and character.

As for the tumor, it did exist in a critical area of the brain. Although, when finally removed, it was found to be benign, the walnut-sized mass was growing in the part of the brain that helps mediate emotions. It is possible that the Reverend Gay's ability to deal with frustration and anger were impaired by its presence. In a way, it did for him what he could not do for himself: it freed his emotions from the tightly bound control he forced upon himself all his life. Tragically, wrapped up in that rigid bundle of emotions was a deadly rage that focused on his son.

I believe that no single element in either the father's or the son's life resulted in the catastrophe. All together, however—the cocaine, the alcohol, the tumor, and the powerful struggle between father and son—combined to snuff out the life of a renowned and much-loved performer.

On September 20, 1984, Marvin Gay, Sr., entered a plea of *nolo contendere* to a charge of voluntary manslaughter with the use of a gun. This is equivalent to a guilty plea, with the exception that it cannot be used as evidence in a civil proceeding. Reverend Gay gave the following statement: "I wish I could bring him back —I would. I thought I was going to get hurt. I didn't know what was going to happen. I'm real sorry for everything that happened."

Taken into consideration by the court was the fact that the Reverend Gay had been attacked by a man who, though his son, was twenty-five years younger and seventy pounds heavier. He was placed on probation in a retirement home.

Although the court was satisfied that justice was done, and Marvin Gaye's fans have his music to keep him alive in their hearts, his father has only the bitter knowledge that his relationship with his son was never resolved. Though all concerned— most of all the criminal justice system—try their best to render a neat finish to this kind of story, it is a vain effort.

In this case, as in others, psychiatric testimony was introduced into the judicial equation to clarify and explain. More often than not, psychiatric input becomes a "battle of experts" based on a maze of technicalities, expanded definitions for mental elements of a crime, and attempts to exculpate an individual either partially or fully for his behavior. Interest in the individual's mental condition is often secondary, and unfortunately the legal results are sometimes illogical despite the term "justice" that is attached. How else can one explain some of the judicial results. Richard Chase, one of the more psychotic individuals depicted in this book paid for his killings with the most severe sentence available, the death penalty, while Orlando Camacho, also psychotic, was sentenced to five years for his murder conviction. And Arlyne Genger, whose condition was equally severe, and whose crime equally chilling, was found not guilty be reason of insanity. Surely, Richard Chase's actions produce a greater revulsion in our collective conscience, but can this justly explain the broad discrepancy in the sentencing result? Kevin Green was sentenced to a minimum of fifteen years for the *murder* of a friend, while John Sweeney spent only a few years in custody for the *manslaughter* of his female companion. And Laura Schindler was confined for less than one year before she was released on probation, while Torran Meier will remain incarcerated for a major portion of his twelve-year sentence. By definition, "justice" prevailed in all instances. Is it logically possible to explain a ten-year distinction between the acts of Kevin Green and John Sweeney? Why did society extract a greater penalty for Torran Meier's behavior than for the acts of Laura Schindler? These are the compromises made in the system and our society at large has reluctantly accepted the results. However, talk to the victims and their families, who feel abandoned by the system. It simply depends on whose ox is being gored. Recall the family letters written by relatives and friends supportive of Lou Schindler, the assailant, pleading for mercy. When he became Lou Schindler, the victim, these same individuals displayed only vengeance toward Laura Schindler, his assailant. The system is not perfect, but to paraphrase Winston Churchill, it's better than any other system out there. This does not mean that we should not strive for improvement, particularly in the use of psychiatric testimony by the legal system.

The legal profession prides itself on objectivity. Improved objectivity in psychiatric involvement within that same legal system is certainly an attainable and realistic goal.

When I was a law student, I noticed what great pains were taken to keep the law library scrupulously clean, neat, and well organized. You might have thought it was going to be used as an operating room. However, the more inside knowledge I got about the law and the criminal justice system, the more I realized that the orderliness of the library was little more than a facade. For once you pulled down a book from those sterile shelves and opened the cover, you were plunged into a world of chaos. For every statement you could find a contrary one, for every decision or point of law that said one thing you could find one that said the opposite.

I soon realized that the law library was, after all, a lot like an operating room, where surgeons often open up a patient and find the chaos of disease. Beneath its placid, orderly surface raged the same turbulent sea of conflicts and contradictions that a psychiatrist finds within the human psyche.

But we do the best we can to apply some order to what, at least to our human eyes, appears to be bedlam. We try to answer the questions, resolve the conflicts, and find a clear, calm channel through the storm. The problem with death, especially violent death at the hands of another human being, is that we are inevitably left with more questions than answers, questions about the nature of madness, murder, and death itself.

Psychiatry cannot answer all those questions. Neither can the law.

But life doesn't wait for the answers. And that can be the greatest mystery of all: how life heals itself and goes on.

Marvin Gay's story makes it a little easier to understand Jason Nelson's, whose story begins and ends this book.

We left Jason lying on a hospital gurney, bleeding from his self-inflicted stab wounds, arrested for the murder of his son.

Doctors found that he had sliced his intestines, so they performed emergency surgery and repaired the wounds in his abdomen and neck. A temporary colostomy was also performed. And while the doctors were patching him up, the authorities were charging Jason Nelson with second-degree murder.

When his wounds were healed, Jason was released into the custody of his family. Within weeks of the death of his son Jason was evaluated by physicians at the Utah State Hospital. On the immediate issue of whether he was competent to stand trial, they concluded that he was. On the issue of his sanity at the time of the offense, their diagnosis was that Jason suffered from "atypical psychosis," which is a psychosis that erupts suddenly from far beneath the normally placid surface of the mind.

When I evaluated Jason, I agreed with that diagnosis. While it was obvious, now, that Jason was psychotic, there had been no evidence of a mental disorder in his previous behavior. This was not to say that after Jason was followed for several weeks or months that a chronic mental illness might not become evident, one reaching back several years that he had somehow managed to keep hidden. But there was little evidence of that when I examined him.

Nor was I saying that he was only "temporarily insane." However sudden and unpredictable had been the turbulence that had loosed itself upon him and his family, Jason was still a profoundly sick man, and in need of further supervision and treatment. Based on Utah law at the time, it was my opinion that he was insane at the time he killed Paul.

That explanation may have been enough for the court, which accepted my evaluation, but there was more to the story. In the case of Marvin Gaye, it was obvious that his father acted in a fit of anger. Jason Nelson also acted in anger. Whereas the Reverend Gay's rage was overt and sparked by a confrontation with his drug-abusing, contentious, middle-aged son, Jason Nelson focused his anger upon his helpless, innocent, infant son. In the Reverend Gay's case, it is relatively easy to understand how the emotions and resentments he failed to express all his life could burst forth in a violent act.

But Jason Nelson was apparently even more successful than Reverend Gay in maintaining a calm surface despite his turbulent inner storms. Following what he believed to be the strictures and requirements of his religious faith, he cultivated powerful frustrations and resentments. Yet he could neither acknowledge nor express them. And when they ultimately found expression, the event diabolically took the form of one of the principal dramas of the very religious traditions Jason was struggling so painfully to epitomize. Jason Nelson, who was so tormented by what he felt were the unattainable demands of his faith, would show the world once and for all that he could be as faithful as Abraham.

Jason Nelson was found not guilty by reason of insanity. He was sent to the Utah State Hospital, where he responded very well to treatment. He was released quite often on temporary furloughs. Finally, after almost three years, he was discharged.

Today, Jason Nelson lives with his wife Ruth and their second child in Logan, Utah.

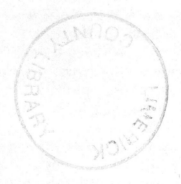